Primary Care Medicine: Evaluation and Management

Primary Care Medicine: Evaluation and Management

Editor: Danna Carson

AMERICAN
MEDICAL PUBLISHERS
www.americanmedicalpublishers.com

AMERICAN
MEDICAL PUBLISHERS
www.americanmedicalpublishers.com

Cataloging-in-Publication Data

Primary care medicine : evaluation and management / edited by Danna Carson.
p. cm.
Includes bibliographical references and index.
ISBN 978-1-63927-451-2
1. Primary care (Medicine). 2. Medical care. 3. Primary health care. I. Carson, Danna.
RC46 .P75 2021
616--dc23

American Medical Publishers,
41 Flatbush Avenue,
1st Floor, New York,
NY 11217, USA

ISBN 978-1-63927-451-2 (Hardback)

Contents

Preface

The main aim of this book is to educate learners and enhance their research focus by presenting diverse topics covering this vast field. This is an advanced book which compiles significant studies by distinguished experts in the area of analysis. This book addresses successive solutions to the challenges arising in the area of application, along with it; the book provides scope for future developments.

The day to day healthcare given by a healthcare provider is referred to as primary care medicine. It includes health promotion, diagnosis and prevention of chronic and acute illness, counseling and patient education in various healthcare settings, etc. The four different areas of primary care are family medicine, pediatrics, internal medicine, and obstetrics and gynecology. Family medicine provides medical care to the entire family and internal care provides primary medical care to adults. There are a few more specialized areas of healthcare which can be dealt with under family medicine such as eating disorders, hepatitis C and infertility. Pediatrics focuses on the primary care of infants, children and adolescents. Obstetrics and gynecology is concerned with the reproductive health of women in addition to offering family planning services. This book unfolds the innovative aspects of primary care medicine which will be crucial for the progress of this field in the future. Such selected concepts that redefine this field have been presented herein. This book attempts to further enlighten the readers about the new aspects in this area.

It was a great honour to edit this book, though there were challenges, as it involved a lot of communication and networking between me and the editorial team. However, the end result was this all-inclusive book covering diverse themes in the field.

Finally, it is important to acknowledge the efforts of the contributors for their excellent chapters, through which a wide variety of issues have been addressed. I would also like to thank my colleagues for their valuable feedback during the making of this book.

Editor

1

Validation of an instrument for the assessment of patient-centred care among patients with multimorbidity in the primary care setting: the 36-item patient-centred primary care instrument

Jane Murray Cramm* and Anna Petra Nieboer

Abstract

Background: Validated instruments are needed to assess the delivery of patient-centred care (PCC) to patients with multimorbidity in the primary care setting. Eight dimensions of PCC have been identified: respect for patients' preferences, access to care, emotional support, information and education, involvement of family and friends, continuity and secure transition between health care settings, physical comfort, and coordination of care. The main objective of this study was to validate an instrument for the assessment of PCC among patients with multimorbidity in the primary care setting: the 36-item patient-centred primary care (PCPC) instrument.

Methods: We included patients with multimorbidity from seven health care practices in the region of Tilburg, the Netherlands. All patients enrolled in at least two chronic care programmes (involving diagnosis of and treatment for combinations of diabetes, asthma and/or chronic obstructive pulmonary disease, cardiovascular diseases and conditions, and age-related frailty) were selected from the practices' data registries and included as eligible participants. A total of 216 patients with multimorbidity filled in the study questionnaire (55% response rate). We tested the instrument using structural equation modelling, and examined its validity and reliability.

Results: Confirmatory factor analyses revealed good indices of fit and overall internal consistency, as represented by Cronbach's alpha values. All eight dimensions of PCC were related positively to satisfaction with care (all $p \leq 0.001$). Patients with multimorbidity who experienced joint decision making and responsibility taking in the primary care setting also had significantly higher scores for all eight PCC dimensions, indicating the instrument's construct validity.

Conclusions: We conclude that the psychometric properties of the 36-item PCPC instrument are good. Based on these results the PCPC instrument seems a promising tool for the assessment of PCC among patients with multimorbidity in the primary care setting.

Keywords: Patient-centred care, Multimorbidity, Primary care, Instrument development, PCPC instrument

* Correspondence: cramm@eshpm.eur.nl
Erasmus School of Health Policy & Management, Erasmus University, Rotterdam, The Netherlands

Background

The number of people with chronic diseases is increasing at an astonishing rate, making millions of patients reliant on primary care systems. As a consequence, such systems throughout the world are struggling to find the best way to deal with large numbers of chronically ill patients while keeping costs low and quality high [1]. Patients with multimorbidity are known to report even worse well-being and health outcomes than do individuals with single chronic conditions [2]. Furthermore, they are more likely to be hospitalised and are at greater risk of premature death than are patients with single chronic diseases [3, 4]. The prevalence of multimorbidity in Europe is currently about 65% among people aged ≥60 years and 85% among those aged ≥85 years [5–7]. Thus, 50 million people in Europe have at least two chronic diseases, and this number is expected to grow as populations age.

Providing optimal care for older patients with (multiple) chronic diseases is actually among the greatest challenges of the healthcare spectrum today [8]. Health professionals clearly express the concern that they often missed the opportunity to engage with multimorbidity patients as true partners in their care and really help them to manage their conditions at home. This situation represents a missed opportunity, as the outpatient primary care setting is precisely the context identified as most appropriate to effectively deal with ageing populations [6–8]. The complexity of many chronic diseases and frailty profiles that come with multimorbidity demands Patient Centred Care (PCC), such that multimorbidity patients are equipped with the information and skills necessary to act as co-producers or co-creators of their care and where abilities to maintain overall well-being are optimised [7–9]. Such care supports active involvement of patients in the design of new care models and in decision making about individual treatment options. Decisions need to be based on personal preferences, needs and circumstances of each patient in every aspect of their live beyond physical health and clinical outcomes only [9–13].

The Harvard School of Medicine collaborated with the Picker Institute to conduct a very comprehensive study of the constituents of PCC [14, 15]. These researchers identified the following eight dimensions of PCC: respect for patients' values, preferences and expressed needs, provision of information and education, access to care, emotional support to relieve fear and anxiety, involvement of family and friends, continuity and secure transition between health care settings, physical comfort, and coordination of care [14–16]. A consultation of additional PCC literature [17–21] revealed no additional aspect or dimension of PCC. Table 1 provides detailed descriptions of the eight PCC dimensions in general [14–21] and describes them for patients with multimorbidity receiving primary care in particular as derived from the literature [22–25].

In a systematic review, Rathert and colleagues [16] showed that organisations which perform well in multiple PCC dimensions report better organisational and patient outcomes (e.g. improved care processes, clinical outcomes, cost reduction). For example, care that is well coordinated, easily accessible, providing physical comfort and attending patients' emotional needs is known to increase patients' satisfaction with care as well as improve joint decision making and responsibility taking [16, 26–29]. Organisations implementing interventions falling into several PCC dimensions reported better outcomes than did those aiming to improve single PCC dimensions, indicating that a constellation of interventions in multiple PCC dimensions leads to better outcomes [16].

Although we have considerable evidence for the benefits of investing in the improvement of the eight PCC dimensions [14–16] to achieve better organisational and patient outcomes, we lack instruments and research investigating the effects of these eight dimensions, especially among patients with multimorbidity in the primary care setting. A broader understanding of patients' experiences with these PCC aspects is important as they could help to improve the organisation and provision of care for this population, which is expected to lead to better outcomes (e.g. improved satisfaction with care, enhanced self-management abilities and well-being) [16, 22–25]. The measurement of levels of PCC among patients with multimorbidity is the first step. Therefore, the main objective of this study is to validate an instrument for the assessment of PCC among patients with multimorbidity in the primary care setting: the 36-item patient-centred primary care (PCPC) instrument. Based on earlier research we expected that investment in the eight dimensions of PCC would be associated positively with satisfaction with care [16]. In addition, we expected that the occurrence of joint decision making and responsibility taking, as perceived by patients with multimorbidity, would align with their experiences with PCC.

Methods

We included adult patients with multimorbidity from seven health care practices in the region of Tilburg, the Netherlands. All patients enrolled in at least two chronic care programs (involving diagnosis of and treatment for combinations of diabetes, asthma and/or chronic obstructive pulmonary disease, cardiovascular diseases and conditions, and age-related frailty) were selected from the data registries of the practices and included as eligible participants. All adult patients with at least two registered chronic conditions ($n = 413$) were eligible to participate. No additional inclusion criterion was applied. Exclusion criteria were too ill to participate and no longer a patient of the health care practices under study. First, these selected patients received questionnaires at home via post. Three weeks later, reminder

Table 1 The eight dimensions of patient-centred care in the primary care setting for patients with multimorbidity

Dimension	Description
1) Patients' preferences	Patients with multimorbidity have indicated that they need to be seen as a whole person instead of a sum of certain diseases. It is, for example, not sufficient to complete a standard template of a care plan for a patient with COPD and another template for the same patient's diabetes. Whole-person care is a concept requiring professionals' understanding of each patient as a whole by taking the time to really get to know the patient and his/her values and preferences, thereby improving the patient's well-being. To enhance PCC, health care professionals should involve chronically ill and multimorbidity patients in decisions about their care and support them in setting and achieving their own treatment and life goals. Preference-sensitive decisions include therapy that may improve one condition but make another worse (e.g., corticosteroids for chronic obstructive pulmonary disease may exacerbate osteoporosis); therapy that may confer long-term benefits but cause short-term harm (e.g., preventive agents, such as statins, frequently have adverse effects); and multiple medications, each with benefits and harms that must be balanced. Finally, preferences may change over time and should be re-examined, particularly with a change in health status.
2) Information and education	The provision of complete information to patients about all aspects of their care is necessary. Patients should have access to their care records (e.g. via e-health applications) and be in charge of their care. Open communication between patients and health care professionals, which requires professionals to possess high-quality communication skills, is also necessary. Although healthcare professionals may often feel that some adverse effects are less important than expected benefits, patients with multimorbidity often consider them to be highly significant given that they often use multiple medicines and treatments. Multimorbidity disproportionally affects those from lower socio-economic groups, which calls for information suitable for patients from all educational levels.
3) Access to care	Access to care refers to waiting times (to schedule an appointment as well as waiting time during the visit), an accessible building (including those with physical limitations and mobility problems) as well as medicine access (patients can easily request a repeat recipe). Research unfortunately shows older patients with (multiple) chronic diseases experience many difficulties when it comes to access to care and find it difficult to make an appointment with their general practitioner and specialist. Obstacles include overloaded telephone lines and the inability to schedule an appointment less than several months in advance. Furthermore, special attention is needed for (im)migrant and illiterate patients.
4) Emotional support	Multimorbidity patients often experience anxiety about the impact of their multiple illnesses on their lives as a whole not just their physical health outcomes. Being in constant pain and feeling tired also limits the ability to invest in social relationships and to keep your job, which may cause a lot of worries and anxieties. Proper support is needed to help patients with multimorbidity in their abilities to achieve social and mental well-being, which is currently a major challenge in the primary care setting.
5) Family and friends	In the case of chronical diseases and especially multimorbidity (depending on the seriousness of the conditions), these illnesses not only affect the patient, but also his/her family and friends. In such cases, PCC may be improved by the involvement of relatives in decisions about the patient's care, and attention to the role and needs of informal caregivers. Furthermore, optimal care of older adults with multimorbidity is best achieved by a collaborative effort that involves patients, family members, and health care providers. Family members, especially spouses, often play a leading role in sharing responsibility for some of the care. A person-centred approach begins by gathering specific information about a person's preferences in light of health circumstances, with input from family members and other caregivers if the person wishes. Added to a comprehensive health and functional assessment within the patient preferences dimension, this information is used to help a person shape and articulate his or her health and life goals. These goals are driven first and foremost by how a person wants to function and what he or she envisions for future well-being.
6) Continuity and transition	Continuity and secure transition between health care settings have been identified as important aspects of PCC for patients with multimorbidity. Smooth transitions require the transfer of all relevant patient information; ensuring that patients are well informed about where they are going, what care they will receive, and who their contact person will be; and the provision of skilled advice about care and support at home after discharge from a hospital for example. Involvement of various healthcare professionals, numerous treatments and taking multiple medications is known to have adverse effects. A complex regimen is associated with non-adherence, adverse drug events, economic burden, and informal caregiver stress. These risks can worsen with impairments in cognitive and physical function. Thus, it is recommended to periodically evaluate the patient's capability to manage medications. Continuity and smooth transition can help simplifying the regimen as well as carefully monitoring the patient with feedback if needed. Older patients with more complex health and psychosocial issues indeed are known to benefit from comprehensive evaluation by geriatricians, psychiatrists, social workers, and home care providers, who continuously work well together.
7) Physical comfort	Multimorbidity patients' physical comfort should be supported effectively in order to support their ability to achieve physical well-being. Pain should be managed effectively, patients have to sleep well and healthcare professionals should take patients' needs about support and their daily living needs into account. Not just physical comfort in the daily life of patients matters, but they should also be provided with comfort during their visit to the healthcare professional; areas should for example be clean and comfortable and patients' privacy must be respected.
8) Coordination of care	Patient care should be well coordinated among professionals (teamwork in care delivery). Health care professionals should be well informed so that patients do not have to repeat their stories over and over again. Given the involvement of multiple professionals in the case of patients with multimorbidity, this becomes increasingly important.

PCC patient-centred care

notices were sent to non-respondents. Another three weeks later, second reminder notices with duplicates of the questionnaire were sent. Finally, when telephone numbers were available, we called non-respondents to ask them to fill in the questionnaire. Nineteen respondents appeared not eligible to participate due to incorrect addresses ($n = 5$), recent moves ($n = 2$), death ($n = 4$), admission to a hospice or nursing home due to terminal illness ($n = 2$), poor cognitive function preventing questionnaire filling ($n = 2$), recent stroke ($n = 1$), and poor eyesight ($n = 3$). Of the remaining 394 patients a total of 216 patients with multimorbidity filled in the questionnaire. Thus, the final response rate was 55%.

The medical ethics committee of Erasmus Medical Centre, Rotterdam, the Netherlands determined that the rules stipulated in the Medical Research Involving Human Subjects Act did not apply to this study (protocol no. MEC-2018-021). Written informed consent to participate in the study was obtained from all participants.

Measures

Patient-centred primary care

The eight dimensions of PCC identified by the Picker Institute were used as a framework for the development of an instrument to assess PCC in the primary care setting for patients with multimorbidity. The development of the patient-centred primary care (PCPC) instrument also builts on our earlier work [30–32], in which we investigated the eight dimensions of PCC in hospital and long-term care settings, as well as adjusting them based on literature describing primary care for patients with multimorbidity (e.g. [22–25]) and consulting experts in the primary care setting when it comes to care for patients with multimorbidity (i.e., general practitioners, practice nurses, and patients with multimorbidity, who were consulted on item adjustment, removal, and addition). General practitioners ($n = 4$) and practice nurses ($n = 3$) known for delivering high levels of PCC in the area of Tilburg and patients dealing with multimorbidity (n = 3) for several years were selected as experts. First, they received the questionnaire via mail. All experts commented on the items via mail followed by a telephone meeting. Both authors discussed the comments and suggestions, which led to an adjusted version we send back to the experts. This was followed by another telephone meeting (with a selection of experts) and a personal meeting (with a patient expert) after which we reached agreement on a final set of 36 items, with responses structured by a five-point scale ranging from 1 (totally disagree) to 5 (totally agree).

Satisfaction with care

We used an adjusted version of the Satisfaction with inpatient Stroke Care (SASC) scale to assess satisfaction with care. Although the 8-item SASC was originally developed for use among stroke patients, it investigates experiences with care in general, not those related specifically to stroke care. Therefore, the SASC has been used widely in various patient populations to assess general satisfaction with care (e.g. [33–36]). The items were adjusted slightly for the primary care setting (e.g. 'The doctors have done everything they can to make me well again' was changed into 'The staff has done everything they can to make me well again'), with removal of irrelevant or overlapping items (e.g. the hospitalization process went smoothly and I have been treated with kindness and respect by the staff at the hospital), resulting in a final set of 6 items: 'I have received all the

Table 2 Characteristics of patients with multimorbidity in the study sample and their experiences with care

Characteristic		Percentage or mean (SD) range
Gender	Male	40.9%
Marital status	Single	43.2%
Educational level	Low	40.0%
Age (years)		74.46 (10.64) 47–94
Patient-centred care	Patients' preferences	3.94 (0.64) 1–5
	Physical comfort	3.91 (0.56) 1–5
	Coordination of care	3.89 (0.61) 1–5
	Emotional support	3.43 (0.75) 1–5
	Access to care	4.03 (0.56) 1–5
	Continuity and transition	3.97 (0.58) 1–5
	Information and education	3.89 (0.56) 1–5
	Family and friends	3.62 (1.00) 1–5
	Overall patient-centred care	3.83 (0.47) 1–5
Satisfaction with care		3.13 (0.45) 1–4

Results are based on list-wise deletion of missing cases. Results based on imputed data ($n = 216$) were similar. SD = Standard Deviation

Table 3 Characteristics of responses to the 36 patient-centred care items ($n = 216$)

Item	Valid n	Not applicable	Missing	Mean	SD	λ
Patients' preferences						
1. I felt taken seriously	214	–	2 (1%)	4.16	0.77	0.779
2.My wishes and preferences were taken into account when choosing a treatment	209	–	7 (3%)	3.93	0.75	0.870
3.I was involved in decisions about my treatment	209	–	7 (3%)	4.01	0.74	0.854
4.The influence that the treatment can have on my life was taken into account	209	–	7 (3%)	3.92	0.81	0.894
5. I was helped to determine my own treatment goals	211	–	5 (2%)	3.82	0.78	0.877
6.I felt supported to achieve my treatment goals	209	–	7 (3%)	3.89	0.78	0.825
7. I received advice that I really could use	209	–	7 (3%)	3.90	0.85	0.869
Physical comfort						
8. Attention was given to my physical comfort (such as the management of pain, shortness of breath)	190	19 (9%)	7 (3%)	4.10	0.83	0.736
9. Attention was paid to fatigue and insomnia	148	58 (27%)	10 (5%)	3.64	0.93	0.788
10. The (waiting) rooms were clean	210	–	6 (3%)	4.13	0.68	0.650
11. The (waiting) rooms were comfortable	211	–	5 (2%)	3.85	0.77	0.528
12. In the treatment room(s) and at the counter there was sufficient privacy	211	–	5 (2%)	3.77	0.89	0.681
Coordination of care						
13. Everyone was well informed; I only had to tell my story once	189	24 (11%)	3 (1%)	3.98	0.80	0.791
14. The care was well attuned between the practitioners involved		38 (18%)	3 (1%)	3.99	0.72	0.849
15. I knew who was coordinating my care	210	–	6 (3%)	3.75	0.82	0.753
16. I could easily contact someone with questions	209	–	7 (3%)	3.88	0.74	0.874
Continuity and transition						
17. When being referred to another care provider (specialist/dietician/physiotherapist) I was well informed about where to go and why	157	54 (25%)	5 (2%)	4.05	0.72	0.727
18. With a referral, all my information was passed on correctly	163	48 (22%)	5 (2%)	4.00	0.75	0.791
19. Advice (such as medication) from different practitioners (medical specialists and family doctor) was well attuned to each other	174	36 (17%)	6 (3%)	3.92	0.79	0.741
20. The treatment of the family doctor is in line with the treatment of other care providers	169	42 (19%)	5 (2%)	3.98	0.68	0.870
Emotional support						
21. Emotional support was also provided	202	–	14 (7%)	3.47	0.84	0.831
22. Attention was paid to possible feelings of fear, gloom and anxiety	98	–	18 (8%)	3.46	0.85	0.841
23. I was made aware of the possibilities for more intensive emotional support	146	61 (28%)	9 (4%)	3.30	1.03	0.851
24. Attention was paid to the impact of my health on my private life (family, relatives, work, social life)	202	–	14 (7%)	3.43	0.83	0.921
Access to care						
25. It was no problem to go from my home to my family doctor and back again	209	–	7 (3%)	3.92	1.03	0.700
26. The general practice was easily accessible	209	–	7 (3%)	4.24	0.63	0.817
27. I could easily schedule an appointment quickly	209	–	7 (3%)	4.00	0.72	0.778
28. On a visit I didn't have to wait long before it was my turn	206	–	10 (5%)	3.73	0.85	0.639
29. I could easily request a repeat recipe	207		9 (4%)	4.24	0.62	0.851
Information and education						
30. I was well informed	209	–	7 (3%)	4.02	0.65	0.883
31. The information I received was well explained	208	–	8 (4%)	3.99	0.67	0.889
32. I had easy access to my own data (lab results, medication overview, referrals)	203	–	13 (6%)	3.47	0.95	0.706
33. I could ask all the questions I wanted	211	–	5 (2%)	4.08	0.60	0.794

Table 3 Characteristics of responses to the 36 patient-centred care items ($n = 216$) *(Continued)*

Item	Valid *n*	Not applicable	Missing	Mean	SD	λ
Family and friends						
34. With my consent, relatives were involved in my treatment	105	103 (48%)	8 (4%)	3.74	1.03	0.954
35. Attention was given to care and support provided by family members	101	108 (50%)	7 (3%)	3.49	1.11	0.906
36. Attention was given to possible questions from my family members	98	110 (51%)	8 (4%)	3.69	0.94	0.903

information I want about the causes and nature of my illness(es)', 'The staff has done everything they can to make me well again', 'I am satisfied with the type of treatment they have given me (e. g. physiotherapy, occupational therapy)', 'I have had enough therapy (e.g. physiotherapy, occupational therapy)', 'I am happy about the effect treatments had on my disease progression', and 'I am satisfied with the treatment provided by the general practitioner who I visit'. Responses are structured by a four-point scale ranging from 1 (strongly disagree) to 4 (strongly agree), with higher mean scores indicating greater satisfaction. In this study among patients with multimorbidity, the Cronbach's alpha value for this adjusted 6-item instrument was 0.89, indicating good reliability.

Joint decision making and responsibility taking: Relational co-production of care

The 7-item relational co-production instrument was used to assess joint decision making and responsibility taking, as perceived by patients with multimorbidity [10, 37, 38]. Relational co-production refers to joint decision making and responsibility taking achieved through open communication, co-operation, and respect for each other, with negotiation of treatment options to accomplish mutually defined goals. Gittell (e.g. [39–42]) identified this concept as "relational coordination" when talking about the quality of relationships and communication among professionals and "relational coordination" if it concerns the quality of relationships and communication between patients and their health care professionals. High-quality relationships reinforce high-quality communication, encouraging professionals and patients with multimorbidity to listen to each other and to take account of the impacts of their actions on those engaged in different parts of the process, thereby helping them to react to new information in a co-ordinated way [43]. This questionnaire measures four aspects of communication (frequent, timely, accurate, and problem-solving) and three aspects of relationships (based on shared knowledge, goals, and mutual respect) between professionals and patients with multimorbidity. Responses are structured by a five-point Likert scale ranging from 1 (never) to 5 (always). This instrument has proven to be reliable and valid (based on structural and content validity, internal consistency and interrater agreement) in assessing the quality of communication and relationships [44, 45]. Higher mean scores indicate better realisation of joint decision making and responsibility taking, with scores ≥4 considered to represent success and scores < 4 considered to represent the lack of success perceived by patients with multimorbidity [46]. In this study, the Cronbach's alpha value for this instrument was 0.87, indicating good reliability.

Analysis

To validate the 36-item PCPC instrument, we first used descriptive statistics to characterise the study population with regard to age, gender, marital status, educational level, and experiences with primary care delivery (the eight dimensions of PCC and satisfaction with care). Second, we calculated the mean, standard deviation, number of missing responses, and lambda value for each

Table 4 Scale characteristics and (inter-)correlations of the 36-item patient-centred primary care instrument

	Cronbach's *α*	1	2	3	4	5	6	7	8
1. Patients' preferences	0.92								
2. Physical comfort	0.72	0.57***							
3. Coordination of care	0.82	0.60***	0.52***						
4. Emotional support	0.87	0.46***	0.37***	0.50***					
5. Access to care	0.74	0.45***	0.54***	0.53***	0.30***				
6. Continuity and transition	0.80	0.63***	0.59***	0.67***	0.43***	0.53***			
7. Information and education	0.78	0.56***	0.48***	0.57***	0.57***	0.53***	0.58***		
8. Family and friends	0.92	0.31***	0.37***	0.36***	0.43***	0.33***	0.42***	0.36***	
9. Overall patient-centred care	0.89[a]	0.77***	0.73***	0.80***	0.71***	0.68***	0.80***	0.76***	0.66***

***$p < 0.001$ (two-tailed). Results are based on list-wise deletion of missing cases. Results based on imputed data ($n = 216$) were similar. [a] Based on the eight dimensions (the value for the 36 items was 0.96)

PCPC item. Third, we used LISREL to conduct confirmatory factor analyses and verify the factor structure of the instrument. Fourth, we assessed model fit using the following cut-off criteria of Hu and Bentler [47]:

- standardised root mean square residual (SRMR) < 0.08,
- root mean square error of approximation (RMSEA) < 0.06, and
- comparative fit index (CFI) > 0.95.

Fifth, we used Cronbach's alpha values to assess the internal consistency of the subscales and examined inter-correlations to verify conceptual relatedness among (sub)-scales. Finally, we assessed the construct validity of the instrument overall and its eight dimensions by analysing associations with satisfaction with care. In addition, we examined whether scores for the eight dimensions of PCC were higher among patients who perceived the successful establishment of joint decision making and responsibility taking with their health care professionals than among those who perceived a lack of success.

Results

The mean age of the patients was 74.46 ± 10.64 (range 47–94) years (Table 2). Of the respondents, 40.9% were male, 43.2% were single, and 40% had lower educational levels.

PCPC item characteristics

Table 3 displays statistics for the 36 PCPC items. Item non-response rates ranged from 1 to 8%. Respondents gave considerable numbers of not-applicable responses in the family and friends dimension (about 100 per item), continuity and transition ($n = 36–54$), and coordination of care (item 14, $n = 38$; item 13, $n = 24$) dimensions. In addition, 61 respondents rated item 23 in the emotional support dimension as not applicable, and 19 and 58 respondents rated items 8 and 9, respectively, in the physical comfort dimension as not applicable.

All items had loadings on the intended factors > 0.50.

Model fit

The model showed good fit, meeting cut-off criteria (CFI = 0.987, SRMR = 0.079, RMSEA = 0.0548).

Internal consistency and inter-correlations

Internal consistency values for the PCPC subscales ranged from 0.72 (physical comfort) to 0.92 (family and friends; Table 4). The internal consistency value for the overall instrument was 0.89. All (sub)scales were correlated significantly and positively (all $p \leq 0.001$), indicating that they were conceptually related.

Construct validity

All eight dimensions of PCC were related positively to satisfaction with care (all $p \leq 0.001$), indicating construct validity (Table 5). In addition, scores in all dimensions were higher among patients with multimorbidity who experienced joint decision making and responsibility taking (Table 6).

Discussion

This study clearly showed that the 36-item PCPC instrument is valid and reliable for the assessment of PCC among patients with multimorbidity in the primary care setting. Given that multimorbidity is becoming the leading threat to population health and the greatest challenge for primary care systems worldwide, such an instrument can help to improve levels of patient centredness for this vulnerable population. Findings from several countries indicate that the prevalence of chronic diseases and multimorbidity is especially high in the primary care setting [8, 48–51]. Primary care providers are currently not equipped to deal with the complexities of ageing populations [51]. Health professionals clearly express the concern that they often missed the opportunity to engage chronically ill older patients as true partners in their care and really help them to manage their conditions at home. Identification of levels of patient centredness according to patients with multimorbidity provides insight in how well organizations are doing regarding the eight dimensions of PCC and helps identify the areas which need improvement (the dimensions with lower scores). Confirmatory factor analyses revealed good indices of fit for the instrument. As indicated by the high reliability coefficient, the scale showed good internal consistency. We found support for construct validity through significant positive correlations between PCPC scores and satisfaction with care. These findings are in line with earlier research showing positive associations between the eight dimensions of PCC and satisfaction with care [16]. This research also showed that patients with

Table 5 Correlations of patient-centred care dimension scores with satisfaction with care

Dimension	Satisfaction with care
Patients' preferences	0.45***
Physical comfort	0.38***
Coordination of care	0.49***
Emotional support	0.32***
Access to care	0.46***
Continuity and transition	0.51***
Information and education	0.46***
Family and friends	0.34***
Overall person-centred care	0.53***

***$p < 0.001$ (two-tailed). Results are based on list-wise deletion of missing cases. Results based on imputed data ($n = 216$) were similar

Table 6 Relationships between joint decision making and responsibility taking (relational co-production of care) and patient-centred care

Dimension	No joint decision making/ responsibility taking (score ≥ 4; 37%)	Joint decision making/ responsibility taking (score < 4; 63%)	*p* value
Patients' preferences	4.16 (0.57)	3.81 (0.65)	≤0.001
Physical comfort	4.09 (0.60)	3.81 (0.51)	≤0.001
Coordination of care	4.11 (0.55)	3.76 (0.62)	≤0.001
Emotional support	3.69 (0.65)	3.30 (0.76)	≤0.001
Access to care	4.22 (0.47)	3.91 (0.57)	≤0.001
Continuity and transition	4.21 (0.55)	3.82 (0.56)	≤0.001
Information and education	4.14 (0.53)	3.82 (0.56)	≤0.001
Family and friends	3.93 (0.94)	3.41 (0.98)	0.009
Overall patient-centred care	4.05 (0.45)	3.71 (0.44)	≤0.001

Results are based on list-wise deletion of missing cases. Results based on imputed data ($n = 216$) were similar

multimorbidity who perceived joint decision making and responsibility taking with their health care professionals also reported higher levels of all eight dimensions of PCC.

Several psychometric properties of the PCPC instrument could not be evaluated in this study and thus remain undefined. They include the instrument's responsiveness, sensitivity to change, predictive value (e.g. clinical outcomes), relationship to other PCC instruments, and different modes of administration. Secondly, we included patients enrolled in at least two chronic care programmes (involving diagnosis of and treatment for combinations of diabetes, asthma and/or chronic obstructive pulmonary disease, cardiovascular diseases and conditions, and age-related frailty). Given that these patients were enrolled in at least 2 or more chronic care programmes we were able to identify and select them from the data registries of the health care practices. As a consequence patients who are dealing with a chronic illness other than diabetes, asthma and/or chronic obstructive pulmonary disease, cardiovascular diseases and conditions, and age-related frailty (which are the most prevalent chronic conditions) were not included. Further research is needed to assess the validity of this instrument among patients with (a combination of) other chronic illnesses as well as the general patient population in the primary care setting. Thirdly, some items had high numbers of 'non-applicable' responses. Although these aspects may not be applicable to all patients with multimorbidity in the primary care setting (e.g., emotional support and attention paid to fatigue and insomnia is only needed for those who struggle in these areas and transition of care is only relevant for those who are referred to another health care professional), if they are applicable they are crucial for their outcomes [22–24]. Fourthly, while after four iterative rounds we reached agreement on a final set of 36 items, we did not use a formal consensus method. Fifthly, while the original SASC to assess satisfaction with care has been validated among patients in the hospital we slightly adjusted the instrument to assess satisfaction with care among patients with multimorbidity in the primary care setting (e.g. replacing 'doctor' with 'staff'). Although the Cronbach's alpha (0.89) shows the instrument is reliable in this setting this adjusted 6-item SASC has not been formally validated yet. This may have limited testing concurrent construct validity of the PCC instrument. Finally, we tested the Dutch version of the 36-item PCPC instrument; we recommend testing of the English version in other countries to ensure international validity using adequate translation procedures such as forward-translations and back-translations recommended by the World Health Organisation [52].

Conclusion

We conclude that the psychometric properties of the 36-item PCPC instrument are good. Based on these results the PCPC instrument seems a promising tool for the assessment of PCC among patients with multimorbidity in the primary care setting.

Abbreviations

CFI: Comparative fit index; PCC: Patient-centred care; PCPC instrument: Patient-centred primary care instrument; RMSEA: Root mean square error of approximation; SASC: Satisfaction with inpatient stroke care; SD: Standard deviation; SRMR: Standardised root mean square residual

Acknowledgements

The authors thank all patients for taking the time to fill in the questionnaires.

Funding

We received funding from CZ and VGZ (Dutch health care insurance companies). They provided funding for this study only, the results are based on the findings of the research only.

Authors' contributions

JC and AN drafted the design for data collection. JC was involved in subject recruitment and data collection, AN performed the statistical analysis, and JC and AN interpreted the data. JC and AN drafted the manuscript and contributed equally to its refinement. Both authors have read and approved the final version.

Consent for publication
Not applicable.

Competing interests
The authors declare that they have no competing interest.

References

1. World Health Organization. People-centred and integrated health services: an overview of the evidence. Interim report. Geneva: World Health Organization; 2015.
2. Fortin M, Lapointe L, Hudon C, Vanasse A, Ntetu AL, Maltais D. Multimorbidity and quality of life in primary care: a systematic review. Health Qual Life Outcomes. 2004;2:51.
3. Vogeli C, Shields AE, Lee TA, Gibson TB, Marder WD, Weiss KB, et al. Multiple chronic conditions: prevalence, health consequences, and implications for quality, care management, and costs. J Gen Intern Med. 2007;22(Suppl 3):391–5.
4. Menotti A, Mulder I, Nissinen A, Giampaoli S, Feskens EJ, Kromhout D. Prevalence of morbidity and multimorbidity in elderly male populations and their impact on 10-year all-cause mortality: the FINE study (Finland, Italy, Netherlands, elderly). J Clin Epidemiol. 2001;54:680–6.
5. van Oostrom SH, Picavet HS, van Gelder BM, Lemmens LC, Hoeymans N, van Dijk CE, et al. Multimorbidity and comorbidity in the Dutch population: data from general practices. BMC Public Health. 2012;12:715.
6. Glynn LG, Valderas JM, Healy P, Burke E, Newell J, Gillespie P, et al. The prevalence of multimorbidity in primary care and its effect on health care utilization and cost. Fam Pract. 2011;28:516–23.
7. Fortin M, Bravo G, Hudon C, Lapointe L, Almirall J, Dubois MF, et al. Relationship between multimorbidity and health-related quality of life of patients in primary care. Qual Life Res. 2006;15:83–91.
8. Osborn R, Moulds D, Squires D, Doty MM, Anderson C. International survey of older adults finds shortcomings in access, coordination, and patient-centered care. Health Aff. 2014;33(12):2247–55.
9. Wagner EH, Bennett SM, Austin BT, Greene SM, Schaefer JK, Von Korff M. Finding common ground: patient-centeredness and evidence-based chronic illness care. J Altern Complement Med. 2005;11:S7–15.
10. Cramm JM, Nieboer AP. Longitudinal study to identify the influence of quality of chronic care delivery on productive interactions between patients and (teams of) healthcare professionals within disease management programs. BMJ Open. 2014;4:e005914.
11. Cramm JM, Nieboer AP. Is "disease management" the answer to our problems? No! Population health management and (disease) prevention require "management of overall well-being". BMC Health Serv Res. 2016;16:500.
12. Cramm JM, Nieboer AP. Chronically ill patients' self-management abilities to maintain overall well-being: what is needed to take the next step in the primary care setting? BMC Fam Pract. 2015;16:123.
13. Cramm JM, Nieboer AP. Disease management: the need for a focus on broader self-management abilities and quality of life. Population Health Management. 2015;18(4):246–55.
14. Gerteis M, Edgman-Levitan S, Daley J, Delbanco TL. Through the patient's eyes: understanding and promoting patient-centered care. San Francisco: Jossey-Bass; 1993.
15. Gerteis M, Edgman-Levitan S, Walker JD, Stokes DM, Cleary PD, Delbanco TL. What patients really want. Health Manage Q. 1993;15(3):2–6.
16. Rathert C, Wyrwich M, Boren S. Patient-centered care and outcomes: a systematic review of the literature. Med Care Res Rev. 2013;70(4):351–79.
17. Bechtel C, Ness DL. If you build it, will they come? Designing truly patient-centered health care. Health Aff (Millwood). 2010;29(5):914–20.
18. Berwick DM. (2009). What patient-centered should mean: confessions of an extremist. Health Aff. 2009;28:555–65.
19. Greene SM, Tuzzio L, Cherkin D. A framework for making patient-centered care front and center. Perm J. 2012;16(3):49–53.
20. Kitson A, Marshall A, Bassett K, Zeitz K. What are the core elements of patient-centred care? A narrative review and synthesis of the literature from health policy, medicine and nursing. J Adv Nurs. 2013;69(1):4–15.
21. Mead N, Bower P. Patient-centredness: a conceptual framework and review of the empirical literature. Soc Sci Med. 2000;51(7):1087–110.
22. Duguay C, Gallagher F, Fortin M. The experience of adults with multimorbidity: a qualitative study. J Comorbidity. 2014;4:11–21.
23. Sturmberg JP, Botelho RJ, Kissling B. Integrated multimorbidity management in primary care: why, what, how, and how to? Journal of Comorbidity. 2016;6(2):114–9.
24. AGS (American Geriatrics Society) Expert Panel on the Care of Older Adults with Multimorbidity. Patient-centered Care for Older Adults with multiple chronic conditions: a stepwise approach from the American Geriatrics Society. J Am Geriatr Soc. 2012;60(10):1957–68.
25. Kim DH, Rich MW. Patient-centred care of older adults with cardiovascular disease and multiple chronic conditions. Can J Cardiol. 2016;30:1097–107.
26. Delaney LJ. Patient-centred care as an approach to improving health care in Australia. Collegian. 2018;25(1):119–23.
27. Ekman I, Wolf A, Olsson L, Taft C, Dudas K, Schaufelberger M, Swedberg K. Effects of person-centred care in patients with chronic heart failure: the PCC-HF study. Eur Heart J. 2012;33:1112–9.
28. Kinmonth AL, Woodcock A, Griffin S, Spiegal N, Campbell MJ. Randomised controlled trial of patient centred care of diabetes in general practice: impact on current wellbeing and future disease risk. The diabetes care from diagnosis research team. BMJ. 1998;317:1202–8.
29. Wolf D, Lehman L, Quinlin R, Rosenzweig M, Friede S, Zullo T, Hoffman L. Can nurses impact patient outcomes using a patient-centered care model? J Nurs Adm. 2008;38(12):532–40.
30. Cramm JM, Leensvaart L, Berghout MA, van Exel J. Exploring views on what is important for patient-centred care in end-stage renal disease using Q methodology. BMC Nephrol. 2015;16:74.
31. Berghout MA, Leensvaart L, van Exel J, Cramm JM. (2015). Healthcare professionals' views on patient-centered care in hospitals. BMC Health Serv Res. 2015;15:385.
32. Cramm JM, Nieboer AP. Validation of an instrument to assess the delivery of patient-centred care to people with intellectual disabilities as perceived by professionals. BMC Health Serv Res. 2017;17:472.
33. Baumann C, Rat AC, Mainard D, Cuny C, Guillemin F. Importance of patient satisfaction with care in predicting osteoarthritis-specific health-related quality of life one year after total joint arthroplasty. Qual Life Res. 2011;20(10):1581–8.
34. Brédart A, Robertson C, Razavi D, Batel-Copel L, Larsson G, Lichosik D, et al. Patients' satisfaction ratings and their desire for care improvement across oncology settings from France, Italy, Poland and Sweden. Psychooncology. 2003;12(1):68–77.
35. Pöder U, Von Essen L. Perceptions of support among Swedish parents of children on cancer treatment: a prospective, longitudinal study. Eur J Cancer Care (Engl). 2009;18(4):350–7.
36. Von Essen L, Larsson G, Oberg K, Sjödén PO. 'Satisfaction with care': associations with health-related quality of life and psychosocial function among Swedish patients with endocrine gastrointestinal tumours. Eur J Cancer Care (Engl). 2002;11(2):91–9.
37. Gittell JH, Douglass A. Relational bureaucracy: structuring reciprocal relationships into roles. Acad Manag Rev. 2012;37:709–33.
38. Van der Meer L, Nieboer AP, Finkenflügel HJM, Cramm JM. The importance of person-centred care and co-creation of care for the well-being and job satisfaction of professionals working with people with intellectual disabilities. Scandinavian J of Caring Sci. 2017; https://doi.org/10.1111/scs.12431.
39. Gittell JH. Organizing work to support relational coordination. Internat J Human Resource Management. 2000;11:517–39.
40. Gittell JH. Coordinating mechanisms in care provider groups: relational coordination as a mediator and input uncertainty as a moderator of performance effects. Management Sci. 2002;48(11):1408–26.
41. Gittell JH, Fairfield K, Bierbaum B, Jackson R, Kelly M, Laskin R, Lipson S, Siliski J, Thornhill T, Zuckerman J. Impact of relational coordination on quality of care, postoperative pain and functioning, and length of stay: a nine-hospital study of surgical patients. Med Care. 2000;38(8):807–19.
42. Weinberg DB, Gittell JH, Lusenhop RW, Kautz CM, Wright J. Beyond our walls: impact of patient and provider coordination across the continuum on outcomes for surgical patients. Health Serv Res. 2007;42(1):7–24.
43. Gittell JH. Relationships between service providers and their impact on customers. J Serv Res. 2002;4:299–311.
44. Gittell JH, Seidner R, Wimbush J. A relational model of how high-performance work systems work. OrganizationScience. 2010;21(2):490–506.
45. Valentine MA, Nembhard IG, Edmondson AC. Measuring teamwork in health care settings. A review of survey instruments. Med Care. 2015;53(4):e16–30.
46. Relational Coordination Analytics Inc. Overview and analysis: relational coordination data (memo). Cambridge: Relational Coordination Analytics Inc; 2016.

47. Hu L, Bentler PM. Cutoff criteria for fit indexes in covariance structure analysis: conventional criteria versus new alternatives. Struct Equ Modeling. 1999;6:1–55.
48. Fortin M, Stewart M, Poitras ME, Almirall J, Maddocks H. A systematic review of prevalence studies on multimorbidity: toward a more uniform methodology. Ann Fam Med. 2012;10:142–51.
49. Schneider KM, O'Donnell BE, Dean D. Prevalence of multiple chronic conditions in the United States' Medicare population. Health Qual Life Outcomes. 2009;7:82.
50. Barnett K, Mercer SW, Norbury M, Watt G, Wyke S, Guthrie B. Epidemiology of multimorbidity and implications for health care, research, and medical education: a cross-sectional study. Lancet. 2012;380:37–43.
51. Korownyk C, et al. Competing demands and opportunities in primary care. Can Fam Physician. 2017;63(9):664–8.
52. WHO: Process of translation and adaptation of instruments http://www.who.int/substance_abuse/research_tools/translation/en/. Accessed 27 May 2018.

2

Novel oral anticoagulants in primary care in patients with atrial fibrillation: a cross-sectional comparison before and after their introduction

Simon Schwill[1*], Katja Krug[1], Frank Peters-Klimm[1], Jan van Lieshout[2], Gunter Laux[1], Joachim Szecsenyi[1] and Michel Wensing[1]

Abstract

Background: Novel oral anticoagulation (NOAC) has been introduced in recent years, but data on use in atrial fibrillation (AF) in primary care setting is scarce. In Germany, General Practitioners are free to choose type of oral anticoagulation (OAC) in AF. Our aim was to explore changes in prescription-rates of OAC in German primary care before and after introduction of NOAC on the market.

Methods: Data of a representative morbidity registration project in primary care in Germany (CONTENT) were analysed. Patients with AF in 2011 or 2014 were included (before and after broad market authorization of NOAC, respectively). We defined three independent groups: patients from 2011 without follow-up (group A), patients from 2014 but without previous record in 2011 (group B) and patients with AF and records in 2011 and 2014 (group C).

Results: 2642 patients were included. Group A ($n = 804$) and B ($n = 755$) were comparable regarding patient characteristics. 87.3% of group A and 84.8% of group B had CHA_2DS_2-VASc-Score ≥ 2, indicating a need for oral anticoagulation (OAC). Prescription of OAC increased from 23.1% ($n = 186$) to 42.8% ($n = 323$, $p < .01$) with stable use of vitamin-k-antagonist (22.6–24.9%). NOAC increased from 0.6 to 19.2% ($p < .01$). Monotherapy with Acetylsalicylic acid (ASA) decreased from 15.3% ($n = 123$) to 8.2% ($n = 62$, $p < .01$). In group C ($n = 1083$), OAC increased from 35.3 to 55.4% ($p < .01$), with stable prescription rate of vitamin-k-antagonist (34.4–35.7%). NOAC increased from 0.9 to 21.5% ($p < .01$).

Conclusions: In summary, our study showed a significant increase of OAC over time, which is fostered by the use of NOAC but with a stable rate of VKA and a sharp decrease of ASA. Patients on VKA are rarely switched to NOAC, but new patients with AF are more likely to receive NOAC.

Keywords: Atrial fibrillation, Stroke prevention, Oral anticoagulation, Vitamin K antagonists, Novel oral anticoagulants

* Correspondence: simon.schwill@med.uni-heidelberg.de
[1]Department of General Practice and Health Services Research, University Hospital Heidelberg, Heidelberg, Germany
Full list of author information is available at the end of the article

Background

Atrial fibrillation (AF) is the most common cardiac arrhythmia, with an estimated prevalence of 1.5 to 2% of the general population, which is increasing worldwide, driven by an ageing population [1–3]. Nearly 10% of people above 75 years suffer from AF [4]. Patients have an almost fivefold higher risk of stroke [5] and mortality is up to 2.5 times higher compared with age-matched individuals [2].

Regardless of causal treatment, prophylaxis of stroke by use of oral anticoagulation (OAC) was shown to reduce risk of stroke and therefore is recommend in patients with AF by international guidelines [6, 7]. The CHA_2DS_2--VASc-Score has been recommended for risk stratification [6–8]. For decades vitamin-K antagonists (VKA) had been the only OAC in AF, accompanied by prescription of acetylsalicylic acid (ASA), which is no longer recommended [6, 7]. In recent years novel-oral-anticoagulants (NOAC) such as Apixaban, Dabigatran, Edoxaban and Rivaroxaban offered an alternative OAC to prevent stroke in non-valvular AF. Use of NOAC is increasing and recently updated guidelines on AF by the European Society of Cardiology advocate use of NOAC over VKA [6]. Clinical guidelines on AF for primary care physicians present NOAC as a valid option, but do not necessarily recommend changing patients from VKA to NOAC [9].Data on use of (N)OAC in AF in routine primary care setting is scarce [10–14]. In Germany, NOAC were licensed for the indication of oral anticoagulation for the prevention of stroke in non-valvular atrial fibrillation between November 2011 and June 2015: Dabigatran in 11 /2011, Rivaroxaban in 12/2011, Apixaban in 12/2012 and Edoxaban in 06/2015 [15–18]. The aims of this study were to document changes in prescription-rates of OAC (VKA and NOAC) in primary care patients with AF in Germany before and after introduction of NOAC on the market, and to explore whether known patients with AF were switched onto NOAC.

Methods

Study design

We performed a retrospective epidemiological study in primary care practices including a cross-sectional comparison of two independent samples and a cross-sectional comparison of same patients at two points of time.

Setting

Data were derived from the CONTinuous-morbidity-registration-Epidemiologic-NeTwork (CONTENT) in South-Germany, which started in 2005 [19]. A total of 43 general practices were involved in this study. CONTENT provides representative data in terms of social, ethnic and economic backgrounds as well as urban, suburban and rural areas. The quality of data is high due to constant education of participating teams as well as continuous feedback on recording quality to participating physicians.

Sample

In 2016, data of CONTENT starting in 2005 up to 31.12.2014 was included in the study and analysed retrospectively. We performed a before and after comparison on the prescription of OAC, which compared data from 2011, when there was little experience with NOAC and data from 2014, when Apixaban, Dabigatran and Rivaroxaban were broadly available. Edoxaban was not licensed in Germany in 2014. Out of all patients with diagnosed AF (ICD I48.0) we included patients with AF from 01.01.2011–31.12.2011 or 01.01.2014–31.12.2014. Afterwards, we, defined three independent groups: patients with AF in 2011 but without follow-up in 2014(group A), patients with AF in 2014 but without previous record in 2011 (group B) and patients with AF and records in 2011 and 2014 (group C). Difference between groups A and B was related to newly diagnosed AF, mortality and patient change of practice. Patients of group C were not included in other groups neither A nor B.

Measures

Relevant data were extracted from the CONTENT database. For each patient age, gender as well as prescription of medication, diagnoses and specialist referrals were determined. Age was calculated from the year of birth. Gender and age were used for measurement of CHA_2DS_2-VASc-Score. Diagnoses were given as ICD-10 codes. Prescriptions were given as ATC-codes (Anatomical Therapeutical Classification for medication, World Health Organization). Secondly, prescriptions were analysed for VKA [Phenprocoumon = ATC-B01AA04] and NOAC [Apixaban = ATC-B01AX08, Dabigatran = ATC--B01AE07, Rivaroxaban = ATC-B01AX06] and ASA [acetylsalicylic-acid = ATC-B01AC06]. We extracted diagnoses needed for the CHA_2DS_2-VASc-Score. Congestive heart failure (I50.*), Hypertension (I10.*) Diabetes (E10.-E11.*, E14.*), Stroke (I63.*) and Vascular disease (I70.*). At time of study CHA_2DS_2-VASc-Score ≥ 2 indicated OAC in patients with AF[7]. If data of hypertension or diabetes were not encoded, prescription of an antidiabetic [ATC-A10] or antihypertensive [angiotensin-converting-enzyme-inhibitor = ATC-C09AA, Angiotensin-II-receptor-antagonists = ATC-C09CA, Nifedipine = ATC-C08CA05, Hydrochlorothiazide = ATC-C03AA03] medication was accepted instead.

To address potential contraindications we extracted diagnoses renal insufficiency (N17.*-N19.*), coagulopathy (D68.-D69.*), intracranial bleeding (I60.-I62.*, S06.4-S06.6.*, S06.9), epistaxis (R04.0-R04.2), gastrointestinal bleeding

(K92.0-K92.2, K62.5) and stroke (I63.-I64.*). We recorded specialist referrals only to cardiologists.

Data analysis

Patient-characteristics were summarized in terms of frequencies of categories, means with standard deviation and medians with interquartile range for continuous variables. Differences between independent groups A and B were tested in Chi-squared-tests for frequencies, Fishers exact test, t-tests for independent samples or MannWhitney-U-tests for continuous data, dependent on data distribution. Changes over time (group C) were analysed with McNemar's-tests for frequencies and t-tests for dependent samples or Wilcoxon-signed-rank-tests for continuous data, dependent on data distribution. *P*-values < 0.05 were considered to indicate statistical significance. Due to the exploratory character of the analysis, there was no correction for multiple testing. All analyses were performed with IBM SPSS version 21.0.

Results

Patient characteristics

Total number of patient in CONTENT in 2011 was n = 145,461 (point-prevalence of AF on 31.12.2011: 1.51%), in 2014 n = 207,253 (point-prevalence of AF on 31.12.2014: 1.85%).In total, data of n = 2642 patients from 43 general practices was obtained in this study. We included n = 804 in Group A, n = 755 in Group B and n = 1083 in Group C. In two-sample comparison, presented in Table 1, groups A and B did not differ regarding sex or comorbidities, but group B was younger than group A ($p < 0.01$). Number of patients > 75 years, contributing to CHA_2DS_2-VASc-Score twice, was 66.3% in group A (n = 533) which was comparable to 61.9% in group B (n = 467). 87.3% of patients in group A (n = 702) and 84.8% of patients in group B (n = 640) presented with CHA_2DS_2-VASc-Score ≥ 2, which indicated OAC at time of the study (p = n.s.).

Group C included n = 1083 patients (Table 2), of whom 51.9% were above 75 years in 2011 (n = 562) and 64.4% in 2014 (n = 697). Percentage of patients with CHA_2DS_2--VASc-Score ≥ 2 increased from 81.6% (n = 884) to 83.8% (n = 908, $p < .01$). 91% of patients with diagnosed AF presented with at least one additional diagnosis, such as renal insufficiency (n = 1003).

Prescription of oral-anticoagulation

Two-sample comparison revealed an increase of prescription of OAC from 23.1% in 2011 (n = 186) to 42.8% in 2014 (n = 323, $p < .01$). Prescription-rate of VKA remained stable (22.6%, n = 182 and 24.9%, n = 188). Prescription of NOAC increased from 0.6% (n = 5) to 19.2% (n = 145, $p < .01$), whereas monotherapy with ASA decreased from 15.3% (n = 123) to 8.2% (n = 62, $p < .01$). The majority of patients with NOAC in 2014 received Rivaroxaban (84.8%, n = 121) compared to Dabigatran (9.6%, n = 14) and Apixaban (6.9%, n = 10). In 2014, cardiologists were involved more often compared with 2011 (15.5%, n = 125versus 21.9%, n = 165, $p < .01$).

In group C (involving longitudinal comparison, n = 1083), prescription of OAC increased from 35.3% (n = 382) to 55.4% (n = 600, p < .01) with similar prescription rate of VKA (34.4%, n = 373 and 35.7%, n = 387). Mean annual prescriptions per patient increased from 19.3 to 22.4 (p < .01). Prescription of NOAC in group C increased from 0.9 to 21.5% (p < .01). Prescription of ASA decreased over time (2011:12.6%, n = 136, 2014:9.0%, n = 97, p < .01). 11.9% (n = 44) of patients with VKA were switched to NOAC and in 19.9% OAC (n = 74) was discontinued completely. In 2011, 9 patients received a NOAC, of which 4 were stopped until 2014 and one patient was switched to VKA. 11.9% (n = 44) of patients with VKA were switched to NOAC. In 2014, majority of patients with AF and OAC received VKA: Group B: 56% n = 188/333, Group C: 62.5% n = 387/619.

In group C, 22.6–24.2% of patients attended a cardiologist but involvement of cardiologists did not significantly change over time (2011: 22.6%, 2014: 24.2%, $p < .32$). If cardiologists were involved, prescription of OAC increased over time from 51.6% in 2011 to 67.2% of patients in 2014 ($p < .01$).

Discussion

In patients with recorded AF in German primary care there was in increase in prescription-rate for OAC between 2011 and 2014: A cross-sectional comparison revealed that in 2014 42.8% (n = 323) of patients with AF received OAC compared to 23.1% (n = 186) in 2011. A longitudinal comparison (group C) showed an increase of OAC in AF from 35.3% (n = 383) to 55.4% (n = 600). This increase in prescription-rate was mainly due to new prescription of NOAC, while prescription-rate of VKA remained stable. In longitudinal comparison (group C) use of NOAC increased to 21.4% (n = 232) of patients with AF in 2014, with Rivaroxaban as most frequently prescribed. In 2014, cardiologists were involved in about 25% of patients (Group B: 21.9% (n = 165) and Group C: 24.2% (n = 262) and their involvement increased the likelihood of OAC prescribing. However, analysis showed no difference in cardiologists preference between VKA and NOAC and in 2014 majority of patients with OAC in AF still received VKA (Group B: 56% n = 188/333, Group C: 62.5% n = 387/619). Our analysis showed that patients were rarely switched from VKA to NOAC but were more likely to receive NOAC if diagnosed newly.

Interestingly, over 80% of patients with AF (group A 87.3%, group B 84.8%, group C 81.6%/83.8%) presented with CHADS-VasC Score ≥ 2 indicating OAC (at time of

Table 1 Patient characteristics comparing 2011 and 2014 independently

			GROUP A (2011)	GROUP B (2014)	*p*-value
patients (n)	total		804	755	
	gender (%)	male	374 (46.5%)	388 (51.4%)	.06[a]
		female	429 (53.4%)	367 (48.6%)	
		undetermined	1 (0.1%)	0	
	age (years)	Median (IQR)	79 (71–86)	77 (70–83)	<.01[b]
		Min – Max	19–99	18–103	
		< 65	92 (11.4%)	118 (15.6%)	
		65–74	179 (22.3%)	170 (22.5%)	
		≥75	533 (66.3%)	467 (61.9%)	
	additional diagnosis	at least 1 additional	750 (93.3%)	724 (95.9%)	.02[a]
		renal insufficiency	54 (6.7%)	55 (7.3%)	.66[a]
		coagulopathy	13 (1.6%)	17 (2.3%)	.36[a]
		intracranial bleeding	8 (1.0%)	6 (0.8%)	.68[a]
		epistaxis	7 (0.9%)	10 (1.3%)	.39[a]
		gastrointestinal bleeding	15 (1.9%)	12 (1.6%)	.68[a]
		stroke	43 (5.3%)	34 (4.5%)	.44[a]
	CHA_2DS_2-VASC:	0	48 (6.0%)	56 (7.4%)	.34[a]
		1	54 (6.7%)	59 (7.8%)	
		≥2	702 (87.3%)	640 (84.8%)	
	prescriptions (per year)	patients with at least 1 prescription	684 (85.1%)	677 (89.7%)	<.01[a]
		Md (IQR)	12 (5–25)	15 (6–24)	.31[b]
		Min - Max	1–123	1–123	
		all patients			.02[b]
		Md (IQR)	10 (2–22.8)	13 (3–23)	
		Min - Max	0–123	0–123	
	OAC	VKA or NOAC	186 (23.1%)	323 (42.8%)	<.01[a]
		VKA	182 (22.6%)	188 (24.9%)	.29[a]
		Rivaroxaban	0 (0.0%)	121 (16.0%)	<.01[a]
		Dabigatran	5 (0.6%)	14 (1.9%)	.03[a]
		Apixaban	0 (0.0%)	10 (1.3%)	<.01[c]
	ASA (without additional OAC)[d]		123 (15.3%)	62 (8.2%)	<.01[a]
	consultation of cardiologist		125 (15.5%)	165 (21.9%)	<.01[a]

CONTENT-Patients with diagnosis of atrial fibrillation, which were registered only once, either in 2011 (group A) or in 2014 (group B). *OAC* oral anticoagulation, *VKA* vitamin-k antagonists, *NOAC* novel oral anticoagulation, *ASA* Acetylsalicylic acid
[a]Chi^2-test, [b]Mann-Whitney-U-test, [c]Fisher's exact test
[d]Indication for ASA (100 mg), such as peripheral vascular disease or post-stroke or post-myocardial infarction or else and either as primary or secondary prophylaxis, could not clearly be stated

study). High percentage might be explained by the age, as in our study about two third of patients were 75 years of age or higher, scoring 2 within the CHA_2DS_2-VASc--Score, and thereby had a formal indication for OAC at time of the study. However, this represents the population in primary care.Recently updated guidelines on AF postulate evidence that OAC can prevent majority of ischemic strokes in AF and prolong life [6]. Although our findings suggest suboptimal prescribing-rates of OAC, they should be interpreted carefully. Patient populations in clinical trials of OAC differ regarding age, sex and co-morbidities from those treated in primary care [20, 21].

The benefit-risk-ratio of OAC and NOAC more particularly, may be less positive in primary care patients compared to patients in cardiology trials. In routine data, we miss documentation of reasons for not-prescribing OAC such as increased bleeding risk, alcohol-abuse, liver-failure or uncontrolled hypertension (which could not be accessed). Qualitative studies on prescribing OAC in

Table 2 Patient characteristics over time

			GROUP C (2011)	GROUP C (2014)	*p*-value
patients (n)	total		1083		n/a
	gender (%)	male	584 (53.9%)		n/a
		female	470 (43.4%)		
		undetermined	29 (2.7%)		
	age (years)	Median (IQR)	75 (68–81)	78 (71–84)	n/a
		Min – Max	24–93	27–96	
		< 65	200 (18.5%)	145 (13.4%)	
		65–74	321 (29.6%)	241 (22.3%)	
		≥75	562 (51.9%)	697 (64.4%)	
	additional diagnosis	patients With at least 1	1003 (92.6%)	986 (91.0%)	.13[a]
		renal insufficiency	61 (5.6%)	65 (6.0%)	.77[a]
		coagulopathy	17 (1.6%)	17 (1.6%)	1.0[a]
		intracranial bleeding	4 (0.4%)	5 (0.5%)	1.0[a]
		epistaxis	21 (1.9%)	14 (1.3%)	.30[a]
		gastrointestinal bleeding	13 (1.2%)	17 (1.6%)	.59[a]
		stroke	33 (3.0%)	28 (2.6%)	.58[a]
	CHA_2DS_2-VASC:	0	92 (8.5%)	59 (5.4%)	<.01[a]
		1	100 (9.2%)	87 (8.0%)	
		≥2	884 (81.6)	908 (83.8%)	
		not computable	7 (0.6%)	29 (2.7%)	n/a
	prescriptions (per year)	total	1056 (97.5%)	1064 (98.2%)	n/a
		M (SD)	19.4 (14.6)	22.6 (16.5)	<.01[b]
		Min - Max	1–118	1–115	
		all patients including those without prescription			<.01[b]
		M (SD)	18.8 (14.8)	22.0 (16.7)	
		Min - Max	0–118	0–115	
	OAC[1]	VKA or NOAC	382 (35.3%)	600 (55.4%)	<.01[a]
		VKA	373 (34.4%)	387 (35.7%)	.41[a]
		Rivaroxaban	3 (0.3%)	181 (16.7%)	<.01[a]
		Dabigatran	7 (0.6%)	23 (2.1%)	<.01[a]
		Apixaban	none	28 (2.6%)	n/c
	ASA (without additional OAC)[2]		136 (12.6%)	97 (9.0%)	<.01[a]
	consultation of cardiologist		245 (22.6%)	262 (24.2%)	.32[a]

CONTENT-Patients with diagnosis of atrial fibrillation, which were observed over time including data from 2011 and follow-up in 2014 (group C). OAC = oral anticoagulation, VKA = vitamin-k antagonists, NOAC = novel oral anticoagulation, ASA = Acetylsalicylic acid

[1]Different prescriptions per year such as VKA and NOAC or NOAC and NOAC was possible (*n* = 29)

[2]Indication for ASA (100 mg), such as peripheral vascular disease or post-stroke or post-myocardial infarction or else and either as primary or secondary prophylaxis, could not clearly be stated

[a]McNemar test, [b] t-test for dependent samples

primary care are rare, but it can be assumed that low life expectancy, high risk of falling and bleeding, as well as frailty are reasons to refrain from prescribing OAC in AF. This contrasts with views of experts, such as the European-Primary-Care-Cardiovascular-Society (EPCCS), who claim that a high bleeding-risk-score (such as HAS-BLED, ORBIT or ABC) should generally not result in withholding OAC [6, 22].

Our data showed a significant increase in the prescription-rate of OAC in AF before and after market-share of NOAC. The design of our study does not allow causal attribution so it is not known if this increase might be caused by an alternative medication to VKA general practitioners had awaited, by an update and implementation of guidelines on non-valvular AF, by a generous promotion of NOAC or a mix of it all.

We showed majority of patients with AF and OAC in 2014 received VKA. Until today, whether NOAC or VKA are safer and/or more effective in prophylaxis of stroke in non-valvular AF remains a key-point of experts-discussions as well as on-going trials [23]. In summary, there is a need for further research into the determinants of prescribing OAC in patients with AF in primary care.

Strengths and limitations

Strengths of this study are large number of primary care practices and reasonably high quality of patient records. Participating practices had university affiliation, which is associated with higher involvement in continuous medical education. It may be noted that in the German health care system documentation of AF (ICD48.*) must be confirmed by Electrocardiogram (ECG), as recommend in updated guidelines on AF [6]. All participating practices were well experienced in daily use of ECG, but we could not independently verify the recorded diagnosis of AF. Secondly, due to routine data out of patient charts underreporting of AF (ICD48.*) as well as comorbidities and follow-up might be possible [24]. However, we focussed on the prescriptions of OAC for patients with AF and those with undocumented AF cannot be considered for treatment. Finally, we did not know which patients did not receive anticoagulants due to (relative or absolute) contraindications such as liver dysfunction.

Conclusions

We aimed to document prescription-rates of OAC (VKA and NOAC) in primary care patients with AF in Germany before and after broad market-share of NOAC and to explore whether known patients with AF were switched onto NOAC. In summary, our study showed a significant increase of OAC over time, which is fosterer by the use of NOAC but with a stable rate of VKA and a sharp decrease of ASA. Patients on VKA are rarely switched to NOAC, but new patients with AF are more likely to receive NOAC. In 2014, 45% of patients with CHA2DS2-VASc-Score ≥ 2 were not prescribed OAC, suggesting room for improvement. Further research is needed to identify factors contributing to this.

Abbreviations

AF: Atrial fibrillation; ASA: Acetylsalicylic acid; CHA2DS2-VASc: Congestive heart failure, Hypertension, Age, Diabetes, Stroke, Vascular Disease, Age, Sex category; CONTENT: CONTinuous-morbidity-registration-Epidemiologic-NeTwork; ECG: Electrocardiogram; ICD: International Statistical Classification of Diseases and Related Health Problems; NOAC: Novel oral anticoagulation; OAC: Oral anticoagulation; VKA: Vitamin-K antagonists

Acknowledgements

We want to thank the participating practices for providing high quality of data.

Funding

Not applicable.

Authors' contributions

SS contributed to conception and design of the study, to acquisition, analysis and interpretation of data and to drafting and revising the manuscript. KK contributed to design of the study, to acquisition, analysis and interpretation of data and to drafting and revising the manuscript. FP-K contributed to analysis and interpretation of data and critically revised the manuscript. JvL contributed to analysis and interpretation of data and critically revised the manuscript. GL contributed to conception and design of the study, to acquisition and analysis of data and critically revised the manuscript. JS contributed to conception and design of the study, to interpretation of data and critically revised the manuscript. MW contributed to conception and design of the study, to analysis and interpretation of data and to drafting and revising the manuscript. All authors read and approved the final manuscript.

Consent for publication

Not applicable.

Competing interests

The authors declare that they have no competing interests.

Author details

[1]Department of General Practice and Health Services Research, University Hospital Heidelberg, Heidelberg, Germany. [2]Radboud Institute of Health Sciences, Radboud University Medical Centre, Nijmegen, Netherlands.

References

1. Piccini JP, Hammill BG, Sinner MF, Jensen PN, Hernandez AF, Heckbert SR, et al. Incidence and prevalence of atrial fibrillation and associated mortality among Medicare beneficiaries, 1993-2007. Circ Cardiovasc Qual Outcomes. 2012;5:85–93.
2. Schnabel RB, Yin X, Gona P, Larson MG, Beiser AS, McManus DD, et al. 50 year trends in atrial fibrillation prevalence, incidence, risk factors, and mortality in the Framingham heart study: a cohort study. Lancet. 2015;386: 154–62.
3. Chugh SS, Havmoeller R, Narayanan K, Singh D, Rienstra M, Benjamin EJ, et al. Worldwide epidemiology of atrial fibrillation: a global burden of disease 2010 study. Circulation. 2014;129:837–47.
4. Heeringa J, van der Kuip DA, Hofman A, Kors JA, van Herpen G, Stricker BH, et al. Prevalence, incidence and lifetime risk of atrial fibrillation: the Rotterdam study. Eur Heart J. 2006;27:949–53.
5. Wolf PA, Abbott RD, Kannel WB. Atrial fibrillation as an independent risk factor for stroke: the Framingham study. Stroke. 1991;22:983–8.
6. Kirchhof P, Benussi S, Kotecha D, Ahlsson A, Atar D, Casadei B, et al. 2016 ESC guidelines for the management of atrial fibrillation developed in collaboration with EACTS: the task force for the management of atrial fibrillation of the European Society of Cardiology (ESC)developed with the special contribution of the European heart rhythm association (EHRA) of the ESCEndorsed by the European stroke organisation (ESO). Eur Heart J. 2016; 37(38):2893-962. PMID: 27567408.
7. January CT, Wann LS, Alpert JS, Calkins H, Cigarroa JE, Cleveland JC Jr, et al. 2014 AHA/ACC/HRS guideline for the management of patients with atrial fibrillation: a report of the American College of Cardiology/American Heart Association task force on practice guidelines and the Heart Rhythm Society. Circulation. 2014;130:e199–267.
8. Lip GY, Nieuwlaat R, Pisters R, Lane DA, Crijns HJ. Refining clinical risk stratification for predicting stroke and thromboembolism in atrial fibrillation using a novel risk factor-based approach: the euro heart survey on atrial fibrillation. Chest. 2010;137:263–72.
9. Deutsche Gesellschaft fürAllgemeinmedizin und Familienmedizin. New oral anticoagulants, AWMF-Reg. 053/031. 2013, updated 2017 http://www.awmf.org/fileadmin/user_upload/Leitlinien/053_D_Ges_fuer_Allgemeinmedizin_und_Familienmedizin/053-031ke_S1_Antikoagulantien_NOAK_2017-01.pdf. Accessed June 5th 2018.
10. Mueller S, Pfannkuche M, Breithardt G, Bauersachs R, Maywald U, Kohlmann T, et al. The quality of oral anticoagulation in general practice in patients with atrial fibrillation. Eur J Intern Med. 2014;25:247–54.

11. Ulrich LR, Mergenthal K, Petersen JJ, Roehl I, Rauck S, Kemperdick B, et al. Anticoagulant treatment in German family practices - screening results from a cluster randomized controlled trial. BMC Fam Pract. 2014;15:170.
12. Beyer-Westendorf J, Ehlken B, Evers T. Real-world persistence and adherence to oral anticoagulation for stroke risk reduction in patients with atrial fibrillation. Europace. 2016;18:1150–7.
13. Haeusler KG, Gerth A, Limbourg T, Tebbe U, Oeff M, Wegscheider K, et al. Use of vitamin K antagonists for secondary stroke prevention depends on the treating healthcare provider in Germany - results from the German AFNET registry. BMC Neurol. 2015;15:129.
14. Robson J, Dostal I, Mathur R, Sohanpal R, Hull S, Antoniou S, et al. Improving anticoagulation in atrial fibrillation: observational study in three primary care trusts. Br J Gen Pract. 2014;64:e275–81.
15. Drug Commission of the Germal Medical Association. https://www.akdae.de/Arzneimitteltherapie/NA/Archiv/201303-Eliquis.pdf. Accessed June 5th 2018.
16. Drug Commission of the Germal Medical Association. https://www.akdae.de/Arzneimitteltherapie/NA/Archiv/2011030-Pradaxa.pdf. Accessed June 5th 2018.
17. Drug Commission of the Germal Medical Association. https://www.akdae.de/Arzneimitteltherapie/NA/Archiv/201310-Xarelto.pdf. Accessed June 5th 2018.
18. Drug Commission of the Germal Medical Association. https://www.akdae.de/Arzneimitteltherapie/NA/Archiv/201504-Lixiana-DVT.pdf. Accessed June 5th 2018.
19. Laux G, Koerner T, Rosemann T, Beyer M, Gilbert K, Szecsenyi J. The CONTENT project: a problem-oriented, episode-based electronic patient record in primary care. Informatics in primary care. 2005;13:249–55.
20. Andreotti F, Rocca B, Husted S, Aijan RA, ten Berg J, Cattaneo M, et al. Antithrombotic therapy in the elderly: expert position paper of the European Society of Cardiology Working Group on thrombosis. Eur Heart J. 2015;36:3238–49.
21. Halperin JL, Hankey GJ, Wojdyla DM, Piccini JP, Lokhnygina Y, Patel MR, et al. Efficacy and safety of rivaroxaban compared with warfarin among elderly patients with nonvalvular atrial fibrillation in the rivaroxaban once daily, oral, direct factor Xa inhibition compared with vitamin K antagonism for prevention of stroke and embolism trial in atrial fibrillation (ROCKET AF). Circulation. 2014;130:138–46.
22. Hobbs FR, Taylor CJ, Jan Geersing G, Rutten FH, Brouwer JR. European primary care cardiovascular society Swg. European primary care cardiovascular society (EPCCS) consensus guidance on stroke prevention in atrial fibrillation (SPAF) in primary care. Eur J Prev Cardiol. 2016;23:460–73.
23. Ruff CT, Giugliano RP, Braunwald E, Hoffman EB, Deenadayalu N, Ezekowitz MD, et al. Comparison of the efficacy and safety of new oral anticoagulants with warfarin in patients with atrial fibrillation: a meta-analysis of randomised trials. Lancet. 2014;383:955–62.
24. Last JM, Adelaide MB. The iceberg "completing the clinical picture" in general practice. Lancet. 1963;282:28–31.

3

Effects of primary care clinician beliefs and perceived organizational facilitators on the delivery of preventive care to individuals with mental illnesses

Bobbi Jo H. Yarborough[1*], Scott P. Stumbo[1], Nancy A. Perrin[1], Ginger C. Hanson[2], John Muench[3] and Carla A. Green[1]

Abstract

Background: Although many studies have documented patient-, clinician-, and organizational barriers/facilitators of primary care among people with mental illnesses, few have examined whether these factors predict actual rates of preventive service use. We assessed whether clinician behaviors, beliefs, characteristics, and clinician-reported organizational characteristics, predicted delivery of preventive services in this population.

Methods: Primary care clinicians ($n = 247$) at Kaiser Permanente Northwest (KPNW) or community health centers and safety-net clinics (CHCs), in six states, completed clinician surveys in 2014. Using electronic health record data, we calculated preventive care-gap rates for patients with mental illnesses empaneled to survey respondents ($n = 37{,}251$). Using separate multi-level regression models for each setting, we tested whether survey responses predicted preventive service care-gap rates.

Results: After controlling for patient-level characteristics, patients of clinicians who reported a greater likelihood of providing preventive care to psychiatrically asymptomatic patients experienced lower care-gap rates (KPNW $\gamma = -.05$, $p = .041$; CHCs $\gamma = -.05$, $p = .033$). In KPNW, patients of female clinicians had fewer care gaps than patients of male clinicians ($\gamma = -.07$, $p = .011$). In CHCs, patients of clinicians who had practiced longer had fewer care gaps ($\gamma = -.004$, $p = .010$), as did patients whose clinicians believed that organizational quality goals facilitate preventive service provision ($\gamma = -.06$, $p = .006$). Case manager availability in CHCs was associated with higher care-gap rates ($\gamma = .06$, $p = .028$).

Conclusions: Clinicians who report they are likely to address preventive concerns when their mentally ill patients present without apparent psychiatric symptoms had patients with fewer care gaps. In CHCs, care quality goals may facilitate preventive care whereas case managers may not.

Keywords: Primary care, Prevention, Mental illness, Schizophrenia spectrum disorder, Bipolar disorder, Preventive services, Clinicians

* Correspondence: bobbijo.h.yarborough@kpchr.org
[1]Kaiser Permanente Northwest Center for Health Research, 3800 N. Interstate Avenue, Portland, OR 97227, USA
Full list of author information is available at the end of the article

Background

People with mental disorders are more likely than the general population to die prematurely [1]. Disparity in life expectancy, especially among people with serious mental illnesses like schizophrenia and bipolar disorder, is largely attributable to preventable chronic conditions [2], sometimes caused or exacerbated by higher rates of behavioral risk factors [3–5] or by the metabolic side effects of antipsychotic medications sometimes used to treat these illnesses [6–8]. Though individuals with mental illness diagnoses appear to receive preventive services at rates similar to persons without these diagnoses [9], screening for certain conditions, including colorectal cancer or osteoporosis, and receipt of certain services like influenza vaccinations remain low, particularly among individuals receiving care in federally qualified health centers [9]. Rates of annual screening of cardiometabolic risk factors among people taking antipsychotics [10] are also suboptimal, even in integrated care settings, despite clinical screening guidelines that have existed for more than a decade [11], and evidence that people with serious mental illnesses are at significantly increased risk for metabolic syndrome [12], and cardiovascular disease and related mortality [13].

Past research has used qualitative and survey methods to identify patient and clinician perspectives on barriers to primary care among those with serious mental illnesses. Patient-level barriers identified include psychiatric illness severity [14]; cognitive and communication limitations [15]; fears of having a serious illness or dying [16]; belief that illnesses will resolve without medical care, lack of knowledge of where to seek treatment, doubt that treatment will be effective, and shame [17]; lack of resources [18, 19]; and logistical issues (e.g., time and transportation). Considerably less work has identified clinician- or organizational-level barriers. Perceived barriers include negative biases [15], difficulty coordinating care [14] across separated primary and mental health care systems [15, 19], and lack of basic primary care training among mental health providers who may be de facto primary care providers [19]. Even fewer studies have directly tested the relationship between clinician and organizational factors and observed rates of preventive services. One group found that low rates of metabolic testing were more strongly associated with patient characteristics and frequency of visits than with clinician and practice characteristics (e.g., care setting location, type, size; colocation of medical and mental health services) [20]. Very little is known about the role that other organizational characteristics, including team-based care [21, 22], outreach related to preventive care use [23, 24], and organizational cultures conducive to quality care [25] may play in preventive service completion among this population.

As part of a larger project designed to assess and compare overall preventive service use patterns among individuals with and without mental illness diagnoses, the current study assessed whether specific clinician characteristics, behaviors, and beliefs, and clinician-reported organizational characteristics, predicted delivery of preventive screening and care to individuals with mental illnesses. The project included two large samples of clinicians representing a diverse set of health care settings. As in the parent study [9], we used patient preventive care gaps (needed preventive services which were not completed; see Yarborough et al. [9] for additional detail) derived from electronic health records (EHR), to assess 12 recommended preventive activities [26]. To our knowledge, this is the first study to link clinician and organizational predictors of preventive service delivery to a broad array of EMR-derived preventive service outcomes among individuals with mental illnesses.

Methods

Settings

Settings were Kaiser Permanente Northwest (KPNW) and federally qualified health centers and safety-net community health clinics (CHC) affiliated with the OCHIN health information technology network. KPNW is a not-for-profit, group-model, integrated health system that provided care to approximately 500,000 members in Oregon and Washington during the study period (2012–2013). KPNW members are representative of the service area in terms of age, sex, and race/ethnicity [27]. OCHIN provides a common EHR platform for its member health care systems enabling EHR-based research across these settings. Thirty-four OCHIN-affiliated health systems met eligibility criteria for recruitment to complete the primary care clinician survey (i.e., served adult patients, had an established EHR system by May 1st, 2012). Of those, 27 organizations representing 107 CHCs in California, North Carolina, Ohio, Oregon and Wisconsin agreed to participate in the clinician survey.

Clinician sample

Primary care clinicians from participating organizations were invited to complete a survey if they had been employed ≥ 2 years with their organization, had ≥100 empaneled patients, and ≥10 patients with qualifying mental illness diagnoses (schizophrenia spectrum, bipolar, anxiety, and major depressive disorders). Qualifying clinicians ($n = 489$) were mailed a study invitation letter and a chocolate bar. A week later an email followed, which contained an embedded link to the survey with a unique identifier for each clinician. Non-respondents were telephoned 1–2 weeks later. Two hundred forty-nine surveys were completed, a 51% response rate overall (61% of KPNW clinicians and 45% of CHC clinicians sent a survey link).

Patient sample

Patients empaneled to clinician survey respondents with ≥ two recorded instances of a qualifying mental health diagnosis (schizophrenia spectrum, bipolar, anxiety, and major depressive disorders) were included if they were ≥19 years old and had ≥ one health care visit in 2012 or 2013. Transgender and unknown gender patients were excluded because preventive service recommendations are gender-specific. Also excluded were patients with ≥ two instances of a diagnosis of a serious cognitive or developmental disability and those with a documented preference to be excluded from research. The Kaiser Permanente Northwest Institutional Review Board approved and monitored the study; a waiver of informed consent was granted for analysis of patient-level EHR data, clinicians consented to study participation by returning a survey.

Primary care clinician survey

A brief, online clinician survey was developed to identify barriers or facilitators of preventive care delivery (see Additional file 1). To inform survey development, formative, semi-structured interviews with clinicians in KPNW ($n = 15$) and CHCs (n = 15) were conducted. Interviews addressed clinicians' experiences providing primary care to people with serious mental illnesses and how those experiences differed from experiences with other patients, assessments of the relative importance of preventive medicine topics, approaches to and comfort with conversations about prevention and risk factors with this population, and perceived effectiveness of those conversations. Themes from the interviews were used to construct the clinician survey.

Clinician and organizational variables from the survey

Clinician behaviors, beliefs, characteristics

The survey asked clinicians about their experience, knowledge, and comfort interacting with patients experiencing serious mental health symptoms. We measured clinicians' beliefs about how health-related recommendations could affect patients' mental health, the degree to which stability of mental health affected clinicians' willingness to make recommendations about preventive services, and the amount of additional support patients with serious mental illnesses required to be successful with preventive care. We also measured clinicians' beliefs about whether or not their patients with serious mental illnesses prioritized preventive care, their confidence that these patients would follow their recommendations, and how that level of confidence compared to their confidence in other patients' ability to follow through.

We asked clinicians to report how often they consulted with mental health providers about their patients' physical health, and about their likelihood of making eight specific recommendations: smoking cessation, improving diet/nutrition, increasing exercise, reducing alcohol/drug use, getting a mammogram, getting laboratory work, getting a flu shot, and completing colon cancer screening. Specifically, we asked how likely clinicians were to make these recommendations when they encountered patients who were not experiencing significant mental illness symptoms (i.e., were psychiatrically asymptomatic), and how much less likely they might be to make the same recommendations when patients are experiencing acute symptoms. Finally, we asked clinicians to describe their gender, race, ethnicity, age, and years practicing medicine. Most survey responses were rated on 5-point Likert-type scales. Gender and race (white/non-white [includes Hispanic]) were dichotomized; years practicing medicine (post-training) was a continuous measure.

Clinician-reported organizational measures

Clinicians reported on a number of characteristics of the organizations in which they practiced, including: availability of behavioral health specialists, case managers, care navigators, health coaches, and peer-provided services to assist patients; use of a team-based care model; co-location of medical and mental health services; community outreach services; or Assertive Community Treatment programs.

We assessed the degree to which several potential care facilitators (e.g., use of mobile prevention services, co-location of laboratory services, EHR best practice alerts) and barriers (e.g., lack of time, insufficient reimbursement, lack of patient interest, acuity of patient concerns in the visit) affected delivery of health promotion and disease prevention. We also assessed the degree to which the clinician's practice setting emphasized staying on time with appointments, patient satisfaction, a patient-centered approach to care, cost-effectiveness, and care quality. Finally, the survey included a measure designed to elicit the degree to which respondents believed that clinician screening goals imposed by the organization (i.e., targets associated with process of care performance measures), affected the likelihood of providing preventive care to individuals with serious mental illnesses. The clinician survey is available upon request.

Electronic health record-derived variables

Main outcome: preventive care-gap rate

EHR data was used to examine needed preventive care for 12 preventive services: obesity measured by calculated body mass index (BMI), hypertension, dyslipidemia (lower-density lipoprotein), diabetes (Hemoglobin A1c or fasting plasma glucose), tobacco use status, evidence of annual influenza vaccine, pneumococcal vaccine (aged 65+), colorectal cancer screenings (aged 50–75), and, for women only, screening for osteoporosis (aged 65+ who have ever received a bone density test), chlamydia (aged 16–24), breast cancer (aged 50–74, mammography), and cervical cancer (aged 24–64 with at least one Papanicolao (pap) test in prior 3 years). Both KPNW and the CHCs specifically used a panel support tool that took into account patient characteristics (e.g., age, gender, past medical history) to determine needed preventive services, and which flagged patients with incomplete services ("care gaps"). Using the care gaps, each of the 12 preventive services were dichotomized as 0 (up to date/completed) or 1 (out of date/not completed). The proportion of needed preventive care (care-gap rate) was computed for enrolled patients by dividing the number of out-of-date services for each patient by the number of eligible preventive services, and multiplying by 100.

Statistical analyses

The main analyses were conducted using multi-level regression in HLM 7 [28] to account for the nesting of patients within clinicians. A Poisson linking function accommodated the skewed distribution of care gaps. Samples from KPNW and the CHCs were analyzed separately because the settings used slightly different approaches for identifying patients with overdue preventive services. Responses from clinicians at KPNW and CHCs were compared using chi-square and t-tests to assess differences in clinician and organizational characteristics on survey responses of interest.

We hypothesized that, after controlling for patient-level characteristics, clinician characteristics (female gender [29], years practicing medicine [30]) and certain behaviors (e.g., consulting with mental health clinicians, providing care to psychiatrically asymptomatic patients) as well as organizational facilitators (e.g., access to case managers or navigators, colocation of services, emphasis on quality) would be associated with better care (i.e. lower care-gap rates), whereas endorsing the belief that patients with serious mental illnesses lack interest in prevention would be associated with higher care-gap rates.

We tested each independent variable of interest separately in a model containing all covariates before finalizing each model. The following patient-level covariates were included: diagnosis, age, gender, race, ethnicity, Medicaid status, Medicare status, physical health comorbidity [31], number of primary care visits, and number of non-primary care visits. All variables not significantly related to care gaps in these individual predictor models were excluded from further analyses; dropped variables included: clinician belief that patients lacked interest in prevention, practice emphasis on care quality, team-based care, amount of consultation between medical and mental health clinicians and co-location of medical and mental health or laboratory services. None of these clinician or organizational characteristics showed associations with care-gap rates.

Clinician and organizational variables that were significantly related to the care-gap rate in either the KPNW or CHC sample were included in the final overall model for both samples. These included: clinician gender, years of practice, likelihood of providing care when patients are asymptomatic, availability of case managers, availability of care navigators, and belief that clinician performance measures increase likelihood of providing services.

Results

Patient panel data was unavailable for two clinicians who returned surveys; the remaining 247 clinicians had an average of 6.8 (SD = 6.8) patients with schizophrenia spectrum disorders on their panel, 17.7 (SD = 11.0) patients with bipolar disorder, 36.3 (SD = 22.0) patients with anxiety disorders, and 90.0 (SD = 43.9) patients with unipolar depressive disorders. See Table 1 for additional results.

Differences between clinician populations

Table 1 presents frequencies and means from the clinician survey for the KPNW and CHC samples. While the survey response rate was higher among KPNW clinicians than CHC clinicians, the CHC sample size was larger such that survey respondents were more likely to practice in CHCs (55% of sample) than KPNW. Respondents were predominantly white (75.9%), had a mean age of 46.5 years (SD = 9.7), and had been practicing medicine post-training for an average of 14.1 years (SD = 9.8). The CHC sample had more female clinicians represented than KPNW (65.9% vs. 44.9%, $\chi^2 = 10.65$, $p = .001$). The two groups also differed in how likely they reported they were to make preventive care recommendations when their patients with serious mental illnesses were not experiencing significant mental health symptoms. Specifically, KPNW clinicians were more likely than their CHC counterparts to make recommendations about smoking cessation, exercise, mammogram, or colorectal cancer screening (KPNW mean = 3.53, SD = .49; CHC mean = 3.35, SD = .57; F(1245) = 6.75; $p = .010$). KPNW clinicians were also more likely to report that an emphasis on care quality facilitated preventive service provision (mean = 1.84, SD = .37 compared to mean = 1.54, SD = .50 at CHCs; F(1236) = 26.57, $p < .001$), and that quality-related performance goals increased their likelihood of providing preventive care (mean = 2.54, SD = .57 compared to mean = 1.95, SD = .70 at CHCs; F(1237) = 50.0, $p < .001$). CHC clinicians, however, were more likely than KPNW clinicians to report consulting with mental health providers about their patients' physical health (mean = 2.46, SD = .88; KPNW mean = 2.22, SD = .79, F(1239) = 4.99, $p = .026$); practicing within a team-based care model (85.3% compared to 52.2% at KPNW, $\chi^2 = 32.34$, $p < .001$); and having greater availability of co-located medical and mental health services (77.9% compared to 36.3% at KPNW, $\chi^2 = 44.29$, $p < .001$). In addition

Table 1 Primary care clinician survey respondent characteristics by site, frequencies and means for model variables[a] ($N = 249$)

	KPNW $n = 113$ (45.4%)		CHCs $n = 136$ (54.6%)		p
	Total N	No. (%)	Total N	No. (%)	
Provider characteristics					
Gender (female)	107	44.9	132	65.9	.001[b]
Race/ethnicity (non-White)	107	24.3	128	15.6	.095
		M(SD)		M(SD)	
Age	104	47.83(8.62)	130	45.44(10.39)	.061
Years in practice	107	15.71(9.11)	132	12.76(10.10)	.202
Provider beliefs/behaviors					
Consult with mental health provider[c]	109	2.22(.79)	132	2.46(.88)	.026[d]
Lack of patient interest affects preventive care delivery[e]	108	1.98(.74)	131	1.85(.73)	.160
Likely to make preventive recommendations when patients not experiencing symptoms[f]					
–Smoking	111	3.59(.64)	136	3.32(.78)	.005[g]
–Diet/nutrition	110	3.30(.71)	136	3.16(.76)	.122
–Exercise	111	3.44(.66)	136	3.18(.80)	.005[g]
–Alcohol/drug use	111	3.44(.75)	135	3.48(.70)	.665
–Getting a mammogram	111	3.62(.52)	135	3.33(.72)	.001[b]
–Getting laboratory work	110	3.62(.54)	136	3.54(.62)	.325
–Getting a flu shot	111	3.62(.57)	136	3.63(.58)	.964
–Completing colon cancer screening	111	3.62(.56)	135	3.19(.81)	<.001[b]
Likelihood of providing care absent symptoms (composite)[f]	111	3.53(.49)	136	3.35(.57)	.010[g]
Organizational characteristics		No. (%)		No. (%)	
Availability of co-located of medical and mental health services	113	41 (36.3)	136	106 (77.9)	<.001[b]
Team-based care approach	113	59 (52.2)	136	116 (85.3)	<.001[b]
Availability of a case manager	113	72 (63.7)	136	86 (63.2)	.937
Availability of a care navigator	113	9 (8.0)	136	60 (44.1)	<.001[b]
		M(SD)		M(SD)	
Co-located laboratory services facilitates care[h]	107	2.23(.95)	131	2.47 (.83)	.046[d]
Emphasis on quality of care[i]	107	1.84(.37)	131	1.54(.50)	<.001[b]
HEDIS screening increases likelihood of delivering care[j]	107	2.54(.57)	132	1.95(.70)	<.001[b]
Provider panel characteristics	Total N	M(SD)	Total N	M(SD)	P
Number of patients					
Schizophrenia spectrum disorder	105	3.78(2.08)	131	9.75(7.93)	<.001[b]
Bipolar disorder	113	16.48(6.91)	134	18.75(13.47)	.090
Major depressive disorder	113	121.05(32.59)	134	63.81(34.06)	<.001[b]
Anxiety disorder	113	50.65(19.48)	134	24.25(16.06)	<.001[b]
Total number of patients represented	19,782		14,551		
Mean patient care gap score[k]					
Schizophrenia spectrum disorder	105	16.12(10.65)	131	25.24(9.49)	-
Bipolar disorder	113	16.15(4.34)	134	28.05(7.08)	-
Major depressive disorder	113	14.84(3.02)	134	29.25(5.98)	-
Anxiety disorder	113	17.95(3.04)	134	29.65(6.47)	-

[a]For a description of patient characteristics, please see Yarborough et. al. [9]
[b]$p \le .001$
[c]Coded1 = not at all, 2 = a little, 3 = a moderate amount; 4 = a great deal
[d] $p \le .05$
[e]Coded1 = not at all/a little, 2 = a moderate amount; 3 = a great deal
[f]Coded 1 = not at all likely, 2 = somewhat likely, 3 = very likely, 4 = extremely likely
[g]$p \le .01$
[h]Coded 0 = not available, 1 = not at all/a little, 2 = a moderate amount; 3 = a great deal
[i]Coded1 = not at all/a little/a moderate amount; 2 = a great deal
[j]Coded 1 = greatly decreases likelihood, 2 = decreases likelihood, 3 = increase likelihood, 4 = greatly increases likelihood
[k]Gap scores were computed differently in each organization therefore statistical comparisons are inappropriate

they were more likely to report that co-located medical and laboratory services facilitated prevention efforts (mean = 2.47, SD = .83 in CHCs; mean = 2.23, SD = .95 at KPNW, F(1236) = 4.03, $p = .046$).

Characteristics that predict preventive services

To assess which variables influenced care, we first estimated variance in care-gap rates, within clinicians, separately for each sample using a fully unconditional model. There was sufficient variability within clinicians in both the KPNW sample ($\tau_{00} = .03$, $p < .001$) and in the CHC sample ($\tau_{00} = .04$, $p < .001$) that could be explained by patient predictors. The intraclass correlation, or proportion of variance in care gaps between clinicians, was 2.9% for KPNW and 3.8% for the CHCs. Put another way, less than 4% of the variance in care-gap rates was explained by clinician factors; the larger remaining proportion of variability was accounted for by patient-level differences.

Next we combined all of the provider-level predictors with significant bivariate relationships with care gaps into overall models for each of our populations (KPNW and CHC). In the KPNW sample, after controlling for patient-level characteristics, patients of female clinicians had fewer care gaps ($\gamma = -.07$, $p = .011$) than those of male clinicians. Additionally, the more likely a clinician was to report that s/he makes preventive care recommendations when patients are *not* experiencing acute mental health symptoms, the lower their patients' care-gap rates ($\gamma = -.05$, $p = .041$). Additional results are reported in Table 2.

Clinician gender was not a significant predictor of care gaps in the CHC sample. Consistent with the KPNW sample, however, clinicians in this sample who were more likely to report providing care to patients when they were not experiencing mental health symptoms had patients with fewer care gaps ($\gamma = -.05$, $p = .033$). Additionally, CHC clinicians who stated that performance goals increased their likelihood of providing preventive care also had patients with lower care-gap rates ($\gamma = -.06$, $p = .006$) as did clinicians who had practiced longer ($\gamma = -.004$, $p = .010$). Unexpectedly, having a case manager available in the practice was associated with having higher care-gap rates ($\gamma = .06$, $p = .028$). No other clinician or organizational characteristics were associated with care-gap rates. Additional results are reported in Table 2.

Given the relationship between patient care-gap rates and clinician-reported likelihood of making preventive care recommendations when patients were not experiencing significant mental health symptoms, we conducted post-hoc analyses to see which clinician characteristics and beliefs were associated with clinician response to this survey item. Being female (b = .242, $p = .001$), and believing that the stability or instability of patients' mental health did not influence their own prevention-related behavior (b = .083, $p = .019$), were both positively related to reporting making recommendations to psychiatrically asymptomatic patients. By contrast, self-reported comfort interacting with patients experiencing serious mental illness symptoms (b = .000, $p = .991$), knowledge of how mental health problems and how their treatment affects physical health (b = –.057, $p = .324$), years in practice (b = .000, $p = .988$), and experience with these patients (b = –.047, $p = .446$) did not predict clinicians' ratings of their likelihood to make recommendations to asymptomatic patients.

Discussion

This study linked clinician and organizational predictors of preventive service delivery among individuals with mental illnesses to observed preventive service outcomes. We found that clinicians of patients with lower preventive care-gap rates reported that they were highly likely to make preventive care recommendations to patients when they were psychiatrically asymptomatic. These clinicians were also more likely to be female and to report that the stability or instability of their patients' mental health did not affect their approach to preventive care. Put another way, these mostly female clinicians may have believed that they were equally likely to make recommendations whether their patients had active symptoms or not, and they had the

Table 2 Clinician-Level[a] Coefficients for Provider Characteristics in Final Multi-Level Poisson Regression Models Predicting Care Gaps

Provider-Level Variables	KPNW		CHCs	
	Coeff.	*p*	Coeff.	*p*
Gender (Female)	–.07	*.011*[b]	–.01	.754
Years practice	.00	.756	–.004	*.010*[c]
HEDIS goals increase likelihood of services	.03	.231	–.06	.006
Likelihood of providing care absent symptoms	–.05	*.041*[b]	–.05	*.033*[b]
Case manager	–.02	.444	.06	*.028*[b]
Care navigator	.03	.506	.05	.062

[a]Patient-level covariates controlled for in the model include age, gender, race, Hispanic ethnicity, comorbidity, [32] number of primary care visits, number of non-primary care, Medicare status and Medicaid status. For frequencies and further details on patient-level covariates, please see Yarborough et. al. [9]
[b]$p \leq .05$
[c]$p \leq .01$

patients with the lowest care gap rates. Patients of female clinicians in the KPNW sample had lower care gaps than patients of male KPNW clinicians overall. Potential practice differences between female and male physicians may have important clinical implications for patient outcomes. There is evidence that, compared to male physicians, female physicians may be more likely to systematically advise patients about prevention [29], adhere to guideline recommendations [32], and provide higher quality care [33–36].

While KPNW clinicians were more likely than CHC clinicians to report an organizational emphasis on care quality and to believe that quality goals increased likelihood of providing preventive care, the latter belief only predicted actual reduced care gaps in CHC clinics. It is possible that population characteristics moderate the effectiveness of performance goals. For example, a substantially higher proportion of CHC patients are economically disadvantaged, homeless, Medicaid beneficiaries, or under- or uninsured compared to KPNW members [9], potentially making timely preventive screening harder to achieve. Indeed, rates of guideline-concordant care tend to be lower among Medicaid beneficiaries compared to the U.S. general population [37]. Performance goals and supports to achieve them may be more powerful for clinicians working with patients in these circumstances.

The finding that access to case managers predicted higher care gaps in the CHC settings is inconsistent with past research demonstrating the positive benefits of case managers in preventive medicine settings [38]. However, as suggested above, it is possible that this finding also reflects the nature of the CHC patient population. In health care settings, case managers are often invoked to help manage complex situations that interfere with adequate medical care (e.g., homelessness). It may be that the need for access to case managers is an indicator of greater unmet needs of the CHC populations and what appears to be poor preventive care may actually be the necessary prioritization of competing demands. It is also possible that unlike the trained case managers in the study of integrated preventive care cited above [38], case managers in the CHCs had less clear roles and diffusion of responsibility resulted in care gaps.

Interestingly, few of the hypothesized clinician and organizational predictors were associated with care-gap rates. For example, clinician perception that patients with serious mental illnesses are uninterested in prevention has been documented in previous studies [15, 18, 20], however, we found no relationship between endorsing this belief and actual care gaps. Neither did we observe relationships between care-gap rates and an organizational emphasis on care quality; use of team-based care models; availability of care navigators; amount of mental health consultation; or co-location of services. This is consistent with prior work suggesting that patient characteristics are more strongly associated with screening completion than clinician or practice characteristics [20].

Limitations and strengths

Generalizability of our findings is limited to individuals with at least minimal health services use because of our decision to require at least one health care visit for inclusion in the analyses of care gaps. We were unable to determine the representativeness of our clinician sample because we could not collect data on non-responders. However, more than half of the clinicians we contacted returned a completed survey, a rate substantially higher than reported in other studies linking clinicians to patient outcomes, enabling a much larger empaneled patient sample [39]. The KPNW and CHC settings were purposefully chosen for their differing health care delivery models, including a private health plan and publicly funded safety-net clinics, and because of the economic, geographic, and racial/ethnic diversity of each setting's population characteristics.

Conclusions

Clinicians who report they are likely to address preventive concerns when seriously mentally ill patients present without apparent mental health symptoms had patients with fewer care gaps. Clinician performance goals related to care quality may facilitate preventive care, especially in CHCs. Availability of case managers in CHCs was unexpectedly associated with greater preventive service gaps, warranting additional study.

Abbreviations

BMI: Body mass index; CHC: Community health centers; EHR: Electronic health record; KPNW: Kaiser Permanente Northwest

Acknowledgments

The authors would like to extend a special thank you to the clinicians who took time to participate in the study interviews and/or survey.

Funding

This work was supported by the National Institute of Mental Health (MH096795); the sponsor had no role in the study design, data collection, analysis or interpretation, manuscript preparation, nor in the decision to publish the paper.

Authors' contributions

BY contributed to the study design and was responsible for manuscript preparation; she had access to all data elements included in this publication. SS assisted with analyses, analytic interpretation and manuscript preparation. NP oversaw all analyses and contributed to the manuscript preparation. GH conducted the analyses and contributed to the manuscript preparation. JM helped design the study and contributed to the manuscript preparation. CG designed the study, and contributed to the analytic interpretation and manuscript preparation. All authors have read and approved the final version of this manuscript.

Consent for publication
Not applicable.

Competing interests
The authors declare that they have no competing interests.

Author details
[1]Kaiser Permanente Northwest Center for Health Research, 3800 N. Interstate Avenue, Portland, OR 97227, USA. [2]Johns Hopkins School of Nursing, 525 N. Wolfe Street, Baltimore, MD 21205, USA. [3]Oregon Health & Science University, 3181 S.W. Sam Jackson Park Road, Portland, OR 97239, USA.

References

1. Walker ER, McGee RE, Druss BG. Mortality in mental disorders and global disease burden implications: a systematic review and meta-analysis. JAMA Psychiat. 2015;72(4):334–41.
2. De Hert M, Correll CU, Bobes J, Cetkovich-Bakmas M, Cohen D, Asai I, Detraux J, Gautam S, Moller HJ, Ndetei DM, et al. Physical illness in patients with severe mental disorders. I. Prevalence, impact of medications and disparities in health care. World Psychiat. 2011;10(1):52–77.
3. Casagrande SS, Anderson CA, Dalcin A, Appel LJ, Jerome GJ, Dickerson FB, Gennusa JV, Daumit GL. Dietary intake of adults with serious mental illness. Psychiat Rehab J. 2011;35(2):137–40.
4. Janney CA, Ganguli R, Richardson CR, Holleman RG, Tang G, Cauley JA, Kriska AM. Sedentary behavior and psychiatric symptoms in overweight and obese adults with schizophrenia and schizoaffective disorders (WAIST study). Schizophr Res. 2013;145(1–3):63–8.
5. LeCook B, Wayne G, Kafali E, Liu Z, Shu C, Flores M. Trends in smoking among adults with mental illness and association between mental health treatment and smoking cessation. JAMA. 2014;311(2):172–82.
6. McIntyre RS, McCann SM, Kennedy SH. Antipsychotic metabolic effects: weight gain, diabetes mellitus, and lipid abnormalities. Can J Psychiatr. 2001;46(3):273–81.
7. Daumit GL, Clark JM, Steinwachs DM, Graham CM, Lehman A, Ford DE. Prevalence and correlates of obesity in a community sample of individuals with severe and persistent mental illness. J Nerv Ment Dis. 2003;191(12):799–805.
8. Daumit GL, Goff DC, Meyer JM, Davis VG, Nasrallah HA, McEvoy JP, Rosenheck R, Davis SM, Hsiao JK, Stroup TS, et al. Antipsychotic effects on estimated 10-year coronary heart disease risk in the CATIE schizophrenia study. Schizophr Res. 2008;105(1–3):175–87.
9. Yarborough BJH, Perrin NA, Stumbo SP, Muench J, Green CA. Preventive service use among people with and without serious mental illnesses. Am J Prev Med. 2018;54(1):1–9.
10. American Diabetes Association, American Psychiatric Association, American Association of Clinical Endocrinologists, North American Association for the Study of Obesity. Consensus development conference on antipsychotic drugs and obesity and diabetes: consensus statement. Diabetes Care. 2004; 27(2):596–601.
11. American Diabetes Association, American Psychiatric Association, American Association of Clinical Endocrinologists, North American Association for the Study of Obesity. Consensus development conference on antipsychotic drugs and obesity and diabetes. J Clin Psychiat. 2004;65(2):267–72.
12. Vancampfort D, Stubbs B, Mitchell AJ, De Hert M, Wampers M, Ward PB, Rosenbaum S, Correll CU. Risk of metabolic syndrome and its components in people with schizophrenia and related psychotic disorders, bipolar disorder and major depressive disorder: a systematic review and meta-analysis. World Psychiat. 2015;14(3):339–47.
13. Correll CU, Solmi M, Veronese N, Bortolato B, Rosson S, Santonastaso P, Thapa-Chhetri N, Fornaro M, Gallicchio D, Collantoni E, et al. Prevalence, incidence and mortality from cardiovascular disease in patients with pooled and specific severe mental illness: a large-scale meta-analysis of 3,211,768 patients and 113,383,368 controls. World Psychiat. 2017;16(2):163–80.
14. Mangurian C, Giwa F, Shumway M, Fuentes-Afflick E, Perez-Stable EJ, Dilley JW, Schillinger D. Primary care providers' views on metabolic monitoring of outpatients taking antipsychotic medication. Psychiatr Serv. 2013;64(6):597–9.
15. Kaufman EA, McDonell MG, Cristofalo MA, Ries RK. Exploring barriers to primary care for patients with severe mental illness: frontline patient and provider accounts. Issues Ment Health Nurs. 2012;33(3):172–80.
16. Ye J, Shim R, Rust G. Health care avoidance among people with serious psychological distress: analyses of 2007 health information national trends survey. J Health Care Poor Underserved. 2012;23(4):1620–9.
17. Andersson LM, Moore CD, Hensing G, Krantz G, Staland-Nyman C. General self-efficacy and its relationship to self-reported mental illness and barriers to care: a general population study. Community Ment Health J. 2014;50(6):721–8.
18. Ross LE, Vigod S, Wishart J, Waese M, Spence JD, Oliver J, Chambers J, Anderson S, Shields R. Barriers and facilitators to primary care for people with mental health and/or substance use issues: a qualitative study. BMC Fam Pract. 2015;16:135.
19. McDonell MG, Kaufman EA, Srebnik DS, Ciechanowski PS, Ries RK. Barriers to metabolic care for adults with serious mental illness: provider perspectives. Int J Psychiatry Med. 2011;41(4):379–87.
20. Morrato EH, Campagna EJ, Brewer SE, Dickinson LM, Thomas DS, Miller BF, Dearing J, Druss BG, Lindrooth RC. Metabolic testing for adults in a state medicaid program receiving antipsychotics: remaining barriers to achieving population health prevention goals. JAMA Psychiat. 2016;73(7):721–30.
21. Dorr DA, Wilcox A, Burns L, Brunker CP, Narus SP, Clayton PD. Implementing a multidisease chronic care model in primary care using people and technology. Dis Manag. 2006;9(1):1–15.
22. Druss BG, von Esenwein SA. Improving general medical care for persons with mental and addictive disorders: systematic review. Gen Hosp Psychiatry. 2006;28(2):145–53.
23. Somkin CP, Hiatt RA, Hurley LB, Gruskin E, Ackerson L, Larson P. The effect of patient and provider reminders on mammography and Papanicolaou smear screening in a large health maintenance organization. Arch Intern Med. 1997;157(15):1658–64.
24. Pham HH, Schrag D, Hargraves JL, Bach PB. Delivery of preventive services to older adults by primary care physicians. JAMA. 2005;294(4):473–81.
25. Williams ES, Manwell LB, Konrad TR, Linzer M. The relationship of organizational culture, stress, satisfaction, and burnout with physician-reported error and suboptimal patient care: results from the MEMO study. Health Care Manag Rev. 2007;32(3):203–12.
26. Published Recommendations. http://www.uspreventiveservicestaskforce.org/BrowseRec/Index. Accessed 27 Dec 2017.
27. Sukumaran L, McCarthy NL, Li R, Weintraub ES, Jacobsen SJ, Hambidge SJ, Jackson LA, Naleway AL, Chan B, Tao B, et al. Demographic characteristics of members of the vaccine safety Datalink (VSD): a comparison with the United States population. Vaccine. 2015;33(36):4446–50.
28. Raudenbush SW, Bryk AS, Congdon R. HLM 7.01 for windows [computer software]. Skokie: Scientific Software International, Inc; 2013.
29. Frank E, Harvey LK. Prevention advice rates of women and men physicians. Arch Fam Med. 1996;5(4):215–9.
30. Choudhry NK, Fletcher RH, Soumerai SB. Systematic review: the relationship between clinical experience and quality of health care. Ann Intern Med. 2005;142(4):260–73.
31. Gagne JJ, Glynn RJ, Avorn J, Levin R, Schneeweiss S. A combined comorbidity score predicted mortality in elderly patients better than existing scores. J Clin Epidemiol. 2011;64(7):749–59.
32. Baumhakel M, Muller U, Bohm M. Influence of gender of physicians and patients on guideline-recommended treatment of chronic heart failure in a cross-sectional study. Eur J Heart Fail. 2009;11(3):299–303.
33. Kim C, McEwen LN, Gerzoff RB, Marrero DG, Mangione CM, Selby JV, Herman WH. Is physician gender associated with the quality of diabetes care? Diabetes Care. 2005;28(7):1594–8.
34. Franks P, Clancy CM. Physician gender bias in clinical decisionmaking: screening for cancer in primary care. Med Care. 1993;31(3):213–8.
35. Berthold HK, Gouni-Berthold I, Bestehorn KP, Bohm M, Krone W. Physician gender is associated with the quality of type 2 diabetes care. J Intern Med. 2008;264(4):340–50.
36. Andersen MR, Urban N. Physician gender and screening: do patient differences account for differences in mammography use? Women Health. 1997;26(1):29–39.
37. McGinty EE, Baller J, Azrin ST, Juliano-Bult D, Daumit GL. Quality of medical care for persons with serious mental illness: a comprehensive review. Schizophr Res. 2015;165(2–3):227–35.

4

Assessing predictors of intention to prescribe sick leave among primary care physicians using the theory of planned behaviour

Yogarabindranath Swarna Nantha[1*], Lei Hum Wee[2] and Caryn Mei-Hsien Chan[2]

Abstract

Background: Providing sickness certification is a decision that primary care physicians make on a daily basis. The majority of sickness certification studies in the literature involve a general assessment of physician or patient behaviour without the use of a robust psychological framework to guide research accuracy. To address this deficiency, this study utilized the Theory of Planned Behaviour (TPB) to specifically gauge the intention and other salient predictors related to sickness certification prescribing behaviour amongst primary care physicians.

Methods: A cross-sectional study was conducted among $N = 271$ primary care physicians from 86 primary care practices throughout two states in Malaysia. Questionnaires used were specifically developed based on the TPB, consisting of both direct and indirect measures related to the provision of sickness leave. Questionnaire validity was established through factor analysis and the determination of internal consistency between theoretically related constructs. The temporal stability of the indirect measures was determined via the test-retest correlation analysis. Structural equation modelling was conducted to determine the strength of predictors related to intentions.

Results: The mean scores for intention to provide patients with sick leaves was low. The Cronbach α value for the direct measures was good: overall physician intent to provide sick leave (0.77), physician attitude towards prescribing sick leave for patients (0.77) and physician attitude in trusting the intention of patients seeking sick leave (0.83). The temporal stability of the indirect measures of the questionnaire was satisfactory with significant correlation between constructs separated by an interval of two weeks ($p < 0.05$). Attitudes and subjective norms were identified as important predictors in physician intention to provide sick leave to patients.

Conclusion: An integrated behavioural model utilizing the TPB could help fully explain the complex act of providing sickness leave to patients. Findings from this study could assist relevant agencies to facilitate the creation of policies that may help regulate the provision of sickness leave and alleviate the work burden of sickness leave tasks faced by physicians in Malaysia.

Keywords: Theory of planned behaviour, Sick leave prescribing, Intention, Primary care physicians

* Correspondence: yogarabin@gmail.com
[1]Non-Communicable Disease Clinic, Seremban Primary Care Clinic, Jalan Rasah, 70300 Seremban, Negeri Sembilan, Malaysia
Full list of author information is available at the end of the article

Background

The act of providing sickness leave to patients is a decision faced by most medical practitioners during routine consultations, especially in primary care settings [1–4]. Studies in various countries indicate that general practitioners are reluctant in their role as gatekeepers of sickness leave tasks [5–13]. Considerable dissonance has been documented between patients who consider themselves worthy of sickness leave and the examining physician who fails to detect an objective clinical finding that is consistent with the history that is given [14]. Consequently, studies have shown that the task and process of providing sickness leave can be a source of emotional strain for physicians as they experience conflict with patients and other stakeholders [6–13, 15].

Worldwide, few studies have examined how physicians routinely prescribe sickness leave [16, 17], particularly when this is compared to the widely available literature focusing on the motivations and behaviour patterns of patients obtaining sick leave. Large variations have been found in the way that physicians regularly prescribe sickness leave [18]. Most studies related to sickness certification appear to focus on the descriptive or epidemiological aspects of physician or patient behaviour and lack theoretical grounding [15, 19]. Fewer studies still have attempted to frame an understanding of the attitudes that underlie actual prescribing behaviours on the part of physicians using theories related to health behaviour [20].

An in-depth understanding and skillful application of a theoretical framework is essential to any research intervention designed to change patient or physician behaviour [15, 21]. The Theory of Planned Behaviour (TPB) is ideally suited to help acquire valuable information on potential areas for behavioural interventions through this study. The strength of the TPB is that it provides a framework to decipher individuals' action and allows the researcher to understand the reasons that motivate the behavior under investigation [21].The TPB by Ajzen [22] posits three constructs that determine behaviour intentions: attitude towards behaviour, subjective norm and perceived behavioural control (Fig. 1) [21].

The current study focuses on how these three constructs influence intention to provide sickness certification and actual sick leave prescribing behaviour in clinical practice. This can be measured using both direct and indirect measures. Direct measures are used to obtain a general assessment or opinion of the respondents with either a semantic differential scale or a bipolar disagree-agree scale. Indirect measures serve to examine the respondent's underlying specific beliefs and outcome evaluations. We hypothesize that attitude, subjective norm or perceived behavioural control are significant predictors of primary care physicians' intent to provide sickness certification. The objective of this study is to identify the factors that influence physician behaviour in providing sickness leave to patients in a primary care setting.

Methods

Study design

A cross-sectional study design was implemented using data from 86 primary health care clinics in two states (Negeri Sembilan and Selangor) in Malaysia consisting of seven and nine districts respectively between February 2014 and March 2015.

Study population

The suggested sample size for studies using the TPB framework should be more than 160 participants [23]. General practitioners from the clinic can be divided into primary care physicians and family medicine specialists. A total of 329 primary care physicians (out of the 666 physicians who were invited to participate in the study) were recruited. Primary care physicians from all participating primary health care clinics with at least one year

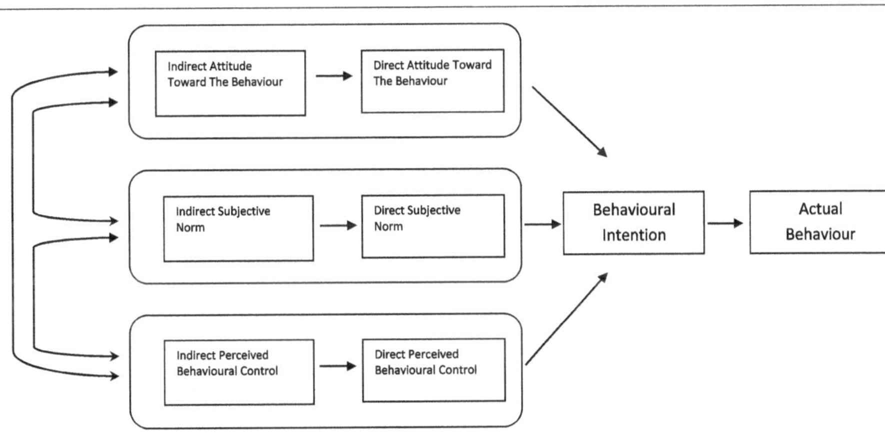

Fig. 1 The constructs in the Theory Of Planned Behaviour as proposed by Ajzen (2006)

of compulsory internship were eligible to participate in the study. Family medicine specialists (consultants) and junior house officers were excluded for two reasons: 1) the frequency of providing sickness certification to patients are vastly minimal compared to all other physicians at the clinic and 2) they attend to a very select number of patients per day and represent a small subset of the primary care physician population in most primary care clinics.

Survey procedure

A meeting involving representatives from all participating primary health clinics was held to explain the nature of the study. Sets of three envelopes containing instructions and questionnaires for each time point were handed to physicians in charge/clinical administrators during the meeting in a sealed envelope. All questionnaires were self-administered. Written informed consent was obtained from all participating physicians prior to the first data collection.

There were two sets of questionnaires (Q1 and Q2). Q2 was administered two weeks after Q1 was first administered. Additional document file shows these questionnaires in detail (see Additional file 1 and Additional file 2). After a lapse of another two weeks, Q2 was re-administered to gauge temporal stability [23]. Each questionnaire had coded numbers for each participant to ensure de-identification and confidentiality. All answered questionnaires were collected in person by the principal investigator. This project was approved by the Medical Research and Ethics Committee of Malaysia (NMRR 12–1422-14,535).

Questionnaire design and development

Testing of direct measures and elicitation phase

Figure 2 summarizes the steps taken in conducting the pilot and main study. The development and reliability analysis of the questionnaire was based on guidelines designed for assessments at a primary care setting [23]. In accordance with the general and specific TPB questionnaire guidelines for health services [22, 23] a pilot study was conducted at a single primary care clinic with a sample size of 30 participating physicians.

Items related to the direct measures of TPB were tested during the pilot stage of questionnaire development. Open-ended questions were used to obtain salient beliefs in relation to the TPB constructs. These elicitation questions assessed instrumental attitude, normative attitude, normative influence and perceived behavioural control [21]. This formed the basis to generate the questions related to indirect measures.

Participant feedback was solicited. Each participant was encouraged to state whether, 1) items in the questionnaire were ambiguous or difficult to answer, 2) the questionnaire felt too repetitive or too long, or 3) the questionnaire had less than ideal wording or format. Open responses were likewise solicited from participants. Participants' response were then categorized according to relevant themes. The extraction of specific themes related to the study was jointly established between authors (YSN and WLH). The two authors obtained consensus on themes derived from the open-ended questions. YSN confirmed the categorization of the identified themes through feedback from individual participants. The preliminary results (recurring themes) were then used to design the indirect measures relevant to the TPB constructs.

Description of constructs and questions involving direct and indirect measures

Standard guidelines for TPB were utilized to generate the questionnaire for direct measures [22, 23]. The intention to act or not to act depends on 3 main constructs. These three constructs of TPB are attitude, subjective norm and perceived behavioural control [22].

Intentions on providing sickness leave

Three items were used to measure intention to provide sickness leave to patients: 'I plan to provide patients sickness leave during an outpatient consultation; 'I want to provide patients with sickness leave during an outpatient consultation, 'I intend to provide patients with sickness leave during an outpatient consultation'. The mean of the response of these three items served as the measure of intention. The scores for this measurement ranged from 1 to 7 (1 = strongly disagree, 7 = strongly agree).

Attitudes toward providing sickness leave

Two items were utilized in this category: 'Providing patients with sickness leave is harmful/beneficial, good/bad, pleasant /unpleasant (for me), worthless/useful; I trust the intentions of patients who request for sickness leave during outpatient consultations (strongly disagree/strongly agree). The scores for both measurements ranged from 1 to 7 (1 = strongly disagree, 7 = strongly agree).

The indirect measure of attitude was designed from the themes derived from the open-ended questions during the pilot study. The arithmetic sum of the belief-based measure (seven-point likely/unlikely dimension) and corresponding outcome evaluations (seven-point extremely undesirable/desirable and not important/important dimension) determined the indirect measure of attitude. The scores for this measurement ranged from −84 to 84.

Subjective norm

The direct measure of subjective norm involved inquiry using four items in the TPB construct: 'Most people who are important to me think that (1 = should not to 7 =

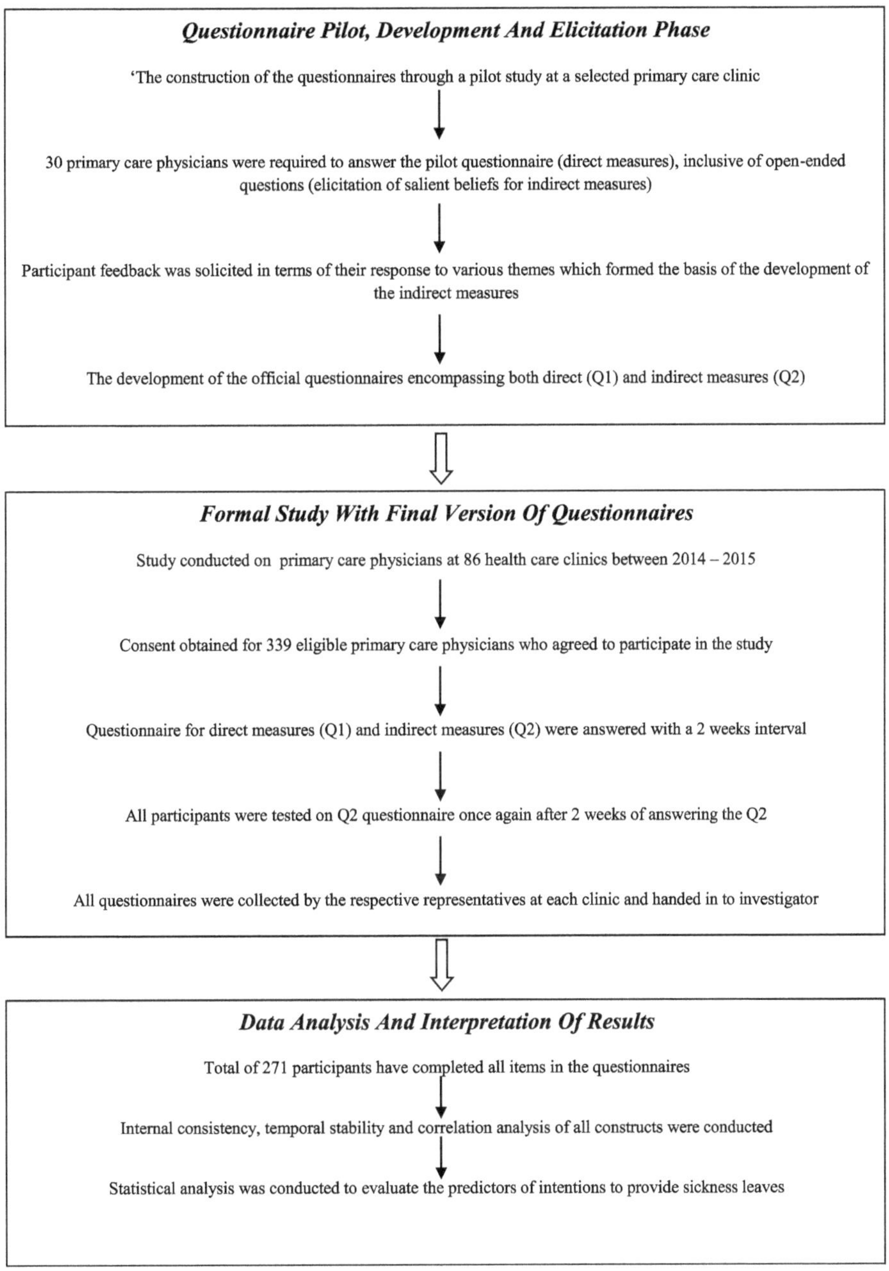

Fig. 2 Flow chart of the study design and process of data collection

should) be strict in providing sickness leave to patients coming for outpatients clinic consultation; 'It is expected of me to provide sickness leave to patients seeking outpatient clinic consultations' 'I feel under social pressure to provide sickness leave to patients who have come for outpatient; 'People who are important to me recommend to be strict in providing sickness leave to patients who have come for outpatient consultations'. The scores for this measurement ranged from 1 to 7 (1 = strongly disagree to 7 = strongly agree).

A belief-based measure of subjective norm was derived from the summed response of 6 normative beliefs (4 injunctive and 2 descriptive) and motivations to comply. The items in the normative belief construct analyzed the factors that significant others would feel about the idea of providing sickness leave to patients. Motivation to comply was assessed based on willingness to provide sickness leave relative to the opinions of others. All items had a seven-point dimension (disapprove/approve, should not/should, avoid giving/do not avoid giving, not at all/very much). The scores for this measurement ranged from −84 to 84.

Perceived behavioural control

The direct measure of perceived behavioural control was obtained by summing up responses to four items under the construct. These included a seven-point dimension assessment of self-efficacy: 'The decision for me to provide my patients with sickness leave is easy or difficult (1 = difficult, 7 = easy)', 'I am confident that I could provide patients with sickness leave appropriately based on the consultation' and controllability: 'The decision to provide sickness leave is beyond my control', 'Whether I provide sickness leave or not is entirely up to me'. The scores for this measurement ranged from 1 to 7 (1 = strongly disagree to 7 = strongly agree).

A belief-based measure of perceived control was derived from the summed response of six beliefs influencing performance and ability to perform. The items for the influencing performance construct analyzed external factors that determined the respondent's act of providing sickness leave to patients. The ability to perform construct assessed the willingness to provide sickness leave under the influence of the external factors. All items had a seven-point dimension (unpleasant/pleasant, disagree/agree). The scores for this measurement ranged from −84 to 84.

Statistical analysis

Data management

All acquired data were entered into the Statistical Package for the Social Sciences program (SPSS version 20; IBM Corp., USA) and Statistics and Data Analysis program (STATA version 13.0; STATA Corp. USA). The items with negative endpoints were recoded to reflect actual scores [22, 23]. The data set was examined to account for missing or invalid values to ensure correct administration.

Reliability and validity

An exploratory factor analysis (EFA) was conducted to evaluate the loading variables using the principal component analysis (PCA) method. The oblique method of rotation (Direct Oblimin) was utilized for extraction of factors of the theoretical components via PCA. With the results of the exploratory factor analysis, the optimal number of factors to retain was obtained using parallel analysis. Subsequently, a confirmatory factor analysis (CFA) and structural equation modelling (SEM) was performed to assess the overall goodness of fit of the structural model.

Internal consistency and construct validity was determined in phases. Firstly, the internal consistency between items in the scales measuring behavioural intentions and the direct measures of attitude, subjective norm and perceived control was examined. A Cronbach's alpha value above 0.7 was considered acceptable [24]. Once the reliability analysis had been completed, the themes were recoded into one composite variable measuring each construct (in total for variables) with a possible range of 1–7 [23].

Subsequently, the relationship between the theoretical constructs were explored using bivariate correlations (Pearson R test). It is hypothesized that the direct TPB measures would positively correlate with intention and are inter-related as they are not seen as categories independent of each other [22].

The relationship between indirect and direct measurements of the same constructs were then determined. By weighting belief statements based on the score of the relevant outcome evaluation, new variables were created into a new set of weighted beliefs by multiplying each behavioural statement with the corresponding behavioural outcome evaluation. In contrast to the direct measures, the indirect measures consist of both negative and positive beliefs because 'people can quite logically hold negative and positive beliefs for the same behavior' [23]. We performed a test-retest reliability to determine the temporal stability of the indirect measures [23].

Finally, we measured correlations between each individual indirect item and direct measurements of the same construct in order to determine if the beliefs had been identified and appropriately measured. Overall composite scores were then summed for each of the three variables. The results were reported as Pearson's R, with a p-value <0.05 considered statistically significant.

Descriptive statistics

Descriptive analysis was undertaken to describe background characteristics (age, gender, and experience at work) and the distribution (mean and standard deviation) of the measures.

Predictability of the developed model

SEM was performed to examine the overall potential of the questionnaire to predict intentions and to identify the predictive strength of each direct and indirect measurement in the form of regression weights. For all outcomes, a p-value <0.05 was considered statistically significant. The explanatory power of the model was obtained from the R^2 squared value of the model through an equation level goodness-of-fit test.

Results

Descriptive statistics

Out of 666 invited participants, 327 primary care physicians did not take part in the study. Therefore the dropout rate was at 49.1%. Of 339 eligible physicians, a total of 271 (79.9%) completed the questionnaires. The mean age of the respondents was 31.8 years (SD ± 4.47; range 26–55 years).There was an over-representation of female participants (74.2%) but this is consistent with the proportion of the study population. The primary care physicians had an average of 5.97 years of service experience (including prior experience in hospital setting). About half (48.7%) recorded 3–5 years of professional experience and about one-third (29.2%) had 6–10 years of experience. The physicians had an average of 2.84 (SD ± 1.29) years of working in a primary care setting. One-third (30.3%) of physicians had at least 1–2 years of primary care working experience.

The mean scores for intention to provide patients with sickness leave was low with a value of 3.2 (SD ± 1.2). For the direct measures, the mean for perceived behavioural control recorded the highest score (4.9) in comparison with other constructs. As for indirect measures, the mean for attitudes recorded the highest score (26.4) followed by subjective norm (24.0) and perceived behavioural control (14.6).

Reliability of the constructs in the direct measure questionnaire

The Cronbach α values for intentions to provide sickness leave to patients and direct measurements (Table 1) ranged from poor to very good across the sample. The Cronbach α values were 0.68 for intentions, 0.77 for attitude 1, 0.83 for attitude 2, 0.35 for subjective norms, 0.53 for perceived behavioural control. The Cronbach α value of the intention scale increased to 0.77 when item 1 was removed. Similarly, the internal consistency of the subjective norm scale increased to 0.62 when items 13 and 14 were removed from the construct.

Table 1 Reliability and items statistics for the constructs of direct measures

Constructs and items of direct measures	Mean (SD)	Cronbach Alpha	Item total correlation
Construct A: Generalized Intention		0.68	
Item 1	3.71(1.73)		0.38
Item 2	3.04(1.44)		0.65
Item 3	2.87(1.51)		0.50
Construct B1: Attitude ATT1 (attitude of physicians providing sickness leaves to patients)		0.77	
Item 4	4.25(1.21)		0.70
Item 5	4.08(1.71)		0.60
Item 6	3.55(1.36)		0.42
Item 7	4.34(1.33)		0.60
Construct B2: Attitude ATT2 (attitude of physicians trusting the intention of patients)		0.83	
Item 8	3.70(1.39)		0.73
Item 9	3.68(1.38)		0.67
Item 10	3.36(1.34)		0.59
Item 11	3.86(1.35)		0.65
Construct C: Subjective Norms		0.35	
Item 12	3.08(1.58)		0.33
Item 13	3.33(1.66)		0.19
Item 14	4.44(1.73)		0.05
Item 15	3.62(1.57)		0.20
Construct D: Perceived Control		0.53	
Item 16	5.67(1.30)		0.40
Item 17	4.22(1.56)		0.23
Item 18	4.74(1.82)		0.32
Item 19	5.04(1.71)		0.34

Dimensionality of the developed model

In the primary EFA, 6 factors with Eigenvalues above 1 were found and explained 67% of the variance. Then, the numbers of factors were limited to 5 as determined via parallel analysis. This model explained 61% of the variance. The KMO measure of sampling adequacy was 0.706 and the Bartlett's test of sphericity was statistically significant ($p < 0.01$). Consistent with the reliability analysis, items 13 and 14 had cross loadings and therefore requires removal from the scale (Table 2).

Fitness of the model

By performing CFA, the TPB model for direct measures fulfilled the indices required for a goodness of fit [root mean square error of approximation (RMSEA) < 0.01; comparative fit index (CFI) = 1.00; Tucker-Lewis index (TLI) = 1.00].

Correlation between direct and indirect measures of the questionnaire

The correlation between indirect and direct constructs were statistically significant with a *p*-value of <0.01 (Table 3).

Predictive strength of direct measures on intention to provide sickness leave

The path analysis conducted via SEM for direct measures (Fig. 3) showed that attitude ATT1 was the strongest predictor of intention to provide sickness leave to patients ($\beta = 0.35$, $p < 0.01$), followed by subjective norms ($\beta = 0.24$, $p < 0.01$). The regression weights for attitude ATT1 and subjective norm were statistically significant. However, this was not statistically significant for perceived behavioural control. An equation level of goodness-of-fit revealed that the three direct measurements

Table 2 Pattern matrix for exploratory factor analysis for direct measures

Constructs and items of direct measures	Factor 1	Factor 2	Factor 3	Factor 4	Factor 5	Extraction communalities
Construct A: Generalized Intention						
Item 1	0.597					0.415
Item 2	0.767					0.662
Item 3	0.723					0.571
ConstructB1: Attitude ATT1 (attitude of physicians providing sickness leaves to patients)						
Item 4		−0.820				0.761
Item 5		−0.834				0.660
Item 6		−0.541				0.423
Item 7		−0.768				0.652
Construct B2: Attitude ATT2 (attitude of physicians trusting the intention of patients)						
Item 8			0.843			0.729
Item 9			0.825			0.677
Item 10			0.768			0.592
Item 11			0.792			0.651
Construct C: Subjective Norms						
Item 12				0.762		0.625
Item 13				–		0.400
Item 14				–		0.290
Item 15				0.830		0.692
Construct D: Perceived Control						
Item 16					0.725	0.527
Item 17					0.556	0.433
Item 18					0.565	0.495
Item 19					0.688	0.512

accounted for 14.8% of the variation in the intention to provide sickness leave.

Temporal stability of indirect measures

The correlation between composite scores for all three constructs (attitude, $r = 0.334$; subjective norm, $r = 0.490$; perceived norm, $r = 0.370$) of the indirect measures after a 2 week interval was adequate with a p-value of less than 0.05.

Correlation with demographics

Only years of professional experience as a physician correlated with the intention to provide sickness leave ($p < 0.05$). Perceived behavioural control was found to be correlated to age ($p < 0.01$), professional years of experience ($p < 0.01$) and clinical years in primary care ($p < 0.05$).

Table 3 Correlation coefficients (Pearson R) of intentions, direct and indirect measures

	Population ($n = 271$) Correlation coefficient (Pearson R)				
	Direct measures				
	Intentions	ATT1	ATT2	SN	PBC
Direct measures					
Direct attitude (ATT1)	0.32[a]	–			
Direct attitude (ATT2)	0.17[a]	–	–		
Direct subjective norm (SN)	0.20[a]	0.04	−0.10	–	
Direct perceived behavioural control (PBC)	−0.08	0.02	−0.02	−0.14[b]	–
Indirect measures					
Indirect attitude (ATT)	0.21[a]	0.30[a]	0.22[a]		
Indirect subjective norm (SN)	0.25[a]			0.15[b]	
Indirect perceived behavioural control (PBC)	−0.11				−0.21[a]

[a]Correlation is significant at the 0.01 level (2-tailed)
[b]Correlation is significant at the 0.05 level (2-tailed)

Discussion

Main findings and comparison with literature

This study is the first attempt in this region to address the provision of sickness leave among primary care physicians using the TPB model. From a regional perspective, a thorough literature review reveals only two other studies pertaining to sickness leave in Malaysia [25, 26]. These studies lack the utilization of a robust psychological framework and focused primarily on descriptive evaluations of sickness absenteeism among employees [25, 26]. Similarly, most studies were also devoid of a suitable theoretical framework to enhance research accuracy [2–4, 11, 13, 27]. A core strength of this study lies in the basis of its theoretical approach to examine the intentions of primary care physicians in terms of providing sickness leave.

The total variance explained of the 5-factor solution of the TPB model for sickness certification behaviour amongst primary care physicians was good (>60%) [28]. Loading of all items in the model was optimal (>0.5) [29]. The model also demonstrated goodness of fit as evidenced by the RMSEA index (<0.06) and CFI (>0.95) [29]. The internal reliability of intentions and direct measures were adequate except for the perceived behavioural control construct. Consequently, the correlations between the constructs that were hypothesized to be theoretically-related were satisfactory except for perceived behavioural control. Therefore, the scale for perceived behavioural control should be omitted from

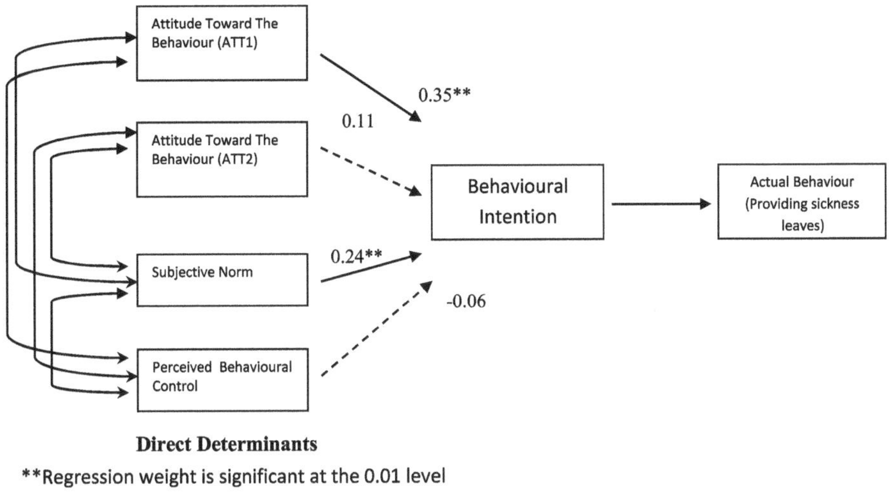

Fig. 3 Path diagram of TPB model of intention to provide sickness certification to patients amongst primary care physicians

the TPB theoretical model. On the other hand, the regression weight between intentions and the direct measures of subjective norm showed statistical significance despite a low Cronbach value of 0.62. This evidence suggests that although the subjective norm construct fits well with the TPB model of sickness leave provision by primary care physicians, items 13 and 14 were not relevant to the current set of participants in this study (as evidenced by poor total item correlation).

The results of this study indicate that the TPB variables, namely, attitude towards the behaviour and subjective norm are important factors associated with the primary care physician's intention to provide sickness leave for patients. Perceived behavioural control poorly predicted behavioural intentions. One probable explanation for this is that most primary care physicians are confident in providing sickness leave to patients as this occurs on a daily basis in their practice. As the provision of sickness leave to patients becomes habitual, actual physician intent may play a lesser role.

Strengths and limitations

In this study, bivariate correlations between direct and indirect measures were statistically significant but had low to average *r* values. Therefore it can be deduced that although the indirect measures was adequately constructed and covered the breadth of all measured constructs in the TPB model, these composites scores only had modest influence (based on effect size) on direct measures.

Although our study showed theoretical support for the use of the TPB model in the analysis of sickness leave in primary care, the study was limited by the low variance of overall explanation of the intentions to provide sickness leave ($r^2 = 14.8\%$). Therefore, we hypothesize that intentions could also be influenced by several factors not gauged in this study, 1) knowledge and skills to provide sickness leave, 2) salience of the act of providing sickness leave, 3) environmental constraints and 4) habitual aspect of providing sickness leave [21]. Thus, an integrated behavioural model [21] could be used to help elicit responses of latent variables that possibly remained unaddressed.

Another limitation of the study was that the data were cross-sectional. However, the reliability of the questionnaire was strengthened by conducting test-retest reliability which demonstrated adequate temporal stability. Future research endeavours should focus on a prospective study design using the TPB framework to allow the assessment of actual behaviour of providing sickness to patients not assessed in this study.

Conclusion

Attitude was a strong predictor of intentions to provide sickness leave in this study, followed by subjective norm. Thus, attitudes and subjective norm should be considered as potential constructs for possible behavioural intervention. As TPB serves only to identify targets for intervention, other methods should be utilized to increase the likelihood of behaviour performance. This can be undertaken in the form of persuasive communication strategies that could help reduce conflict and aid decision making to provide sickness leave to patients among primary care physicians [21]. For example, one method of intervention would be the identification and training of popular opinions leaders (state/district health administrators, family medicine specialists or clinic administrator) to have conversations with peers (primary care physicians) and to model themselves as having adopted the behaviour changes being advocated from the results of the study (in this case beliefs based on the attitude and subjective norm construct) [21].

This study identifies predictors of intentions in providing sickness leave. However, intentions alone may be insufficient to determine behaviour due to an intention-behaviour gap [30]. Future studies should assess the efficacy of intention implementations strategies in increasing actual behaviour of performing an intention [30]. Finally, a larger study should be conducted in various other clinical settings to provide greater understanding of the variation that exists in physician intent to provide sickness leave to patients.

This findings could assist relevant agencies to facilitate the creation of policies that may help regulate the provision of sickness leave. This initiative can be achieved by adhering to a set of guidelines or organizational directives to alleviate the work burden of sickness leave tasks faced by physicians in Malaysia.

Abbreviations

ATT1: Direct measures of attitude of physicians providing sickness leaves to patients; ATT2: Direct measures of attitude of physicians trusting the intention of patients; CFI: Comparative fit index; EFA: Exploratory factor analysis; KMO: Kaiser-Meyer-Olkin test for sampling adequacy; PCA: Principal confirmatory analysis; Q1: Questionnaire 1 (Direct measures); Q2: Questionnaire 2 (Indirect measures); RMSEA: Root mean square error of approximation; SEM: Structural equation modelling; SPSS: Statistical Package for the Social Sciences program; STATA: Statistics and Data Analysis program; TLI: Tucker-Lewis index; TPB: Theory of Planned Behaviour

Acknowledgements

We would like to convey our special thanks to the National Clinical Research Centre, Malaysia (NCRC) and the staff of the State Health Office of Selangor and Negeri Sembilan for their assistance during the formation stage of the research. We would also like to extend our appreciation to Clinical Statistician Ms. Lena Yap for her insightful input.

Funding

This study has no funding source.

Authors' contributions

YSN contributed to the conception and the design of the study. YSN contributed to data collection. YSN and WLH worked on analysis and interpretation of the data. YSN wrote the first draft. YSN, WLH and CMHC assisted in the literature review and revision of the manuscript. All authors approved the final version of the manuscript, all persons designated as authors qualify for authorship, and all those who are eligible for authorship are listed.

Consent for publication

Not applicable

Competing interests

The authors declare that they have no competing interests

Author details

[1]Non-Communicable Disease Clinic, Seremban Primary Care Clinic, Jalan Rasah, 70300 Seremban, Negeri Sembilan, Malaysia. [2]Faculty of Health Sciences, Universiti Kebangsaan Malaysia, 50586 Kuala Lumpur, Malaysia.

References

1. Wahlström R, Alexanderson K. Swedish council on technology assessment in health care (SBU): chapter 11 - physicians' sick-listing practices. Scand J Public Health Suppl. 2004;63:222–55.
2. Winde LD, Alexanderson K, Carlsen B, Kjeldgård L, Wilteus AL, Gjesdal S. General practitioners' experiences with sickness certification: a comparison of survey data from Sweden and Norway. BMC Fam Pract. 2012;13:10.
3. Lindholm C, Arrelöv B, Nilsson G, Löfgren A, Hinas E, Skånér Y, et al. Sickness-certification practice in different clinical settings; a survey of all physicians in a country. BMC Public Health. 2010;10:752.
4. Foley M, Thorley K, Von Hout MC. Sickness certification difficulties in Ireland – a GP focus group study. Occup Med. 2013;63:369–72.
5. Hussey S, Hoddinott P, Wilson P, Dowell J, Barbour R. Sickness certification system in the United Kingdom: qualitative study of views of general practitioners in Scotland. BMJ. 2004;328:88.
6. Swartling MS, Hagberg J, Alexanderson K, Wahlstrom RA. Sick-listing as a psychosocial work problem: a survey of 3997 Swedish physicians. J Occup Rehabil. 2007;17:398–408.
7. Roope R, Parker G, Turner S. General practitioner's use of sickness certificates. Occup Med. 2009;59:580–5.
8. Meershoek A, Krumeich AVR. Judging without criteria? Sickness certification in Dutch disability schemes. Soc Heal Illn. 2007;29:497–514.
9. Bollag U, Rajeswaran A, Ruffieux C, Burnand B. Sickness certification in primary care – the physician's role. Swiss Med Wkly. 2007;137:341–7.
10. Krohne K, Brage S. New rules meet established sickness certification practice: a focus-group study on the introduction of functional assessments in Norwegian primary care. Scand J Prim Health Care. 2007;25:172–7.
11. Engblom M, Nilsson G, Arrelöv B, Löfgren A, Skånér Y, Lindholm C, et al. Frequency and severity of problems that general practitioners experience regarding sickness certification. Scand J Prim Health Care. 2011;29:227–33.
12. Löfgren A, Hagberg J, Arrelöv B, Ponzer S, Alexanderson K. Frequency and nature of problems associated with sickness certification tasks: a cross-sectional questionnaire study of 5455 physicians. Scand J Prim Health Care. 2007;25:178–85.
13. Von Knorring M, Sundberg L, Löfgren A, Alexanderson K. Problems in sickness certification of patients: a qualitative study on views of 26 physicians in Sweden. Scand J Prim Health Care. 2008;26:22–8.
14. Chew CA. Benefits of back pain. Fam Pract. 1997;14:461–5.
15. Wynne-Jones G, Mallen CD, Main CJ, Dunn KM. What do GPs feel about sickness certification? A systematic search and narrative review. Scand J Prim Health Care. 2010;28:67–75.
16. Shiels C, Gabbay M, Hillage J. Recurrence of sickness absence episodes certified by general practitioners in the UK. Eur J Gen Pract. 2016;19:1–8.
17. Hubertsson J, Englund M, Hallgårde U, Lidwall U, Löfvendahl S, Petersson IF. Sick leave patterns in common musculoskeletal disorders–a study of doctor prescribed sick leave. BMC Musculoskelet Disord. 2014;15:1–9.
18. Kankaanpää AT, Putus TM, Tuominen RJ. Factors affecting sick leave prescribing in occupational health care: a survey based on hypothetical patient cases. BMC Health Serv Res. 2014;14:1–7.
19. Tellnes G. Sickness certification in general Practice : a review. Fam Pract. 1989;6:58–65.
20. Grol RP, Bosch MC, Hulscher MEJL, Eccles MP, Wensing M. Planning and studying improvement in patient care: the use of theoretical perspectives. Milbank Q. 2007;85:93–138.
21. Glanz K, Rimer BKVK. Health behaviour: theory, research and practice. 5th ed. San Francisco: Jossey-Bass; 2015.
22. Ajzen I. The theory of planned behavior. Organ Behav Hum Decis Process. 1991;50:179–211.
23. Francis J, Eccles MP, Johnston M, Walker A, Grimshaw J, Foy R, et al. Constructing questionnaires based on the theory of planned behaviour: a manual for health services researchers. 1st ed. Newcastle upon Tyne: Centre for Health Services Research; 2004.
24. Nunnaly JC. Psychometric theory. 2nd ed. New York: McGraw-Hill; 1978.

5

Implementation of the SMART MOVE intervention in primary care: a qualitative study using normalisation process theory

Liam G. Glynn[1*], Fergus Glynn[1], Monica Casey[1], Louise Gaffney Wilkinson[2], Patrick S. Hayes[3], David Heaney[4] and Andrew W. M. Murphy[3]

Abstract

Background: Problematic translational gaps continue to exist between demonstrating the positive impact of healthcare interventions in research settings and their implementation into routine daily practice. The aim of this qualitative evaluation of the SMART MOVE trial was to conduct a theoretically informed analysis, using normalisation process theory, of the potential barriers and levers to the implementation of a mhealth intervention to promote physical activity in primary care.

Methods: The study took place in the West of Ireland with recruitment in the community from the Clare Primary Care Network. SMART MOVE trial participants and the staff from four primary care centres were invited to take part and all agreed to do so. A qualitative methodology with a combination of focus groups (general practitioners, practice nurses and non-clinical staff from four separate primary care centres, $n = 14$) and individual semi-structured interviews (intervention and control SMART MOVE trial participants, $n = 4$) with purposeful sampling utilising the principles of Framework Analysis was utilised. The Normalisation Process Theory was used to develop the topic guide for the interviews and also informed the data analysis process.

Results: Four themes emerged from the analysis: personal and professional exercise strategies; roles and responsibilities to support active engagement; utilisation challenges; and evaluation, adoption and adherence. It was evident that introducing a new healthcare intervention demands a comprehensive evaluation of the intervention itself and also the environment in which it is to operate. Despite certain obstacles, the opportunity exists for the successful implementation of a novel healthcare intervention that addresses a hitherto unresolved healthcare need, provided that the intervention has strong usability attributes for both disseminators and target users and coheres strongly with the core objectives and culture of the health care environment in which it is to operate.

Conclusion: We carried out a theoretical analysis of stakeholder informed barriers and levers to the implementation of a novel exercise promotion tool in the Irish primary care setting. We believe that this process amplifies the implementation potential of such an intervention in primary care. The SMART MOVE trial is registered at Current Controlled Trials (ISRCTN99944116; Date of registration: 1st August 2012).

Keywords: Exercise, Technology, Health behaviour, Qualitative research, Barriers, Facilitators

* Correspondence: Liam.Glynn@ul.ie
[1]Graduate Entry Medical School and Health Research Institute, University of Limerick, Limerick, Ireland
Full list of author information is available at the end of the article

Background

'The current literature demonstrates that there are problematic translational gaps continue to exist between demonstrating the positive impact of a novel healthcare intervention in a research environment and the implementation of this intervention into routine daily practice [1–4]. Implementation science has emerged precipitately as an increasingly influential research field [5] by recognizing that the findings from clinical and health services research have often failed to change population health outcomes. [6] The relative failure to implement what we know mirrors the important imbalance between investment in the development of new drugs and medical technologies versus addressing the fidelity with which care is delivered [5]. We have the evidence that interventions can be effective but high quality evidence with regard to the choice and means of optimizing the elements of complex interventions has been much slower to emerge [7].

A greater role for theoretical approaches in implementation-focused research is one proposed strategy for overcoming translation gaps [5]. The Normalisation Process Theory (NPT) is one such theory which furnishes researchers with a consistent framework that can be used to describe, assess and enhance implementation potential through identifying factors that promote and inhibit the routine incorporation of complex interventions into everyday practice [8, 9].

For example, our research team carried out a randomised controlled trial of an mhealth smartphone application to promote physical activity in primary care (SMART MOVE) which demonstrated a short term and sustained increase in physical activity in the intervention group [10]. The findings from such clinical research cannot change population health outcomes unless health care systems and professionals adopt them in practice [6]. The aim of this study was to conduct a theoretically informed analysis, using NPT, of the potential barriers and levers to the implementation of a mhealth intervention to promote physical activity in primary care.

Methods

SMART MOVE trial

SMART MOVE was an open label randomised controlled trial of a smartphone application to promote physical activity in primary care as part of an International Transnational Telemedicine Solutions (ITTS) project funded by the European Union Northern Periphery Programme [11]. The full study protocol has been published [12]. The trial intervention is summarised in Table 1. The trial demonstrated that the use of a smartphone application successfully promoted physical activity in primary care with a difference in mean improvement of 1029 (95% confidence interval 214 to 1843) steps per day favouring the intervention or approximately a half a mile [10].

Table 1 'SMART MOVE' Randomised Controlled Trial

'SMART MOVE' Trial

Registered with the International Standard Randomised Controlled Trials Register #ISRCTN99944116 and ethical approval obtained.

90 Participants recruited by primary care health professionals or self-referred. Screened by the research team for inclusion suitability.

Inclusion criteria:	Exclusion criteria:
• Adult participants in the community • Over 16 years of age • Active android smartphone participants	• Acute psychiatric illness • Pregnant women • Participants unable to undertake moderate exercise

At baseline screening meeting, participants were given study information, signed consent, were randomised and completed quality of life and mental health score questionnaires. BMI, blood pressure and heart rate were measured. Smartphone application Accupedo-Pro Pedometer was downloaded onto the smartphones but step count display was not made visible.

Week 1: All participants continued their normal activity level while carrying the smartphone during all waking hours so the smartphone application could record their baseline step count while remaining invisible to the participant.

End of week 1: Randomisation code broken and participants assigned to control or intervention groups.

Control Group:	Intervention Group:
• Smartphone application with step count continues to remain invisible • Given information on benefits of exercise • Instructed to increase physical activity with a goal of an additional 30 min walking exercise per day (equivalent to 10,000 steps per day)	• Smartphone application and step count made visible (Fig. 1) • Given information on benefits of exercise • Instructed to increase physical activity with a goal of 10,000 steps per day and encouraged to use the smartphone application to achieve this goal

After completion of eight-week trial:
Quality of life and mental health score questionnaire administered and BMI, blood pressure, heart rate recorded. Quantitative results were analysed with the Statistical Package for the Social Sciences (SPSS) for primary outcome of mean difference in daily step count between baseline and follow-up at eight weeks and also secondary outcomes. After trial completion, all control groups participants were then also shown how to use the App

A qualitative evaluation was then carried out by interviewing a purposeful sample of post-trial participants to explore their experiences within four weeks of finishing the trial.

This study reports a qualitative analysis that followed the trial describing a multi-perspective exploration of the barriers and levers to the implementation of this novel intervention amongst primary care service users and service providers. NPT, a theoretical sociological model from the implementation science domain was used to generate the topic guide, analyse the dataset and subsequently optimize the design of an implementation package to support the utilization and normalization of this novel exercise promotion tool into clinical practice. Ethical approval was obtained from the Clinical Research Ethics Committee at Merlin Park University Hospital, Galway.

Sampling and recruitment

The study took place in the West of Ireland with recruitment in the community from the Clare Primary Care Network within the Western Research and Education Network (WestREN), a network of over 180 family practices covering a mixed urban-rural population of approximately 500,000 patients which has been shown to nationally representative [13]. General practice in Ireland is highly computerised with most practices operating in a paperless fashion with a significant amount of coding of chronic disease but much less coding of each consultation [13]. In regard to primary care service providers, two practices that had, and two practices that had not, participated in the SMART MOVE trial were invited to take part and all consented to do so. Primary care service provider participants are described in Fig. 1. There were general practitioners (GP), practice nurses (PN) and non-clinical staff (NCS) from all four practices included in the study. Staff that had not participated in the trial were included with a view to enriching the discussions after being appraised of the subject matter to enhance their contribution.

As part of the SMART MOVE trial four primary care service users were recruited through purposeful sampling and semi-structured interviews [14] were employed to explore their experiences of using the trial intervention. This cohort of four participants, three from the intervention group and one from the control group were chosen for their capacity to describe in depth their experience of using the intervention, as well as representing diversity in terms of age, gender and control or intervention in the context of the trial (Table 2).

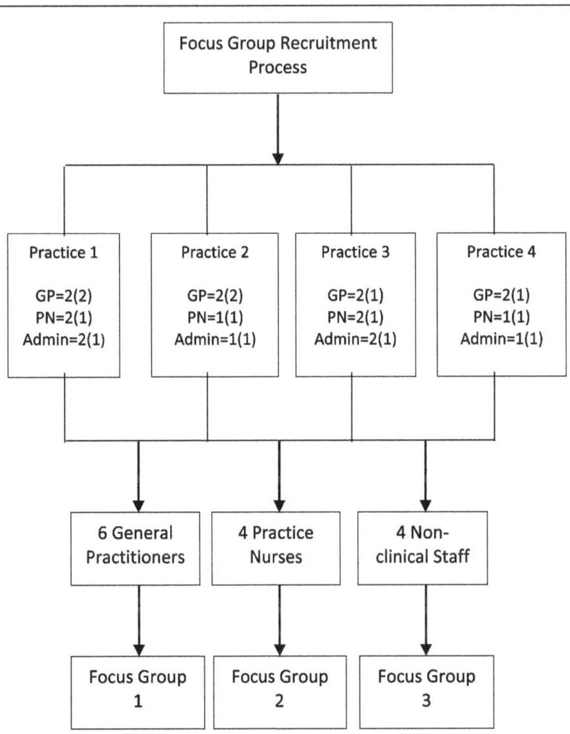

Fig. 1 Recruitment of primary care service providers [*n* = number of staff in each practice (number recruited)]

Data collection

The primary care service providers were invited to participate in focus groups [15] facilitated by the research team. An NPT generated topic guide (Table 3) was used to encourage discussion coherent with the study objectives. Open-ended questions were employed throughout so as not to bias how respondents might express themselves [16]. The format for the focus groups was as follows: (i) a presentation was delivered describing the SMART MOVE trial results and the associated qualitative evaluation of the trial [17] (ii) facilitated group discussion using the NPT generated topic guide and (iii) an open question and answer session. A refinement to the focus group method, the fishbowl technique [18] was employed.

The one-on-one interviews were conducted by the research team with service users who had participated in the SMART MOVE trial. The questions were iterative and evolved accordingly throughout the interview process [19]. An NPT generated topic guide (Table 4) was used to encourage discussion coherent with the study objectives. The audio-taped focus group and individual interviews were professionally transcribed, following which the audio files and transcriptions were correlated as per the demands of reliable analysis [20]. All participants were consented for interview and for the use of anonymous quotations. Continuous observation of the concepts of saturation and sequential analysis appropriately steered the modification of both the individual interviews and the focus group discussions.

Methodological considerations

Specific strategies to successfully address the challenges of implementation focused research include a preeminent role for theoretical approaches [5]. The Normalization Process Theory is one such theory from the field of implementation science offering researchers "a consistent framework that can be used to describe, evaluate and enhance the implementation potential of healthcare interventions" [1]. NPT offers a means of determining factors that help and hinder the successful implementation of

Table 2 Primary care service users interviewed

Participant code	Intervention or Control	Age range	Gender
P1	Intervention	50–60	F
P2	Intervention	50–60	M
P3	Intervention	30–40	F
P4	Control	60–70	F

Table 3 Focus group topic guide for primary care service providers

In the topic guide, the term "App" is used to refer to the smartphone application under study.
Coherence is about sense making.
1. Did you have a clear understanding from the outset of how this intervention would benefit patients?
2. What strategies have you used previously to increase exercise amongst patients in the practice?
3. How does the App differ from previous strategies?
4. Do you think that one of your important professional roles is the discussion and promotion of increased activity levels with your clients/patients?
5. In your opinion, does the promotion of this strategy fit well with the overall goals and activity of your medical practice?
Cognitive Participation is about engagement/'buy in':
1. How did you get involved and who told you about the idea?
2. Why was it right for you to get involved and promote this to your patient/clients?
3. Were you prepared to commit the time and effort to promote its use amongst patients/clients?
4. Who was driving this forward/encouraging involvement in this work?
Collective action is about actions and interactions that are required to use the intervention:
1. Did the promotion of the App fit easily with your daily work practices or did you have to change your usual way of working/ consulting with patients?
2. Can you talk about the training/education you received from the outset ....was this helpful/unhelpful and if so, in what ways?
3. What did you find easy and what did you find difficult about promoting the use of the App to your clients/patients?
4. Did you have to work with others to promote the use of the App – who? What was that experience like?
Reflexive monitoring is about appraisal and evaluation:
1. Do you feel that using the App is an effective and worthwhile way to increase activity levels amongst patients and if so how do you know?
2. Can you tell about some of the feedback you've had from clients/ patients who have used the App.
3. Do you have any suggestions for improving the promotion and use of the App amongst your clients/patients?
4. Is there anything you would do/do differently now in your consultations to promote the use of the application to patients?

interventions into daily practice. Moreover, it examines all stages of this process from early implementation to the point at which it becomes so completely ingrained into routine practice that it becomes 'normalised'. It is important to note that this theory also describes how work practices can also become denormalised (i.e. use of paper notes in general practice) and equally normalisation can often be undesirable (i.e. over-utilisation of antibiotics in respiratory tract infections) [21].

Essentially the work that individuals and groups must undertake to enable an intervention to become normalised is the primary focus of NPT and comprises four main components [22, 23]. These four components are described below with examples from the current study given for illustration purposes:

i) *Coherence* is about sense making. How do stakeholders (primary care service providers whose role it is to promote and support the use of the smartphone application as well as the service users themselves who are the intended users of this novel exercise promotion tool) make sense of the intervention and consider its relevance to their lives?
ii) *Cognitive participation* is about engagement or 'buy in'. Do stakeholders engage with this idea as a means of promoting behaviour change around exercise? For example what roles will service providers have to take on to facilitate or promote its implementation?
iii) *Collective action* is about actions and interactions that are demanded of both service providers and service users for the intervention to be promoted and utilized successfully. For example, do service providers report that promoting and supporting the use of the smartphone application amongst service users is overly burdensome in the context of their usual work demands?
iv) *Reflexive monitoring* is about appraisal and evaluation; how do service providers and service users formally and informally evaluate the use and benefits of the smartphone application in their lives and work environments respectively?

Table 4 Interview topic guide for service users

In the topic guide, the term "App" is used to refer to the smartphone application under study.
Coherence:
1. Can I take you back to the 'life before the trial (!)' can you tell me about other strategies you have used in the past to increase your exercise
2. In what way was the idea of using the App different from these other strategies?
Cognitive participation is about engagement/'buy in':
1. How did you get involved - who told you about the idea?
2. Can you tell me why you thought it was right for you to get involved in the trial and to give this App a go?
Collective action is about actions and interactions that are required to use the intervention:
1. Now let's focus on when you were starting to use the App itself, can you talk to me about starting to use it and the strategies that made it easy to do so and difficult to do so?
2. What was your sense of trust in the App as a device to support/ stimulate your exercise routines?
3. Can you tell me about the different skills you needed to use the App? (develop some prompts here based on your knowledge of the different tasks that people had to perform to use the App)
4. What are your thoughts about using the App once/now that the trial is over?
Reflexive monitoring is about appraisal and evaluation:
1. Was using the application an effective and worthwhile way to improve your exercise?
2. How do you know?
3. Is it worthwhile to keep using the App now that the trial is over?

That NPT can act as a sensitizing tool allowing the researchers to scrutinize implementation issues pertaining to the use of the smartphone application in the particular context studied in the trial. This made it an ideal choice for the detailed examination of the implementation potential of this novel exercise promotion tool.

Data analysis

Coding was undertaken by two researchers from different professional backgrounds (general practitioner and practice nurse). The data was reviewed periodically by the four member research team made of up of two general practitioners (including author) a nurse and a clinical engineer. QSR International NVivo 10 software [24] was employed as a data organisation tool to expedite the analysis and identification of relationships between coded ideas which facilitated understanding and evaluation of the interview information [25].

Quality and rigour

In order to enhance the quality of data generation and analysis, coding was undertaken by two researchers from different professional backgrounds (general practitioner and practice nurse) to facilitate *inter-coder reliability* as well as generating increased reflexivity [26]. *Reflexivity* suggests an awareness of the means by which the researcher and the research process can shape the assembled data and includes the effects of the researcher's personal characteristics and professional status [27] on the collected data and was further ensured by the exploration of themes by a four member research team made of up of two general practitioners (including author) a nurse and a clinical engineer [28]. *Fair dealing* describes the principle whereby the viewpoint of one group is never presented as if it expresses the sole truth about a situation. The research design specifically incorporated a range of different viewpoints which included those of general practitioners, practice nurses, non-clinical practice staff as well as service users [27].

Results

As well as using the Normalisation Process Theory to generate the interviews and focus group topic guides for service providers and service users, it was also used to analyse the resulting dataset. Four themes emerged from the process of framework analysis. This process consists of five stages which included familiarization, thematic framework identification, indexing, charting, mapping and interpretation [29]. The themes were: personal and professional exercise strategies; roles and responsibilities to support active engagement; utilisation challenges; and evaluation, adoption and adherence.

Theme 1: Strategies to promote exercise - personal and professional (sense-making work)

Learning about the smartphone application intervention describes the work service providers had to undertake to develop a complete understanding of this novel exercise promotion tool. It was immediately apparent that usually there was an absence of a formal strategy to promote increased physical activity amongst service providers.

> *"No, again nothing formal, I suppose I might have you know outlined the benefits of weight bearing activities such as walking but I suppose nothing prescriptive or anything like that no."* [Dr 3]

Both service providers and service users described having had no strategy previously to measure how much exercise they were doing nor did they know how much they needed to exercise to be considered active.

> *"I was a bit shocked because I wasn't doing as much running around as I thought I was doing."* [P3]

Many service providers expressed exasperation that previous strategies were rarely successful despite genuine and repeated efforts to encourage the patients to increase their activity levels. Evidence of previous failed strategies were frequently cited. The fact that previous negotiations with service users were often preoccupied with the emotive issue of weight had rendered certain service providers much less inclined to discuss the topic of exercise in their routine work.

> *"I think it's a difficult thing to engage with patients, I've always found it, I've never been particularly comfortable around raising issues around exercise and weight...."* [Dr 1]

In comparison with previous negative experiences when promoting increased exercise to service users with weight problems, service providers who had utilised the smartphone application observed the manner in which promoting the use of the application allowed the focus of the conversation to shift largely towards exercise promotion rather than the weight issues of the individual service user. The novel idea of engaging with the smartphone technology and the step count screen widget and graphs to monitor their progress was a new concept to most, coupled with the convenience that they were already carrying the smartphone. This "depersonalisation" and neutral space offered by the technology seemed to help service providers in dealing with the sensitivities around issues of obesity and sedentary lifestyle and overlaps with theme 3 of collective action.

> *"What was attractive about this was the sort of more neutral conversation you could have, ...didn't have to necessarily be associated with a conversation about them being obese, overweight or anything like that....."* [Dr 1]

Theme 2: Roles and responsibilities to support active engagement with the app (participation work)

Participants had definite expectations in regard to the technology altering their relationship with exercise and being a lever for change.

> *"I hoped to ....incorporate fitness into my lifestyle really ....unless it's the walk with the kids or something like that, (exercise) was incidental....So basically I wanted it to incorporate (the App) so I would have some exercise throughout, a regular exercise during the week and that I'd be able to continue it after the study, that was the aim." [P3]*

Both service providers and service users described new motivation around behaviour change in relation to physical activity as a result of their introduction to, and experience with, this novel exercise promotion tool. It was of interest and well received by service users as it appeared to provide a clear structure for a strategy to increase their exercise levels to a point where they were confident that they were exercising enough to be considered active.

> *"I think it is a good, you know to use because it's quantifiable. You can see the amount of steps, it's measurable. You know there's a definitive guide there."* [PN2]

> *"I think if you're going into a doctor's surgery and it is a wonderful aid and it is a great awareness for someone, you know so you can say yes this is the goal of 10,000, you're back here at 2,000 so in the next few weeks we're going to try and see can you go from 2,000 to maybe 4,000 and 6,000, 8,000 up, give a step by step approach."* [P3]

Service users provided numerous reasons for active engagement with this smartphone application as a means of increasing their activity levels. These included continual awareness of one's step count in relation to daily step count goals through the instant feedback facilitated by the smartphone application visual settings which enabled goal setting and adjustment throughout the day.

> *"I hated going out in the dark but I have gone out as far as the road and back to get my steps and I also had a, there's a stepper upstairs and I went on that a few times.....My behaviour completely changed."* [P1]

Certain service providers, particularly those from the two primary care medical centres that had not participated in the trial were initially apprehensive about promoting the intervention to service users owing to their own limited smartphone literacy. Understandably these service providers were also concerned that it would demand significant extra workload.

> *"My apprehension is that people will come in for their smartphone you know to talk about but then they'll start looking for medication and blood pressure and everything else along with it and then your consultation time is going to run over. So you know that's one fear I have."* [PN2]

In general, while service providers acknowledged its central importance, they frequently struggled with their exercise-promoting role as it often times made the service user uncomfortable.

> *"I find a good barometer of the level of enthusiasm for this type of intervention is the haste with which the patient wants to get off that entire subject."* [Dr 3]

Many of the service providers bought into the concept of it and started increasing their own physical activity and employed it to increase their activity levels.

> *"We all, you know decided to engage with the process and I think it probably changed all our approach to the issues around weight and exercise....we're all raising the topic a bit more and recording BMI... it has changed the way we operate as a team."* [Dr 1]

Non-clinical staff didn't see it as their role to promote the smartphone application directly to service users but suggested that they would be happy to assume a supporting role.

> *"Maybe if a suggestion that a doctor or the nurse could make it known that if the patient had any problems that the admin staff are there to help...but it's not your place to approach them."* [NCS 2]

Theme 3: Utilisation challenges (enacting work)

The actions and interactions required of service providers and service users to use the smartphone application were next considered. Service providers and service users both remarked that the simplicity of using a smartphone application was a significant lever to its utilisation.

> *"You know which is nice, it's very clear, like it's a very accessible app to most people because there isn't much vocabulary involved, there isn't much text involved in it, it's all very clear, so for that reason I think it's very accessible to most people."* [P3]

"Anybody could use it.....if you could dial a number on a phone you could use it because it's on the screen and it just works." [PN2]

Primary care service providers, while doing the necessary work to familiarise themselves with the smartphone applications, remarked frequently on the significant motivational potential offered by the visual appeal and live feedback on step count. Moreover, they were impressed by the motivating influence of a formalized structure offered by step count and daily goals supported by continuous visual feedback in contrast to the relatively unstructured paradigm which characterized previous exercise advice.

"Yeah, well like I've said they liked that they could set goals for themselves, they liked that they could look back and see what the previous day had, how they had done on previous days." [PN1]

Service users also remarked positively about the motivational potential of the smartphone application through its visual appeal and the immediacy of the step count feedback and felt confident that this was a clear advantage over previous strategies.

"The daily graph because there was a kind of recognition of what you were doing a visual recognition of what you were doing." [P1]

However, both primary care service providers and service users reported challenges with the intervention, notably with respect to technological issues observed as a result of the smartphone application. However, in many instances these were quite readily overcome.

"But the negative feedback as I said was all to do with the battery drainage." [PN2]

"Well number one the battery (was) the biggest problem I had so I found myself then having to remember to keep charging it. I bought a charger for the car so that I could do it continuously....when it did get up and going and when you had access to it and were able to handle the technology yourself I found things did work better." [P2]

There were different views about trusting the accuracy of the App in recording physical activity but in general once service users became familiar with the technology, their levels of trust stabilised accordingly....

"I think you have to realise that it is just an app and it is technology and technology isn't going to be 100% the whole time and technology can be manipulated as well ....you just have to have a sense of honesty and trust in yourself, you know where you're at and that's it." [P3]

Service providers opined that now that the trial period was complete, role clarification should be central to the implementation phase. However, they felt that the promotion of the smartphone application fitted easily into their daily work practices and didn't demand important changes to their usual routine or ways of working.

"I think it's simple...as you know a 30 second conversation...oh yeah we're talking about exercise, there's this really good app that I know about that counts your steps and gives you feedback on your exercise, would you be interested in it...ok go and have a conversation with the practice nurse about it..." [Dr 1]

Theme 4: Evaluation, adoption and adherence (reflexive monitoring)

Service users described in detail the increased sense of ownership and control they felt over their relationship with exercise. They also described how the App was a facilitator in this process of change and how the proximity of the technology on their smartphone made it very easy to connect and re-connect with this intervention.

"I just think that because you have full control of it yourself its useful because lots of people don't like to join clubs or they don't like to join weight watchers, or they don't like to join exercise programs or groups. But you have control of this yourself. And you can just do it privately and nobody need know anything about it. And you can motivate yourself with yourself and nobody else. It doesn't cost anything, it's completely free. And even if you fall off and stop working at it today you can always start a month down the line or three weeks down the line or whenever. You can re-start just get yourself into gear and get going again." [P4]

Service users also described the App as an educator which increased their awareness of their exercise patterns. In addition, participants differed in their longer term use of the App with some just using it to stimulate behaviour change while others continued to require the motivational effects of the technology.

"I don't carry it around with me all the time but I'm more aware now, ok I have a sense of right I know roughly how many steps I have now and I really need to go for a walk, or I really need to go for a long walk this evening, you know that type of way." [P3]

"I have to say that that app has... it's kind of changed me.....I don't know how I'd be if I turned it off. I won't turn it off, not for the moment anyway. I am quite happy to have it on because I am much more conscious of going out for that walk." [P1]

Service providers remarked that they were determined to focus on simplifying the process when implementing the smartphone application into routine practice. Moreover, service providers who hadn't been involved in the trial expressed a readiness to utilise this novel exercise promotion tool in routine practice.

"Well I think the way has been simplified ...... the best idea is to keep it simple...it's not a magic pill, it's just something extra to have, another conversation you can have, it's another little prod that you can give in the right direction...non-judgmental way, provides a neutral space to talk about the issue...I think it's just something extra." [Dr1]

"I suppose the confidence that working with it has brought, you know...you feel a bit more enthusiastic and you feel confident about being able to talk to patients about it." [PN 1]

A cascade effect (defined as an unforeseen series of events which can occur due to an action affecting a particular environment) described in previous research on smartphone interventions [17] was also noted. The smartphone application appeared to arouse curiosity and encouraged others to initiate or become involved in other physical activity interventions.

"We saw effects in the community in terms of a walking group and running group that was formed by somebody who was involved, who downloaded the application." [Dr 1]

Primary care service providers offered a number of ideas to promote increased uptake of the smartphone application as an exercise promotion tool.

The need for a specific service provider staff member to drive the utilisation of the smartphone application by other team members was felt to be an essential ingredient in ensuring successful implementation. That all service providers promoting it should have the application initiated on their own smartphones and ideally having experience of utilising it to change their own exercise behaviour was suggested as an additional lever that may increase uptake.

"I think the last thing is that the person who is spearheading the whole thing has to kind of lead by example themselves." [Dr 4]

Discussion

Summary

This qualitative evaluation of the SMART MOVE Trial demonstrates that introducing a new healthcare intervention into an Irish primary health care context demands a comprehensive evaluation of not only the intervention itself but also of the environment in which it is to operate. However, it is evident that despite certain obstacles the opportunity exists for the successful implementation of a novel healthcare intervention. For this to be successful, it must address a hitherto unresolved healthcare need (*structured and measurable strategy to increase activity levels)* in a particular context *(Irish primary health care),* that has strong usability attributes for both disseminators *(primary care service providers)* and target users *(primary care service users)* and coheres strongly with the core objectives and culture of the health care environment in which it is to operate.

Comparison with existing literature

The potential barriers and levers to the implementation of this new healthcare intervention in a primary healthcare context, as identified by examination of the dataset, bear many similarities to those identified in existing literature. In addition, theyhave critically influenced the design of the implementation package, which is in effect a guideline to support the utilisation of the smartphone application by primary care service providers to promote increased activity amongst primary care service users. The decision to utilise the Normalisation Process Theory to evaluate and optimize the implementation potential of this novel exercise promotion tool is strongly reflected in the literature where it is evident that it has already been extensively used to develop and evaluate complex health care interventions [30, 31]. The data generated in this study illustrates the importance of reflecting on the numerous levels at which healthcare is delivered, their respective cultural contexts and how they interplay which is increasingly recognized as guiding precept of implementation research [32].

For this study specific benefits were that NPT was used to generate the focus group and interview topic guides and to analyse the resulting dataset allowed us to identify factors that were likely to promote and inhibit the incorporation of this novel exercise promotion tool into an Irish primary health care environment. As this exercise promotion tool is entirely novel and although the existing literature was therefore unable to fully encompass the experience of service providers and service users in their efforts to utilise this smartphone application as an exercise promotion tool, an important number of similarities with successful implementation experiences elsewhere were identified.

Once technical issues had been addressed, simplicity and ease of use characterised the experience of most disseminators (service providers) and target users (service users) of the smartphone application in this study which is a noted characteristic of health care interventions that have been successfully normalised into routine practice [33]. That the trial provided an evidence base for the effectiveness of the smartphone application in promoting increased activity levels was an additional attribute that was observed to increased implementation potential in other studies [34]. The fact that the implementation package design has been exclusively shaped by primary care service providers and primary care service users who constitute the target group of the implementation strategy is an attribute known to amplify implementation potential [35]. Moreover, promotion of the smartphone application by primary care service providers to potential users is a process that is closely allied to clinical decision making which has been identified as an lever to implementation elsewhere [36]. Negative attitudes from superiors along with poor support reduces implementation while conversely the presence of an identifiable staff member to act as a peer advisor and driver of utilization increases implementation potential [30, 34] and these experiences were also reflected in our results.

Strengths and limitations

The study strengths included the sampling framework which included a balance of views from all stakeholders, namely: primary care service providers including clinical and administration staff along with primary care service users. Within the focus groups the views of those who had experience of the trial in addition to contributions from a wider cohort of primary care service providers that had not yet used the intervention enriched the focus group discussions.

Moreover, the focus groups, which utilised the fishbowl method and were divided along professional lines was deliberately designed with a view to enhance data generation. The use of the Normalisation Process Theory to generate the focus group and interview topic guides and to frame the data analysis was an additional strength, offering as it does a theoretical approach to determining factors that help and hinder the successful implementation of complex interventions into daily practice. The study limitations were the small numbers of service users and the homogenous cultural characteristics of the sample being all Irish Caucasian clinicians, administration staff and participants, which potentially may not be generalizable to other contexts and populations.

Implications for practice

Primary health care service providers, exasperated by the repeated failure of previous attempts to promote exercise, identified certain key attributes of this novel exercise promotion tool that are likely to positively impact its implementation into routine practice. The smartphone application offered a clearly defined and quantifiable plan to increase exercise versus previous unstructured approaches, a strong motivational potential afforded by the continuous visual feedback and strong usability qualities for both primary care service providers and service users. In conjunction with increasing smartphone literacy and growing market penetrance of smartphone devices along with its coherence with the overall goals of the healthcare environment in which it is to be implemented, this solidly positions this novel exercise promotion tool for future implementation. However, implementation challenges do exist including technical concerns such as battery drainage, limited smartphone literacy and ownership amongst elderly populations and incomplete compatibility with iPhone devices. Service providers concerns included having sufficient smartphone literacy to allow effective promotion of the smartphone application, imposition on existing work routines, requirement for a staff member to drive utilization and wider issues such as on-going reductions in funding of the primary health care sector.

Conclusions

We are aware that problematic translational gaps continue to exist between demonstrating the positive impact of healthcare interventions and the implementation and normalisation of such interventions into routine daily practice. Following on from this study, an implementation package will be developed for rollout to primary care using the NPT generated dataset and analysis to inform this process. We believe that the process used to develop this implementation package amplifies the implementation potential of such an intervention in primary care.

Abbreviations

GP: General practitioner; ITTS: International transnational telemedicine solutions; NCS: Non-clinical staff; NPT: Normalisation process theory; PN: Practice nurse; WestREN: Western research and education network

Acknowledgements

The authors are deeply indebted to the practices of the WESTREN Network; the North Clare Primary Care Team and Clare Primary Care Network; staff of the Discipline of General Practice at the National University of Ireland (NUI), Galway (where the study was coordinated); and Anne Macfarlane, University of Limerick, for her expertise in NTP.

Funding

Funding was awarded by the European Union's Northern Periphery Programme through the Implementing Transnational Telemedicine Solutions project (reference number: 7.13). The funder had no role in: the design and conduct of the study; collection, management, analysis, and interpretation of the data; preparation, review, or approval of the manuscript; and decision to submit the manuscript for publication. Corusen, the designers of the Accupedo-Pro Pedometer app, had no involvement in any aspect of the study including design, analysis, or decision to publish and did not provide any funding or apps free of charge for the purposes of the trial.

Authors' contributions

LG, MC, PH and FG conceived this study and along with LW, DH and AM designed the study, analyzed the data and contributed to the discussion and wrote and edited the manuscript. MC PH and FG conducted the interviews. FG and LG wrote the first draft of the manuscript. All authors read and approved the final manuscript.

Consent for publication

Written consent for publication, including publication of anonymous quotes, was undertaken for all participants who were recruited to the study; these procedures formed part of the ethical approval process.

Competing interests

The authors declare that they have no competing interests.

Author details

[1]Graduate Entry Medical School and Health Research Institute, University of Limerick, Limerick, Ireland. [2]Southampton University Medical School, Southampton University, Southampton, UK. [3]Discipline of General Practice, National University of Ireland, Galway, Ireland. [4]Centre for Rural Health, University of Aberdeen, Inverness, Scotland.

References

1. Murray E, Treweek S, Pope C, MacFarlane A, Ballini L, Dowrick C, et al. Normalisation process theory: a framework for developing, evaluating and implementing complex interventions. BMC Med. 2010;8(1):63.
2. Grol R, Grimshaw J. From best evidence to best practice: effective implementation of change in patients' care. Lancet. 2003;362(9391):1225–30.
3. Cooksey D. A review of UK health research funding: TSO shop; 2006.
4. Woolf SH. The meaning of translational research and why it matters. JAMA. 2008;299(2):211–3.
5. Eccles MP, Armstrong D, Baker R, Cleary K, Davies H, Davies S, et al. An implementation research agenda. Implement Sci. 2009;4(18)
6. Pencheon D, Guest C, Melzer D, Muir Gray J, Korkodilos M, Wright J, et al. Oxford handbook of public health practice. Oxford: Elsevier; 2002.
7. Foy R, Eccles M, Jamtvedt G, Young J, Grimshaw J, Baker R. What do we know about how to do audit and feedback? Pitfalls in applying evidence from a systematic review. BMC Health Serv Res. 2005;5(1):50.
8. Presseau J, Sniehotta FF, Francis JJ, Campbell NC. Multiple goals and time constraints: perceived impact on physicians' performance of evidence-based behaviours. Implement Sci. 2009;4(77)
9. Petticrew M, Whitehead M, Macintyre SJ, Graham H, Egan M. Evidence for public health policy on inequalities: the reality according to policymakers. J Epidemiol Community Health. 2004;58(10):811–6.
10. Glynn LG, Hayes PS, Casey M, Glynn F, Alvarez-Iglesias A, Newell J, et al. Effectiveness of a smartphone application to promote physical activity in primary care: the SMART MOVE randomised controlled trial. Br J Gen Pract. 2014;64(624):e384–e91.
11. Casey M, Hayes PS, Heaney D, Dowie L, ÓLaighin G, Matero M, et al. Implementing transnational telemedicine solutions: a connected health project in rural and remote areas of six northern periphery countries: series on European collaborative projects. Eur J Gen Pract. 2013;19(1):52–8.
12. Glynn LG, Hayes PS, Casey M, Glynn F, Alvarez-Iglesias A, Newell J, et al. SMART MOVE-a smartphone-based intervention to promote physical activity in primary care: study protocol for a randomized controlled trial. Trials. 2013; 14(1):157.
13. Kavanagh K, O' Brien N, Glynn L, Vellinga A, Murphy A. WestREN: a description of an Irish academic general practice research network. BMC Fam Pract. 2010;11(1):74.
14. Edwards R, Holland J. What is qualitative interviewing?: Bloomsbury publishing; 2013.
15. Krueger RA, Casey MA. Focus groups : a practical guide for applied research. Thousand Oaks, CA [etc.]: Sage; 2000.
16. Patton MQ. Qualitative research: Wiley online library; 2005.
17. Casey M, Hayes PS, Glynn F, ÓLaighin G, Heaney D, Murphy AW, et al. Patients' experiences of using a smartphone application to increase physical activity: the SMART MOVE qualitative study in primary care. BJGP. 2014; 64(625):e500–e8.
18. The Fishbowl Technique – Gaining Deep Insights with Polarized Participants | Next Step Consulting 2013. Available from: http://nextstepconsult.com/Article_12.php.
19. Grbich C. Qualitative research in health an introduction. London: Sage Publications; 1999.
20. Silverman D. Interpreting qualitative data: methods for Analysing talk, text and interaction. 2nd edition. 2001.
21. Petersen I, Johnson AM, Islam A, Duckworth G, Livermore DM, Hayward AC. Protective effect of antibiotics against serious complications of common respiratory tract infections: retrospective cohort study with the UK general practice research database. BMJ. 2007;335(7627):982–4A.
22. May CR, Mair F, Finch T, MacFarlane A, Dowrick C, Treweek S, et al. Development of a theory of implementation and integration: normalization process theory. Implement Sci. 2009;4(29):29.
23. May C, Finch T. Implementing, embedding, and integrating practices: an outline of normalization process theory. Sociology-the Journal of the British Sociological Association. 2009;43(3):535–54.
24. Software for Qualitative Research – From Content Analysis and Evaluation to Market Research. 2013. Available from: http://www.qsrinternational.com/.
25. Pitney WA, Parker J. Qualitative research in physical activity and the health professions. USA: Human Kinetics; 2009.
26. Pope C, Ziebland S, Mays N. Qualitative research in health care: Analysing qualitative data. Br Med J. 2000;320(7227):114.
27. Mays N, Pope C. Qualitative research in health care: assessing quality in qualitative research. BMJ. 2000;320(7226):50.
28. Grbich C. Qualitative research in health: an introduction: sage; 1999. p. 312.
29. Ritchie J, Spencer L. The Qualitative Researcher's Companion by A. Michael Huberman & Matthew B. Miles published in 2002 by Sage Publications in California; 2002.
30. Tooth S, Ong B, Foster N. eds. Using a conceptual framework to study the introduction of a new approach to the assessment and treatment of low back pain in primary care in. Boston: Report from the International Forum for Low Back Pain Research in Primary Care; 1998.
31. Gallacher K, May CR, Montori VM, Mair FS. Understanding patients' experiences of treatment burden in chronic heart failure using normalization process theory. The Annals of Family Medicine. 2011;9(3):235–43.
32. Ferlie EB, Shortell SM. Improving the quality of health care in the United Kingdom and the United States: a framework for change. Milbank Q. 2001; 79(2):281.
33. Simpson SH, Marrie TJ, Majumdar SR. Do guidelines guide pneumonia practice? A systematic review of interventions and barriers to best practice in the management of community-acquired pneumonia. Respir Care Clin N Am. 2005;11(1):1–13.
34. Saillour-Glenisson F, Michel P. Individual and collective facilitators of and barriers to the use of clinical practice guidelines by physicians: a literature review. Rev Epidemiol Sante Publique. 2003;51(1):65–80.
35. Sachs M. Successful strategies and methods of nursing standards implementation. Pflege. 2006;19(1):33–44.
36. Grimshaw J, Freemantle N, Wallace S, Russell I, Hurwitz B, Watt I, et al. Developing and implementing clinical practice guidelines. Quality in health care : QHC. 1995;4(1):55–64.

6

Influences on the adoption of patient safety innovation in primary care: a qualitative exploration of staff perspectives

Ian Litchfield[1*], Paramjit Gill[2], Tony Avery[3], Stephen Campbell[4], Katherine Perryman[4], Kate Marsden[3] and Sheila Greenfield[1]

Abstract

Background: Primary care is changing rapidly to meet the needs of an ageing and chronically ill population. New ways of working are called for yet the introduction of innovative service interventions is complicated by organisational challenges arising from its scale and diversity and the growing complexity of patients and their care. One such intervention is the multi-strand, single platform, Patient Safety Toolkit developed to help practices provide safer care in this dynamic and pressured environment where the likelihood of adverse incidents is increasing. Here we describe the attitudes of staff toward these tools and how their implementation was shaped by a number of contextual factors specific to each practice.

Methods: The Patient Safety Toolkit comprised six tools; a system of rapid note review, an online staff survey, a patient safety questionnaire, prescribing safety indicators, a medicines reconciliation tool, and a safe systems checklist. We implemented these tools at practices across the Midlands, the North West, and the South Coast of England and conducted semi-structured interviews to determine staff perspectives on their effectiveness and applicability.

Results: The Toolkit was used in 46 practices and a total of 39 follow-up interviews were conducted. Three key influences emerged on the implementation of the Toolkit these related to their ease of use and the novelty of the information they provide; whether their implementation required additional staff training or practice resource; and finally factors specific to the practice's local environment such as overlapping initiatives orchestrated by their CCG.

Conclusions: The concept of a balanced toolkit to address a range of safety issues proved popular. A number of barriers and facilitators emerged in particular those tools that provided relevant information with a minimum impact on practice resource were favoured. Individual practice circumstances also played a role. Practices with IT aware staff were at an advantage and those previously utilising patient safety initiatives were less likely to adopt additional tools with overlapping outputs. By acknowledging these influences we can better interpret reaction to and adoption of individual elements of the toolkit and optimise future implementation.

Keywords: Patient safety, Primary care, General practice, Health services research, Quality improvement

* Correspondence: I.Litchfield@bham.ac.uk
[1]Institute of Applied Health Research, College of Medical and Dental Sciences, University of Birmingham, Birmingham, UK
Full list of author information is available at the end of the article

Background

Primary care in the UK continues to undergo rapid changes with national initiatives leading to increasing numbers of interventions designed to meet the growing demands of an ageing and chronically ill population [1–3]. However, implementing interventions that are frequently complex and multi-dimensional [4] in an adaptive system such as primary care means change is seldom effected in a linear and prescribed manner [5–7]. In reality, successful implementation is dependent not only on elements intrinsic to the innovation but also a range of organisational and environmental factors specific to each location including existing systems, patient demographics and available resource [8–13]. This complexity has led to calls for more research to clarify the dynamics that underlie the implementation and adoption of successful innovation [14] and a better understanding of the influence of local context particularly in primary care [15].

Research suggests that innovative patient safety activities are amongst those that need to recognise the full range of influences on implementation [16] encouraging acceptability by accounting for the local circumstances of the health care setting [17, 18]. One such patient safety initiative was the NIHR School of Primary Care research funded Patient Safety Toolkit [19, 20] designed to combat the variation in safety awareness and behaviour in a modern primary care environment [21]. The multi-element toolkit was presented on a single platform to meet the challenges presented by the diversities of scale, resource and sophistication of primary care, [21–24] and intended to address shortcomings in patient safety across a range of areas such as communication, medication, and administration [19, 24–28]. Specifically the Toolkit was developed to address patient safety issues within four key areas; identifying patients at specific risk of harm, identifying gaps in safety systems, determining a practice's safety culture, and understanding patient perspectives on safety. It comprises of six tools, a tool for rapid retrospective note review to detect patient safety incidents (the Trigger Tool), an on-line survey to assess the safety climate amongst staff (PC-SafeQuest), a questionnaire to gauge patients' experiences of safety in primary care (PREOS-PC), a software based intervention to prevent medication related injury (Prescribing Indicators Tool), a tool to assess medicines reconciliation for recently discharged patients (Medicines Reconciliation Tool), and a checklist looking at background systems (Concise Safe Systems Checklist for General Practice) [29]. The Toolkit is currently available on the Royal College of General Practitioners' (RCGP) website with accompanying guidance on the use and outputs of each [20].

Here we present our qualitative findings from the final phase of implementation and evaluation of the Toolkit and describe staff experiences of using individual tools alongside their views on the factors influencing the broader adoption of the Toolkit. Our findings help understand the factors that influenced this implementation and how its sustained adoption might be more precisely supported.

Methods

Settings/ recruitment

The Patient Safety Toolkit Project (PST) was a multiphase study conducted across five geographic areas in England [19, 20]. General Practices from the East Midlands, Greater Manchester and North Staffordshire were involved in the development of the Toolkit [19]. These were joined by practices in the West Midlands and the South Coast for the final phase when the Toolkit was implemented and evaluated across all five areas. We set out to recruit ten practices from each area with every practice implementing four of the six tools to ensure that all tools were implemented and evaluated in comparable numbers. Practices were issued an email via their local National Institute for Health Research Primary Care Research Network (latterly the regional Clinical Research Network) requesting if they would like to be involved. If they responded positively a study information pack would be issued and a meeting arranged with the local academic study lead who would discuss the project and answer any queries that emerged.

Distribution of the toolkit

The Toolkit consisted of six individual tools and a summary of the key attributes of each tool and the regions they were introduced can be found in Table 1. All practices distributed the PC PREOS Patient Questionnaire [30] and completed the Trigger Tool [20] (as the maximum amount of data was needed to support their further development). A combination of two of the remaining four tools, as determined by the study team, was then employed by each practice with the intention that each tool would be used at a minimum of ten practices.

Data collection

Semi-structured interviews were conducted with both clinical and non-clinical staff involved in the implementation of the PST. The interview schedule asked staff to describe staff experiences of the tools used, perspectives on the Toolkit as a whole, and its implementation in practice as summarised in Fig. 1. Due to the constraints of time and resource a combination of telephone and face to face interviews were conducted by authors IL, a research fellow employed by the University of Birmingham, KP a research fellow employed by the University of Manchester and Kate Marsden, a research associate at the University of Nottingham. All interviewers were trained and experienced in qualitative research. KP and KM had worked with the practices and interviewees in Greater Manchester and East Midlands respectively during an earlier phase of the PST project [7]. Maximum variation sampling was employed in recruiting

Table 1 Description of patient safety tool kit

Name of tool	Description	Methodology	Participants	Estimated time to completion	Regions participating
Trigger Tool [20]	A system of rapid retrospective note review to allow clinicians to detect episodes of harm and patterns of error which might be occurring undetected in their practices.	Sample created of 25 random patients over the age of 75 to screen for any harm or patient safety incident. The Trigger Tool provides a framework for the case review that highlights any incidents of harm or near misses. The data is summarised to promote reflection on learning points and learning needs on an individual or practice level.	Single or multiple GPs or GP registrars	90 min	All
PC-SafeQuest [20]	An online tool which is intended to be completed by all members of the practice team allowing for a quantitative assessment of the perceived climate of safety within a practice.	Staff are invited to complete an anonymised survey on line. Once completed by a sufficient number of staff, a report can be generated summarising the findings. These are presented as a score in one of four domains, (i) workload; (ii) communication; (iii) leadership; (iv) teamwork; and (v) safety systems. These scores are then used to facilitate discussions around any issues that emerged.	All practice staff. Participation is voluntary.	10–15 min per individual.	West Midlands East Midlands Greater Manchester South Coast
Patient Reported Experiences and Outcomes of Safety in Primary Care (PREOS-PC) [20, 30]	A questionnaire to gather the experience of patients with respect to patient safety in general practice, and on patient reported safety outcomes. Questions are asked within five areas; practice activation; patient activation; experiences of patient safety events; harm; and general perceptions of patient safety.	Practice supplied with 150 envelopes containing the questionnaire, instructions for patients and a reply paid envelope. The practice will then produces the list of recipients and post the questionnaire. Completed questionnaires are returned to the authors at the University of Oxford who produce and distribute a practice specific report.	A sample of 150 patients over the age of 18 generated by the practice. A GP is expected to check that this does not include vulnerable patients.	60 min	All
Prescribing Safety Indicators [20]	Indicators involve the use of CHART (Care and Health Analysis in Real Time) software to extract data on patients at risk of medication-related injury. There are 36 in total and include prescribing related to issues such as cardiovascular and respiratory disease, im munosuppression and laboratory test monitoring.	Install CHART software, download the prescribing safety indicators from PRIMIS Hub, run the computer queries on the GP clinical system and uploading the results to CHART online. The resultant data i dentifies at-risk patients for the practice who then upload an anonymised version to CHART online, aggregated and shared so practices can view their results in relation to other practices.	Various (including member of study team)	60 min	West Midlands North Staffordshire South Coast
Medicines Reconciliation Tool [20]	Used to assess the quality of medications reconciliation process on discharge with a focus on vulnerable patients.	Staff populate a data collection form using the discharge document, the consultation record and the medication record of 20 patients aged 65 and over discharged from emergency hospital between 3 and 6 months ago. This data helps to assess how promptly and how accurately medication changes suggested by the hospital have been made. It also assesses the extent to which changes have been discussed with patients.	Senior staff member collecting data from records	100 min	East Midlands Greater Manchester
Concise Safe Systems Checklist for General Practice [20]	A checklist covering aspects of patient safety not covered by existing tools or legislation. Specifically relates to background systems in practices such as items relating to repeat prescriptions and logs of details of minor operations.	Completion of the checklist form by a practice manager or a senior clinician and used annually.	Senior staff member	30 min	North Staffordshire

The individual tools

1. For each tool used
   a. *What were your expectations of using this tool?*
   b. *What was your experience of using the tool?*
   c. *How easy was the tool to use?*
   d. *Are there any ways you think this tool could be improved?*
   e. *Did you take any action as a result of using the tool?*

General attitudes to the Patient Safety Toolkit

2. What are your opinions of a primary care oriented Patient Safety Toolkit?

3. Which, if any, tool or tools would you use again?
   Prompts: Why?

4. What kind of changes have you or your practice made to the way you work as a result of using the toolkit?
   Prompts: How did the toolkit fit with current work streams?
   Have you made any changes to facilitate the use of the tool/toolkit?

5. Has anything surprised you about using the Patient Safety Toolkit

Implementation

6. Who do you see as the key individual(s) needed to implement this toolkit/tool at your practice?
   Prompts: What length of time was required by these individuals?
   Was capacity an issue?
   What are the training requirements for members of staff using the tools/toolkit?

7. What would encourage you to continue using the toolkit?
   Prompts: Evidence of benefits?
   Financial incentives?
   Supporting website?

Fig. 1 The Topic Guide

practices to the study which meant we could explore influences on patient safety across a broad range of demographically varied cases [31, 32]. Interviews were conducted until data saturation was reached [33] and all were digitally recorded and transcribed verbatim.

Analysis

All data were analysed using thematic analysis [34]. Three transcripts were independently coded by IL who has extensive experience of qualitative research in service delivery research and SG, a professor in medical sociology, a methodologist with expertise in qualitative research as part of mixed methods research. The emerging sub-themes were discussed and agreed upon by IL and SG and used in the subsequent analysis undertaken by IL.

Results

Ultimately 46 practices were recruited with a range of patient characteristics and socio-economic environments [29] reflective of national averages as summarised in Table 2. Practices were predominantly from urban environments with a similar ratio of urban to rural practices found across the UK [31]. A total of 39 interviews were conducted with general practitioners (GP), a GP Registrar, practice managers (PM), practice nurses and one health care assistant (HCA). The interviews lasted between 17 and 46 min. In each case a single practice representative was interviewed except for WM07 where the interview was conducted jointly with a GP and practice manager. A breakdown of those interviewed by job role and geographical area can be found in Table 3.

Table 2 Average characteristics of study practices

	List Size[a]	Under 18[a]	65 + [a]	% Non-White[b]	Deprivation Score[a]	QOF Score (2013)[a]	% Female[b]
Study practice Average/SD[c]	8824 6289	20.4% 4.7%	15.5% 7.4%	17.7% 22.6%	21.8 12.4	976.7 19.6	51.1% 5.0%
English Average	7041[a]	20.8%[a]	16.7%[a]	13%[b]	21.5[a]	961[a]	51%[b]

[a]taken from National General Practice Profiles (Public Health England) [31]
[b]taken from the GP Patient Survey July 2014 [32]
[c]The practice average and standard deviation use values that are weighted by the practice list size but the median and interquartile range use values that are not weighted by the list size

Thematic analysis

Three key themes emerged relating to the implementation of the Toolkit: Tool Design - relating to the utility and usability of each tool; Organisational Factors relating to staff characteristics, practice culture, resource and existing safety systems; and finally Environmental Factors describing the influence of their local Clinical Commissioning Group and the broader influence of central policy. The major themes and sub-themes are summarised in Table 4.

Tool design

Here we describe the prima facie response to the design of the tools in relation to their utility and usability, respectively defined as the relevance and applicability of their individual and combined output, and the ease with which the tool can be used.

Utility The degree to which constituent tools were able to contribute to improving patient safety was the central consideration. Staff commented on how they can be used to raise awareness of the importance of patient safety amongst staff, gain insight into safe practice from patients and non-clinical staff, quantify improvements over time, support the training of junior doctors and produce evidence of safe practice for regulators.

Impact on safe practice Taken as a whole, a Toolkit requiring the input of both clinical and non-clinical staff was seen as a useful means of raising or maintaining awareness of patient safety and creating a culture where the whole work force remained attentive to its importance.

> "It's probably a part of creating this ethos of patient safety as much as anything ... creating an environment where people are mindful of patient safety" *GP Registrar – GM03*

> "...it makes you aware of what could go wrong; you know, what you need to be doing for the patient safety" - *Practice Nurse NS05*

Individual tools provided a range of perspectives on various aspects of patient safety. For example the PREOS-PC questionnaire was seen as offering a useful insight into patients' interpretation of the concept of patient safety.

> "I think probably the learning point here was "What does it mean to patients themselves?" because it may mean something else to them, and something else to us." - *Practice Nurse WM02*

It was also felt that the PC SafeQuest tool was a practical way of supporting interaction between different staff groups, particularly between clinical and non-clinical staff. For example, one practice manager felt it an important means of managers gaining critical feedback from administrative staff that might otherwise have been missed.

> "... as managers we tend to miss out on things because we are so busy with paperwork and this and

Table 3 Job role of those interviewed at each practice

	East Midlands (EM)	Greater Manchester (GM)	South Coast (SC)	North Staffordshire (NM)	West Midlands (WM)	Total
GP	8	4[a]	5	3	1[b]	21
PM	1	2	–	4	8	15
Practice Nurse	–	–	–	1	2	3
HCA	–	–	–	1	–	1
Total number of interviews	9	6	5	9	10	39

[a]including one GP Registrar
[b]Interviewed alongside Practice Manager

Table 4 Summary of themes and sub-themes in relation to individual tools

Theme	Sub-theme 1	Sub-theme 2	Trigger tool	PC-Safe-Quest	PREOS-PC	Prescribing Safety Indicators	Medicines Reconciliation Tool	Concise Safe Systems Checklist for General Practice
1. Tool Design	1.1 Utility	Inform patient safety Training aide Provide evidence of safe practice.	Did not uncover enough learning points for those using SEA.	Provided a useful practice-wide staff perspective.	Provided a novel patient perspective.	Produced useful patient specific information.	Produced useful information.	Produced useful information that prompted reflection on safety issues.
	1.2 Usability	Format Time to completion Integration with existing systems	Was time consuming in the selection of individual records.	Completed online and easy to follow.	Resource intensive due to the addressing and packing of multiple envelopes.	Required either existing IT knowledge or additional help and support.	Straightforward to use.	Easy to use and quick to complete
2. Organisational factors	2.1 Staff training	Existing skill set	Was straightforward to use though a preference for an electronic version was expressed.	No training needed though an email address for each staff member was required.	Issues arose selecting random patients and using 'mail merge' to address letters and envelopes.	Staff training was required to run the software and upload the results.	No formal training required. An electronic version preferred.	No training required
	2.2 Available resource	Staffing levels, Time constraints						
	2.3 Existing patient safety approaches	Comparative effectiveness						
3. Environmental context	3.1 Clinical commissioning group	Existing initiatives	N/A	N/A	N/A	N/A	Repeated the work of a CCG initiative in one area.	N/A
	3.2 Central policy	Financial Incentives Fragmented policy						

> that you forget your staff and it's nice to get a feedback of the staff, of what they think and how they feel, and patient safety, communication and all that kinda stuff. So it does highlight a lot of interesting points." – *Practice Manager WM08*

The scores produced by this tool could be compared over time to provide a quantitative measure of any changes in performance.

> "So the managers obviously think we're doing a great job, the non-managers not so convinced, looking at that [report]. Perhaps that is something we need to address. I suppose that's one of the strengths of using this sort of approach, that you pick up things which you perhaps actually thought you were doing okay, but maybe we're not doing as well as we could... the major utility of something like this is to repeat it and see if there is an improvement." – *GP EM08*

Training aide Staff at several practices felt the whole Toolkit would have real value as a means of training junior doctors, raising their awareness of the issues around patient safety.

> "I think if I could convince a trainee to perhaps do it as a project, which I think could be really useful for them as well, then that might work really well and I think maybe I would consider doing that... in fact it's now a requirement of completion of general practice training that they must have done either an audit or a quality improvement project and this would be ideal." – *GP EM08*

Provide evidence of safe practice In attempting to ensure delivery of care that consistently meets national standards, regulatory bodies such as the UK's Care Quality Commission (CQC) [35] are charged with objectively measuring the performance of practices across a number of criteria. Some we spoke to felt the Toolkit would be useful in providing evidence to regulators of the work the practice do in the area of patient safety.

> "So if I present this report to a [CQC] inspector, he will probably be quite surprised, 'Where the hell did you get this from?' and you'd actually be able to quantify it and provide some kind of qualitative interpretation as to what this actually means. They'll probably consider it as a good or an outstanding, to be honest with you." – *Practice Manager WM07*

Usability Staff described how the design of the tools contributed to their ease of use including their composition, the length of time needed to complete them, and the degree to which they were integrated with existing systems.

Format Each tool had been developed or refined during earlier phases of the study with the intention that by the final phase of evaluation the usability of novel tools such as the Concise Safe Systems Checklist had been optimised.

> "The questions are well laid-out - yes/no answers and any comments that you want to make...very easy to follow." - *Practice Manager NS04*

Time to completion An important consideration was how long it took to use the tool. For example one practice manager commented how the speed with which the online survey of practice safety culture (PC-SafeQuest) could be completed was a distinct advantage.

> "For me the fact that there was a good uptake suggests that it was quite straightforward to access... and the fact that it didn't take long to fill in, I mean, if it was me I, I would just look, 'Oh God, this is taking 25 minutes. I'm not going to do it.' So I think for a lot of people it's doable." - *Practice Manager WM07*

By contrast the Patient Safety Questionnaire was too long for many patients to complete, certainly when they were unsure of its impact as one Practice Manager explained.

> "I think it had more than 40 questions, I thought it was quite a long questionnaire so if I was a patient who had received it I may not complete it because, why would somebody complete such a long survey?" – *Practice Manager WM09*

Level of integration with existing systems Staff described their preference for a tool that could integrate into existing practice software. One example was the reliance of the Trigger Tool on the manual selection of records for review. One practice manager suggested this selection process could be based on an automated algorithm to speed up the process.

> "It might be better if something could be written into the clinical system like, when you go to Sainsbury's, the random person gets a questionnaire, or the random person gets a voucher – if you get a random pop-up after, you know, X amount of patients. 'Oh, right, I've gotta fill this one in, and then look back on

that one.' If it was, more like that and integrated..." – *Practice Manager WM04*

Another example was the paper-based Medicines Reconciliation Tool viewed as anachronistic by a GP Registrar in an era where patient data is increasingly held on integrated electronic systems.

> "there's an expectation amongst GPs that these sorts of tools will be...because the electronic records systems now are so good...I think it just seems a little bit strange - in a way- going back to a pen and paper system where you're having to manually read through lists of medications and then reconcile them with manual lists on the screen." - *GP Registrar GM03*

Organisational Factors

Here we describe how factors relating to individual practice organisations impacted on the attitude toward and implementation of the Toolkit. Specifically the skill set of individual staff and the resources available.

Staff skill set For software based tools or those that relied on a degree of familiarity with the clinical management system the practice employed, it became apparent that a lack of information technology training limited the ability of staff to use some of the tools. One example was the Prescribing Safety Indicators tool that involved downloading and running a software package that interrogated the clinical management system for medication records then uploading the results to a secure third party for analysis. One practice manager felt the tool was too complicated and far removed from the usual roles and responsibilities of their administrative staff to use.

> "I certainly wouldn't expect the staff...they wouldn't have a clue where to start ... No, it's got to be simple and to the point, and relative to their work, their everyday work." - *Practice Manager WM04*

One practice nurse also described how unfamiliarity with the required software allied to the infrequent use of the tool meant they were unlikely to continue to use it.

> "You can't teach an old dog new tricks, so...it's my knowledge of all that, you know, learning new software again and stuff. When you're only using it once or twice, you can't get to grips with it." – *Practice Nurse WM02*

Available resource A number of participants described how limits on staff numbers and increasing demand on staff time impacted on their ability to implement the Toolkit.

Staffing levels Shortages in the number of administrative staff appeared to limit the chance of the long-term adoption of some of the tools. For example one Practice Manager felt that using her relatively expensive time to print and distribute the Patient Safety Questionnaire was not an efficient use of practice resource.

> "I think if we did anything like it again, I'd ask 'the company' to facilitate PREOS you know? When you think what an hourly rate for a practice manager is, stuffing envelopes...because I haven't got the manpower to pass it down." – *Practice Manager WM04*

Time constraints The pressure on the time and resource of practices of implementing a multi-faceted intervention like the Toolkit was a concern. For some, the perception that a large number of tasks required completion meant busy staff would fail to engage with the concept.

> "it's a very big - it's got lots of different dimensions with GPs involved, you've got to send it out to patients, you've got internal ... I think you've got to streamline it in a way... 'Oh, this sounds interesting. How much time and cost is it? I'm not interested now." *Practice Manager WM07*

> "I think you really need one sheet of paper that we can do everything on or try and streamline it down... People aren't going to do lots and lots of different tools...if you ask too much of someone they won't do it." – *GP EM02*

Introducing any tool that took a relatively lengthy time to complete appeared problematic despite potentially valuable outputs. For example the Trigger Tool was one that involved a manual search of patient records and subsequent completion of a paper form.

> "...it's probably helpful and an important way to try and identify some of these incidents that are not...don't lead to complaints, or they don't lead to harm. From a clinical point of view I think it's probably just a bit too cumbersome and time-consuming to be useful and I don't think we're going to continue using it in our practice..." – *GP Registrar GM03*

Existing approaches

The acceptability of individual tools was dependent on the presence and effectiveness of existing patient safety measures.

Comparative effectiveness If a tools outputs were too similar to those derived from existing safety improvement approaches then they risked being judged a poor use of time. For example, one GP felt the small number of novel issues identified by the Trigger Tool in comparison to those highlighted by their Significant Event Analysis [36] were insufficient to warrant the time required for its use.

> "You don't have the time to go through 10/20 sets of notes before you find one learning point because...there will be a pile of complaints, there'll be a pile of SEAs and these are things which are prioritised because they're more likely to lead to learning points than these sorts of trawls of triggers and things like that." - *GP Registrar GM03*

Environmental context

This describes how implementation was influenced by factors relating to both the initiatives of their Clinical Commissioning Group (CCG) and also those stemming from the broader impact of national policies and guidance.

Clinical commissioning group The priorities of the Clinical Commissioning Group (CCG) of each region varied. For example staff at one practice described how improvements to the discharge process orchestrated by their CCG meant the Medicines Reconciliation Tool repeated work already undertaken.

> "...'cause we've already done things like this with the CCG, so I felt a bit like I was redoing the sort of thing that I'd already been doing." *GP GM02*

The importance of the CCG in facilitating the sustained adoption of the Toolkit was recognised.

> "...but I think it needs to go in at the commissioning side and I think we need to tie this in to a better template of use...then it actually does get built in." *Practice Nurse EM05*

Central policy Staff discussed how financial incentives influenced their decision to change ways of working, particularly when attempting to assimilate numerous policies and initiatives that emerged from a variety of sources with different agendas.

Financial incentives Financial incentives have been used in primary care to encourage certain behaviours and have become relied upon as a valuable funding stream by senior staff. For some, the financial rewards of taking part in the study were a significant factor in their decision to participate.

> "To be perfectly honest, it was the GP that picked up on it, from an income point of view - as another income stream. Because, you know, the way they're pulling money off us in all directions, we've got to look at everything. We're running a business, at the end of the day, so we've got to be doing things that are financially rewarding for the practice." – *Practice Manager WM04*

Fragmented policy

Staff described how the quantity of frequently changing policies and initiatives introduced by various local and national bodies impacted on their ability to adopt further innovation.

> "...[adoption is difficult] because you're dealing with CCG, you're dealing with NHS England, City Council, the nurses, you're dealing with the patients, you're dealing with your policies and procedures, you're dealing with an audit. You got the day to day running of the surgery and then you're going back to the action plans and the reports and all that kinda stuff. So there's a whole sort of set of things that you need to do..." – *Practice Manager WM08*

A GP at another practice described how the number of existing work streams meant there might not be the capacity to devote the necessary time to another.

> "There's so many things, ok? That you can't keep going 'yet another'...all the GPs are bombarded with different practices and I don't know, 'ideas' from all this and departments - I'm not sure whether they would be welcoming this. I mean I'm certain it would be useful but how much time anybody is going to spend looking in to it? I'm not certain..." *GP SC03*

Discussion

General findings

The concept of a Patient Safety Toolkit (PST) [20] comprised of a diverse set of tools to address a range of issues proved popular with participants. As a toolkit is was able to provide evidence of safe practice to regulators and could be used as a training aide to raise awareness of patient safety amongst Junior Doctors and the broader staff team. Of the constituent tools those that were favoured either met a distinct need and could be completed quickly and easily, such as the PC SafeQuest survey [20] or the Safety Checklist for General Practice, [20] or otherwise offered novel insights into patient safety as provided by the PREOS-PC [37].

Despite, the apparent benefit of the Toolkit, staff were hesitant about committing to its continued use due to a number of factors linked to both the practice organisation and the broader practice environment these included the need for additional staff training, its relevance in relation to existing approaches to improving patient safety, and the profusion of service initiatives from external bodies. Taken together these contextual factors impacted on the practice's ability, capacity, and willingness to incorporate the PST into existing work streams. This relationship between innovation and the context of individual practice needs to be acknowledged and addressed if sustained adoption of this valuable patient safety resource is to be realised.

Specific findings

Tool design

For any innovation to be successfully adopted it must possess clear applicability, relevance and benefit [38–42]. One tool where this was the case was the PC SafeQuest Survey [20] that provided all practice staff an anonymous platform to share their experiences of, and attitudes toward patient safety. Many previous strategies to improve quality and safety have advocated the democratisation of knowledge, skills and authority in order to successfully change systems and processes [10, 11, 43, 44] recognising the importance of an open, learning culture [45–47] and the identification of managerial "blind spots" [48, 49]. The Survey emerged as a practical and viable solution to engage all staff and increase the visibility of those issues that might have otherwise been missed by senior staff. Another tool which was well received for its' novel perspective was the PREOS-PC patient questionnaire [37]. Though reservations were voiced about its length the resource required in its administration it was judged to provide valuable insights into patient perspectives on safety. The positive role played by patients in improving patient safety has previously been noted [50] and while the most efficient methods of harnessing patient involvement remain undefined, [51] our participants recognised the importance of understanding patient perceptions of safety and harm.

Organisational influences

The primary care landscape is diverse and reflected in the variation of preferences and requirements of individual practices. The skill set of staff can vary and inconsistent levels of training, particularly around IT, directly affected the capability of practices to independently implement the software based Prescribing Safety Indicators. The importance of continuous staff training to support a practice's internal capability to deliver safer care has been described previously [38, 39, 41, 52] and smaller practices in particular can lack IT support [53, 54] limiting their use of software-based innovation [38, 55–58]. Those designing such systems should retain a socio-technical perspective that considers from the earliest design phases not only how the technical features of a system meet demand but also seeks understanding of how they interact with the working healthcare environment [4–6]. However, of larger consequence than the technical ability of staff it seems the single biggest restriction on the implementation of the Toolkit appeared a lack of time and resource. Primary care is experiencing unprecedented demand with consultation rates doubling in recent years [59, 60] in response to increasing numbers of chronically ill multi-morbid patients [61]. In the UK concerns about current and predicted shortages in the primary care workforce, are widely recognised [62] and the growing pressure on practice services not only increases the likelihood of patient safety incidents [63–67] but appears to reduce the willingness of organisations to adopt innovations or additional work streams that require any substantial amount of time or training to complete [68, 69]. For our participants this translated into an unwillingness to engage with a multi-strand toolkit or to utilise individual tools that failed to produce substantial new findings or otherwise overlapped with existing approaches to patient safety.

Environmental influences

Some of the existing safety initiatives being used by participating practices were introduced by their local CCG and their outputs overlapped with those of certain tools. The value of concerted CCG led initiatives may mean that their proactive (including financial) support might be the key factor in helping embed the Toolkit into existing practice systems and sustain adoption at a time when resources in primary care are so stretched [70]. The continuing financial pressures of modern primary care are leading senior staff to explore every opportunity for increasing practice income [71]. For some the financial incentives associated with piloting the Toolkit were the primary motivation for involvement, with suggestions that similar remunerations would need to be in place if they were to use the Toolkit in the future. The reluctance to unilaterally commit to its continued use might in part be attributed to the uncertainty engendered from reconciling numerous and evolving policies alongside local initiatives and directives [1, 3]. Staff described their vulnerability to a stream of frequently incoherent targets and objectives from multiple sources and this type of dynamic and complex health economy has previously been observed to reduce the willingness of senior staff to pursue innovative strategies [72].

There have been previous calls for a greater understanding of how the type of contextual influences we've identified here inform implementation [73–75]. Though unlikely to exist or act in isolation, [76, 77] a better understanding of the range of influences that impacted on the implantation of the Toolkit is an important step if we are to provide targeted support for this valuable patient safety resource.

Conclusions

The experienced research team gathered data from a number of regions interviewing clinical and non-clinical staff at a range of practices until saturation was reached [33]. Not only have we identified the key design attributes of successful tools but also the inter-related contextual factors that influence the sustained implementation of complex interventions of this type. Logistical constraints meant we have so far been unable to explore the level of sustained adoption of the Toolkit by participating practices and it will be interesting to determine how the characteristics of practices and their patients influence the types of tool they continue to use.

Abbreviations

CCG: Clinical Commissioning Group; GP: General Practitioner; HCA: Health Care Assistant; PM: Practice Manager; PST: Patient Safety Toolkit; RCGP: Royal College of General Practitioners

Acknowledgements

Katie Dixon who collected data, Nacho Cabello who developed and distributed the PREOS-PC Safety Questionnaire.

Funding

The 'Development of the NSPCR Patient Safety Toolkit for general practices' was funded by the National Institute for Health Research School for Primary Care Research (NIHR SPCR). The funding body was neither involved in the design of the study nor the collection, analysis, and interpretation of data and writing of the manuscript.

Authors' contributions

PG, AA, SC and SG were responsible for the concept and design of the work of the work including the methodology for the acquisition and analysis of the data. KP, KM, and IL were responsible for collecting the data. IL and SG were responsible for the original idea for the manuscript and undertook the analysis. IL produced an initial draft and numerous iterations were reviewed and amended for content and intellectual rigour by PG, AA, SC, KP and KM. The final version was forwarded to all authors for approval prior to submission.

Competing interests

There are no competing interests financial or otherwise from any of the authors.

Author details

[1]Institute of Applied Health Research, College of Medical and Dental Sciences, University of Birmingham, Birmingham, UK. [2]Warwick Medical School - Social Science and Systems in Health, University of Warwick, Coventry, UK. [3]School of Medicine, Division of Primary Care, University of Nottingham, Nottingham, UK. [4]Centre for Primary Care, Division of Population Health, Health Services Research and Primary Care, University of Manchester, Manchester, UK.

References

1. NHS England. The NHS five year forward view. 2014. https://www.england.nhs.uk/wp-content/uploads/2014/10/5yfv-web.pdf. Accessed Sept 2017.
2. NHS England. Next steps on the NHS five year forward view. 2017. https://www.england.nhs.uk/wp-content/uploads/2017/03/NEXT-STEPS-ON-THE-NHS-FIVE-YEAR-FORWARD-VIEW.pdf Accessed Sep 2017.
3. Health and Social Care Act 2012, c.7. Available at: http://www.legislation.gov.uk/ukpga/2012/7/contents/enacted.
4. Craig P, et al. Developing and evaluating complex interventions: the new Medical Research Council guidance. BMJ. 2008;337:a1655.
5. Miller WL, et al. Understanding change in primary care practice using complexity theory. J Fam Pract. 1998;46:369–76.
6. Miller WL, et al. Practice jazz: understanding variation in family practices using complexity science. J Fam Pract. 2001;50:872–8.
7. Crabtree BF. Primary care practices are full of surprises! Health Care Manag Rev. 2003;28:279–83.
8. Weiner BJ. A theory of organizational readiness for change. Implement Sci. 2009;4(1):67.
9. The King's Fund. Experience-based co-design toolkit. 2014. https://www.kingsfund.org.uk/publications/pressures-in-general-practice. Accessed Sept 2017.
10. Lawrence M, Packwood T. Adapting total quality management for general practice: evaluation of a programme. Qual Health Care. 1996;5:151–8.
11. Baker GR, et al. A conceptual framework for learning continual improvement in health administration education programs. J Health Adm Educ. 1995;13:67–90.
12. Fishbein M, Ajzen I. Belief, attitude, intention, and behavior: an introduction to theory and research. Reading: Addison-Wesley; 1975.
13. Meyer JP, Herscovitch L. Commitment in the workplace: toward a general model. Hum Resour Manag Rev. 2001;11:299–326.
14. Lemiengre MB, et al. Optimizing antibiotic prescribing for acutely ill children in prmiary care (ERNIE2 study protocol, part B): a cluster randomized, factorial controlled trial evaluating the effect of a point-of-care C-reactive protein test and a brief intervention combined with safety net advice. BMC Pediatr. 2014;14:246.
15. Lau R, et al. Achieving change in primary care – causes of the evidence to practice gap: systematic reviews of reviews. Implement Sci. 2016;11:40.
16. Verstappen W, et al. Patient safety improvement programmes for primary care. Review of a Delphi procedure and pilot studies by the LINNEAUS collaboration on patient safety in primary care. Eur J Gen Pract. 2015; 21(Suppl 1):50–5.
17. Bosch-Capblanch X, et al. Guidance for evidence-informed policies about health systems: rationale for and challenges of guidance development. PLoS Med. 2012;9:e1001185.
18. Epstein RM, Peters E. Beyond information: exploring patients' preferences. JAMA. 2009;302:195–7.
19. Spencer R, Campbell SM. Tools for primary care patient safety: a narrative review. BMC Fam Pract. 2014;15:166.
20. Royal College of General Practitioners. Patient Safety Toolkit for General Practice. http://www.rcgp.org.uk/clinical-and-research/toolkits/patient-safety.aspx/ Accessed Sep 2017.
21. The Health Foundation. Evidence scan: Levels of harm. 2011. http://www.health.org.uk/sites/health/files/LevelsOfHarm_0.pdf/ Accessed Sep 2017.
22. Sandars J, Esmail A. The frequency and nature of medical error in primary care: understanding the diversity across studies. Fam Pract. 2003;20:231–6.
23. Ghandi TK, Lee TH. Patient Safty beyond the hospital. N Engl J Med. 2010; 363:1001–3.
24. Zwart DLM, et al. Patient safety culture measurement in general practice. Clinimetric properties of 'SCOPE'. BMC Fam Pract. 2011;12:117.

25. Gaal S, Vertappen W, Wensing M. What do primary care physicians and researchers consider the most important patient safety improvement strategies? BMC Health Serv Res. 2011;11:102.
26. Litchfield I, Bentham L, Lilford R, et al. Test result communication in primary care: a survey of current practice. BMJ Qual Saf. Published Online First: 04 August 2015. https://doi.org/10.1136/bmjqs-2014-003712.
27. Woolf SH, et al. A string of mistakes: the importance of Cascade analysis in describing, counting, and preventing medical errors. Ann Fam Med. 2004;2: 317–26.
28. Makeham MAB, et al. Patient safety events reported in general practice: a taxonomy. Qual Saf Health Care. 2008;17:53–7.
29. Bell BG, et al. Tools for measuring patient safety in primary care settings using the RAND/UCLA appropriateness method. BMC Fam Pract. 2014;15:110.
30. Ricci-Cabello I, et al. Measuring experiences and outcomes of patient safety in primary care: a systematic review of available instruments. Fam Pract. 2015;32:106–19.
31. Public Health England. National General Practice Profiles. http://fingertips.phe.org.uk/profile/general-practice/ Accessed Sep 2017.
32. NHS England. GP Patient Survey. https://gp-patient.co.uk/. Accessed Sept 2017.
33. Fusch PI, Ness LR. Are we there yet? Data saturation in qualitative research. Qual Rep. 2015;20(9):1408–16.
34. Cassell C, Symon G. Essential guide to qualitative methods in organizational research. London: SAGE Publications; 2004.
35. Care Quality Commission. http://www.cqc.org.uk/ Accessed Sep 2017.
36. Bowie P, McNaughton E, Bruce D, et al. Enhancing the Effectiveness of Significant Event Analysis: Exploring Personal Impact and Applying Systems Thinking in Primary Care. The Journal of Continuing Education in the Health Professions. 2016;36(3):195–205. https://doi.org/10.1097/CEH.0000000000000098.
37. Ricci-Cabello I, et al. Measuring patient safety in primary care: the development and validation of the "patient reported experiences and outcomes of safety in primary care" (PREOS-PC). Ann Fam Med. 2016;14: 253–61.
38. Miller WL, et al. Primary care practice development: a relationship-centered approach. Ann Fam Med. 2010;8(Suppl 1):S68–79.
39. Dawda P, Jenkins R, Varnam R. Quality Improvement in General Practice. London: The King's Fund; 2010.
40. Mickan S, Burls A, Glasziou P. Patterns of 'leakage' in the utilization of clinical guidelines: a systematic review. Postgrad Med J. 2011;87:670–9.
41. Dulko D. Audit and feedback as a clinical practice guideline implementation strategy: a model for acute care nurse practitioners. Worldviews Evid-Based Nurs. 2007;4:200–9.
42. Kendall E, et al. When guidelines need guidance: considerations and strategies for improving the adoption of chronic disease evidence by general practitioners. J Eval Clin Pract. 2009;15:1082–90.
43. Deming WE. Out of the crisis. Cambridge: MIT Press; 1986.
44. Jones D, Mitchell A. Lean thinking for the NHS. London: NHS Confederation; 2006. Report No. BOK 56701.
45. Yammarino FJ, Dansereau F, Kennedy CJ. A multiple-level multidimensional approach to leadership: viewing leadership through an elephant's eye. Organ Dyn. 2001;29:149–63.
46. Milligan F, Dennis S. Building a safety culture. Nurs Stand. 2005;20:48.
47. Kaufman G, McCaughan D. The effect of organisational culture on patient safety. Nurs Stand. 2013;27:50–6.
48. Dixon-Woods M, et al. Explaining Michigan: developing an ex pos theory of a quality improvement program. Milbank Q. 2011;89:167–205.
49. Charles K, McKee L, McCann S. A quest for patient-safe culture: contextual influences on patient safety performance. J Health Serv Res Policy. 2011;16: 57–64.
50. Longtin Y, et al. Patient participation: current knowledge and applicability to patient safety. Mayo Clin Proc. 2010;85:53–62.
51. Trier H, et al. Involving patients in patient safety programmes: a scoping review and consensus procedure by the LINNEAUS collaboration on patient safety in primary care. Eur J Gen Pract. 2015;21(Suppl 1):56–61.
52. Broens TH, et al. Determinants of successful telemedicine implementations: a literature study. J Telemed Telecare. 2007;13:303–9.
53. Crossland L, Janamian T, Jackson CL. Key elements of high-quality practice organisation in primary health care: a systematic review. Med J Aust. 2014; 201(3 Suppl):S47–51.
54. Menachemi N, et al. Enviromental factors and health information technology management strategy. Health Care Manag Rev. 2011;36:275–85.
55. Hayward-Rowse L, Whittle T. A pilot project to design, implement and evaluate an electronic integrated care pathway. J Nurs Manag. 2006;14:564–71.
56. Meade B, Buckley D, Boland M. What factors affect the use of electronic patient records by Irish GPs? Int J Med Inform. 2009;78:551–8.
57. Dorr D, et al. Informatics systems to promote improved Care for Chronic Illness: a literature review. J Am Med Inform Assoc. 2007;14:156–63.
58. Ekeland AG, Bowes A, Flottorp S. Effectiveness of telemedicine: a systematic review of reviews. Int J Med Inform. 2010;79:736–71.
59. Royal College of General Practitioners. A Vision for General Practice in the future NHS. 2013. http://www.rcgp.org.uk/campaign-home/~/media/files/policy/a-z-policy/the-2022-gp-a-vision-for-general-practice-in-the-future-nhs.ashx/ Accessed Sep 2017.
60. The Deloitte Centre for Health Solutions. Primary care: Today and tomorrow. Improving general practice by working differently. 2012. http://www2.deloitte.com/uk/en/pages/life-sciences-and-healthcare/articles/primary-care.html/ Accessed Sep 2017.
61. Barnett K, et al. Epidemiology of multimorbidity and implications for health care, research, and medical education: a cross-sectional study. Lancet. 2012; 380(9836):37–43.
62. Health Education England. The future of primary care Creating teams for tomorrow. 2015.https://www.hee.nhs.uk/sites/default/files/documents/The%20Future%20of%20Primary%20Care%20report.pdf. Accessed Sept 2017.
63. Ordonez L, Benson L. Decisions under time pressure: how time constraint affects risky decision making. Organ Behav Hum Decis Process. 1997;71:121–40.
64. Ben Zur H, Breznitz SJ. The effect of time pressure on risky choice behavior. Acta Psyhcologica. 1981;47:89–104.
65. Dror I, Busemeyer J, Basola B. Decision making under time pressure: an independent test of sequential sampling models. Mem Cogn. 1999;27:713–25.
66. Croskerry P. The cognitive imperative: thinking about how we think. Acad Emerg Med. 2000;7:1223–31.
67. Bell BG, et al. Safety climate in English general practices: workload pressures may compromise safety. J Eval Clin Pract. 2016;22:71–6.
68. Holm AL, Severinsson E. Chronic care model for the management of depression: synthesis of barriers to, and facilitators of, success. Int J Ment Health Nurs. 2012;21:513–23.
69. Pereira JA, et al. Barriers to the use of reminder/recall interventions for immunizations: a systematic review. BMC Med Inform Decis Mak. 2012;12:145.
70. Royal College of General Practitioners. 89% of GPs say they worry that lack of resources is putting patient care at risk and 58% plan to leave or reduce their hours within five years. 2016. http://www.rcgp.org.uk/news/2016/april/89-of-gps-say-they-worry-that-lack-of-resources-is-putting-patient-care-at-risk.aspx Accessed Oct 2017.
71. Millett C, et al. Impact of a pay-for-performance incentive on support for smoking cessation and on smoking prevalence among people with diabetes. Can Med Assoc J. 2007;176:1705–10.
72. Layman EJ, Bamberg R. Environmental scanning and the health care manager. Health Care Manag. 2005;24:200–8.
73. Cummings GG, et al. The relationship between characteristics of context and research utilization in a pediatric setting. BMC Health Serv Res. 2010;10:168.
74. Attieh R, et al. Organizational readiness for knowledge translation in chronic care: a review of theoretical components. Implement Sci. 2013;8:138.
75. Fulop N, Robert G. Context for successful improvement: evidence review. London: The Health Foundation; 2015. ISBN 978-1-906461-68-3
76. Kitson A, Harvey G, McCormack B. Enabling the implementation of evidence based practice: a conceptual framework. Qual Health Care. 1998;7(3):149–58.
77. Rycroft-Malone J, et al. Ingredients for change: revisiting a conceptual framework. Qual Saf Health Care. 2002;11(2):174–80.

7

Factors influencing decision of general practitioners and managers to train and employ a nurse practitioner or physician assistant in primary care

Mieke van der Biezen[1*], Emmy Derckx[2], Michel Wensing[1,3] and Miranda Laurant[1,4]

Abstract

Background: Due to the increasing demand on primary care, it is not only debated whether there are enough general practitioners (GPs) to comply with these demands but also whether specific tasks can be performed by other care providers. Although changing the workforce skill mix care by employing Physician Assistants (PAs) and Nurse Practitioners (NPs) has proven to be both effective and safe, the implementation of those professionals differs widely between and within countries. To support policy making regarding PAs/NPs in primary care, the aim of this study is to provide insight into factors influencing the decision of GPs and managers to train and employ a PA/NP within their organisation.

Methods: A qualitative study was conducted in 2014 in which 7 managers of out-of-hours primary care services and 32 GPs who owned a general practice were interviewed. Three main topic areas were covered in the interviews: the decision-making process in the organisation, considerations and arguments to train and employ a PA/NP, and the tasks and responsibilities of a PA/NP.

Results: Employment of PAs/NPs in out-of-hours services was intended to substitute care for minor ailments in order to decrease GPs' caseload or to increase service capacity. Mangers formulated long-term planning and role definitions when changing workforce skill mix. Lastly, out-of-hours services experienced difficulties with creating team support among their members regarding the employment of PAs/NPs.

In general practices during office hours, GPs indented both substitution and supplementation for minor ailments and/or target populations through changing the skill mix. Supplementation was aimed at improving quality of care and extending the range of services to patients. The decision-making in general practices was accompanied with little planning and role definition. The willingness to employ PAs/NPs was highly influenced by an employees' motivation to start the master's programme and GPs' prior experience with PAs/NPs. Knowledge about the PA/NP profession and legislations was often lacking.

Conclusions: Role standardisations, long-term political planning and support from professional associations are needed to support policy makers in implementing skill mix in primary care.

Keywords: Substitution, Supplementation, Skill mix, General practitioner, Nurse practitioner, Physician assistant, Primary care, Implementation

* Correspondence: Mieke.vanderbiezen@radboudumc.nl
[1]Radboud university medical center, Radboud Institute for Health Sciences, IQ healthcare, Scientific Center for Quality of Healthcare, P.O. Box 910, Nijmegen 6500 HB, The Netherlands
Full list of author information is available at the end of the article

Background

With an aging population, more patients with chronic complaints and reforms that shift care from hospitals to the community, the pressure on primary care is high [1–3]. It is not only debated whether there are enough general practitioners (GPs) to comply these increasing demands but also whether specific tasks can be transferred to other care providers. Changing the healthcare workforce skill mix has been applied to improve effectiveness and efficiency of healthcare [4]. Around the world, physician assistants and nurse practitioners (PAs/NPs) have been involved in primary care. Although definitions, education and legislation of PAs/NPs differ per country, there is a common ground that PAs/NPs are trained to diagnose and treat defined patient groups (semi-) independently or under physician supervision [2, 3, 5]. Research has shown that PAs/NPs can substitute for GPs on a wide range of patient care tasks, resulting in at least comparable outcomes to those of GPs and higher patient satisfaction [1, 2, 6]. In addition, PAs/NPs can be involved in specific complementary roles such as preventive care or home visits [2, 7, 8]. Nevertheless, the implementation of PAs/NPs differs between and within countries [9–12]. In the Netherlands, most PAs/NPs work in hospital settings and their implementation in primary care is still at a pioneering stage [13, 14]. The number of PAs/NPs in relation to GPs (headcount) is approximately 1 PA and 2 NPs per 100 GPs [15, 16].

PAs/NPs have worked in the Netherlands since 2001. The education of PAs/NPs in the Netherlands includes a master's programme of respectively 2.5 and 2 years at universities of applied sciences [10]. Their education incorporates a dual work-education model, meaning that students are employed within a practice and receive salary [17]. Although PAs' education is based on a medical model and NPs' education on a nursing model, the position of PAs and NPs in primary care is often regarded as interchangeable [18–20]. In the Netherlands both care providers are allowed to prescribe drugs and perform certain preserved procedures related to diagnosis and treatment independently [10, 21]. However, there is still a lack of clarification regarding their role and value in primary care; a situation observed internationally [2, 22, 23]. So far, the Dutch College of General Practitioners (NHG) and National Association of General Practitioners (LHV) have not proposed a role for PAs/NPs in the basic primary care team in general practice [10].

Currently there is limited insight into the reasons to employ, or not to employ, a PA/NP in primary care. Evidence from European countries is lacking or outdated [4]. To support policy making, more evidence is needed about the reasons and perspectives of GPs and managers to train and employ PAs/NPs in primary care.

Methods

Study aim and design

A qualitative study to provide insight into factors influencing the decision of GPs and managers to train and employ a PA/NP within their organisation.

Setting & cohort

In the Netherlands, GPs are a patient's first point of contact and the 24/7 gatekeepers for secondary care. During office hours, the majority of GPs work in small-scale general practices (eighty percent are duo or solo practices) [24, 25]. To deliver out-of-hours care, GPs from a region are organised in general practitioner cooperatives (GPCs). At those GPCs 40 to 250 GPs take turns on being on duty to take care of populations ranging from 100,000 to 500,000 citizens [26, 27]. In 2013 a project was initiated in the Netherlands that offered both general practices and GPCs additional financial support to train a PA/NP within their organisation. PAs/NPs who were formally employed by GPCs were trained during office hours in general practices in the region. Those organisations whose application for financial support was granted were included in the study cohorts. There was no further selection of participants and all organisations were included. The 2013 cohort included 13 PAs/NPs and the 2014 cohort included 19 PAs/NPs who were either formally employed by a general practice or a GPC (see Fig. 1). We included one GP from all general practices where the PAs/NPs received their training during office hours. In addition, in the case that the PA/NP was formally employed at a GPC, we also included a manager of that GPC. Some GPCs employed more than one PA/NP.

Data collection

Data were collected between September 2014 and January 2015. As there was a lack of previous knowledge and the topic of PAs/NPs in primary care might be considered controversial, individual semi-structured interviews were chosen to obtain in-depth information about the experiences of the participants. Interviews were conducted either face-to-face at the practice site or by telephone. Three main topic areas were covered in the interviews: determinants of the decision-making process, considerations and arguments to train and employ a PA/NP, and PAs'/NPs' tasks and responsibilities. Each topic area included 3 or 4 open-ended questions to encourage participants to discuss their perspectives and considerations. The interview guide was developed by the primary researcher (MB) with guidance from the co-authors (ML, ED). An additional file shows the interview guide in more detail [see Additional file 1]. The interviews were conducted by the primary researcher; a health scientist trained

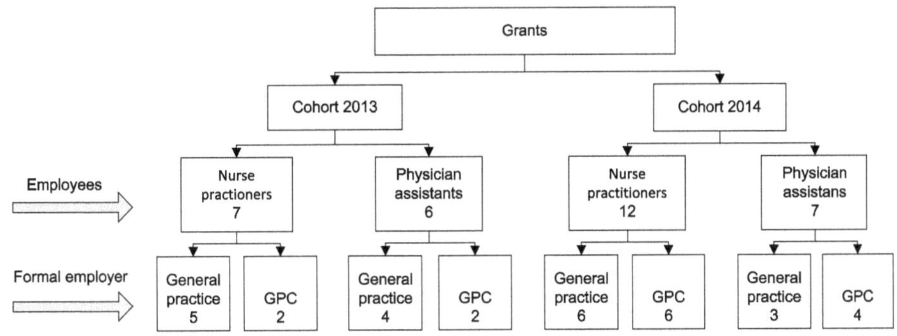

Fig. 1 Overview study cohort

in qualitative research methods. Interviews were audiotaped and then transcribed verbatim.

Data analysis

The transcribed interviews were analysed using content analysis, a qualitative research method to systematically organise data into a structured format [28]. First, two researchers (MB, IM) independently coded the transcripts using an inductive approach. Coding was done with constant comparison of interpretations and the generated list of codes was developed into a shared codebook. During face-to-face meetings the codes of the two researchers were discussed until consensus was reached. Next, coding was followed by a collaborative interpretation in which data was mapped into themes and subthemes. Data was declared to have reached saturation when no new themes were emerging. Lastly, these (sub) themes were discussed for framing of the results and the final refinement of the codes and themes was done by the research team (MB, ML). Atlas.ti software V.7.1.5. was used to facilitate the coding process.

Results

Study population

A total of 32 PAs/NPs started their training in general practices in September 2013 or in September 2014. All GPs owning those practices participated in the interviews. Thirteen of the 32 PAs/NPs were formally employed by a GPC. Therefore, a manager from each GPC was interviewed in addition to the interviews with the GPs. Table 1 provides an overview of the interviewees and there were no refusals to participate. General practices and GPCs were situated across the Netherlands. The first six interviews took place at the practice site and all others were conducted by telephone. The mean duration of the interviews was 51 min (SD 12.71). Only 5 GPs had experience working with a PA/NP in their practice prior to the project.

The analysis resulted in three themes from which 11 categories emerged (see Table 2).

Theme I. Reasons to employ a PA/NP

Three categories emerged from this theme explaining why GPs or GPCs employ a PA/NP: (1) substitution of care; (2) quality improvement; and (3) new/ additional services.

Substitution of care

The main reason for GPs and GPCs to employ a PA/NP was substitution of care. They wanted a professional who is capable and authorised to treat patients independently and take over surgery hours from GPs. This is a response to the increasing workload for GPs due to changes in patient population (e.g. ageing populations, multi-morbidity) and changes in organisation of healthcare (e.g. task shifts from hospital to primary care and an increase in demand to participate in community projects). Some GPs wanted to employ the PA/NP in order to replace a GP, to expand the number of patients in their practice or to create job opportunities for their own professional development (e.g. focussing on more complex patients, more time for study or ancillary activities). Only one GP indicated a shortage of GPs as a reason to employ a PA/NP.

> *"The intention is to get more time for the increase in complex problems we have to deal with in the near future. This is the start of an evolution: ageing, substitution, tasks shifts from hospital care to primary care. I expect that GPs will get larger practices and*

Table 1 Characteristics of interviewees ($N = 39$)

General practitioner solo practice	13	(33.3%)
General practitioner duo practice	8	(20.5%)
General practitioner group practice	11	(28.2%)
Manager general practitioner cooperative	7	(17.9%)
Male	18	(46.2%)
Female	21	(53.8%)
Mean age GPs (years)	48	(SD 8.6)

Table 2 Themes and categories influencing the decision of GPs and managers to train and employ a PA/NP

Theme I. Reasons to employ a PA/NP
Substitution of care
Quality improvement
New/ additional services
Theme II. Influencing factors
Organisational factors
Factors regarding professional relations
Factors regarding GPs' workload and job satisfaction
Experience with the PA/NP profession
Vision about the PA/NP profession
Insecurities regarding the PA/NP profession
Theme III. PAs'/NPs' tasks and responsibilities
Direct patient care
Indirect patient care

cannot comply with the demand for care without support."

(GP group practice, employing a PA)

For the GPCs an important determining factor was the opening of an emergency care access point (ECAP) for out-of-hours emergency care. This new model is expected to increase the number of consultations at the GPC resulting in an increase in number of shifts per GP.

"With the opening of a new ECAP we expect an increase in workload that cannot be answered by the GPs in the region. Therefore, we initiated to work with NPs to meet the increase in patients so that GPs can focus on the complex patients."
(Manager GPC, employing an NP)

Quality improvement

By employing a PA/NP most GPs expected to improve the quality of care provided within their practice. Under quality improvement they mentioned: more continuity of care compared to employing a young doctor (often young doctors start their own practice sooner or later); schedule more time for complex patients; more monitoring of target populations and less waiting time for patients with minor ailments. GPs who employed an NP considered a nursing view complimentary to the medical view of the GP. GPs expected NPs to pursue a mix of cure and care and have better collaboration with other care providers in primary care like community nurses. Other quality improvements are related to new additional services.

"I am experienced with GPs employed by another GP. Yet the downside is that they will leave as soon as they can start their own practice, which causes disturbance among the patients."

(GP solo practice, employing a PA)

"Looking at the NPs at the GPC, I notice they comply even more to guidelines and bring a nursing view into their considerations that is of added value for patient care."

(GP group practice, employing an NP)

New/ additional services

Some GPs considered the employment of a PA/NP an opportunity to implement new services within their practices. Most often these services reflect the current policies of the Ministry of Health, Welfare and Sport, health insurance companies and shifts in populations to treat. For example, increasing monitoring of elderly or participating in community projects for preventive care. Some GPs wanted an expansion in care settings for patients such as offering surgery hours in nursing homes or providing hospital care (e.g. diagnostics) in their practices.

"There are machines to measure the COPD condition, which is something that can easily be delegated to a PA. That would be an improvement in patient care and a lower burden for patients who otherwise have to go to the city."

(GP solo practice, employing a PA)

Quality improvement and new/additional services were not mentioned by GPCs as a reason to employ PAs/NPs.

Theme II. Influencing factors decision-making process

There were several factors influencing the decision to employ a PA/NP. Six categories emerged around this theme: (1) Organisational factors; (2) Factors regarding professional relations; (3) Factors regarding GPs' workload and job satisfaction; (4) GPs' experience with the PA/NP profession; (5) Vision of the PA/NP profession; and (6) Insecurities regarding the PA/NP profession.

Organisational factors

For some GPs financial certainty was an important factor and they let an accountant calculate the financial impact of employing a PA/NP. As a consequence of the implementation of the PA/NP, support staff from practices without prior experience with PAs/NPs needed extra guidance in the triage of patients to the right care provider.

Lastly, having a sufficient number of surgery rooms was a precondition for all GPs.

> *"When you compare practices with GPs only with practices with GPs and NPs, you need a shift in the organisation, for example triage nurses need to decide which patient has to be treated by which care provider."*
>
> *(GP group practice, employing an NP)*

For GPCs, the preparation of implementing a new discipline within the organisation took a lot of effort and had an impact on several departments (e.g. human resources and finances), site managers and support staff. A main issue for GPCs was the fact they offer care out-of-hours. In order to maintain a balanced work-private life, they could only offer small contracts with a maximum of eight hours per week. They therefore rely on general practices' willingness to offer more contract hours to the PA/NP during office hours. However, finding those practices was difficult. GPs often missed the experience and knowledge about PAs/NPs or they criticised their role in primary care. When GPs were positive, a shortage of surgery rooms or financial factors negatively influenced the implementation. Lastly, some GPCs expressed difficulties recruiting PAs/NPs with the proper preliminary training and/or experience, or with a supportive home situation.

> *"It is very hard to find GPs who are willing to offer work during office hours. Often the preconditions cannot be met; not enough surgery rooms, colleagues are not supportive, finances don't fully cover, 'we already have so many employees in our practice'. We have heard all of these arguments before."*
> *(Manager GPC, employing an NP)*

Factors regarding professional relations

For most GPs the primary motive to employ a PA/NP was either a willingness to meet the concerns of GPCs by offering the PA/NP a job opportunity during office hours, or maintaining an appreciated team member. Most often this team member was a practice nurse who already worked within the practice and had the ambition to expand his or her nursing practice by becoming a PA or NP. GPs wanted to meet this ambition in order to keep this employee for their practice. Support among their staff was for almost all GPs a requirement to employ a PA/NP. Another precondition was sometimes the collaboration with another practice.

> *"The PA training was the choice of the PA herself, whereas for me an important factor to approve the training was losing her as an employee if I wouldn't have provided her the opportunity."*
>
> *(GP solo practice, employing a PA)*

For GPCs decisions are made by a management team in consultation with the members council (i.e. GPs who own practices in the region). Creating a support base for the employment of PAs/NPs with their members was therefore of great importance and very time consuming. GPCs experienced that the negative viewpoint of the professional associations made GPs reluctant to employ a PA/NP in their practices during office hours.

> *"You can say, there is no support from GPs' professional associations for the position of PAs in general practices. That makes GPs hesitant to include this profession within their own ranks."*
>
> *(Manager GPC, employing a PA)*

Factors regarding GPs' workload and job satisfaction

As a consequence of the PA/NP treating the less complex patients, all GPs expected a difference in their own caseload. While some GPs considered this an opportunity for their own professional growth and enhancing job satisfaction, others feared a more complex caseload. This included a fear of losing routine in treating minor ailments or an increased work pressure due to more complex complaints during surgery hours. Some GPs expected difficulties in taking proper responsibility for their patients and feared missing out on things in case the PA/NP takes over patient care. Detailed knowledge about the Dutch legislation regarding PAs/NPs was often lacking.

> *"Look, you delegate a great part of the care. That means you partly lose sight. But the same would happen were you to employ another GP."*
>
> *(GP solo practice, employing an NP)*

> *"Maybe a disadvantage is a transformation in GPs' surgery hours in case the number of low complexity problems decreases and the majority of problems become highly complex."*
>
> *(GP group practice, employing an NP)*

GPs' experience with the PA/NP profession

Some GPs previously worked together with a PA/NP, either at a GPC or in a foreign country, which positively influenced their decision to employ a PA/NP. Also positive experiences of colleagues influenced the decision. However, due to the small number of PAs/NPs in primary care in the Netherlands not many GPs had experience with them or knew a colleague with a PA/NP and they made little effort to to get in contact with any colleague.

> *"We experienced working together with NPs at the GPC and my colleague and I were very satisfied with their functioning. That made us curious how it would work out in our practice."*
>
> *(GP group practice, employing an NP)*

> *"I am always eager to innovate, so I thought "why not?". This was also because I had heard from a colleague that they are really happy with their physician assistant."*
>
> *(GP solo practice, employing an NP)*

Vision of the PA/NP profession

In general, GPs had a lack of knowledge regarding the differences between the PA and the NP professions. They often did not know the differences in education and scope of practice. The choice to employ either a PA or an NP was mostly the training preference of the applicant. Some GPs had let themselves be informed by the Foundation for Development of Quality Care in General Practice and one GP made his decision based on scientific literature. GPs considered the PA to be more medically educated and the NP to be more connected with care in general. There were also inaccuracies expressed, for example the belief that a nurse could not apply for a PA training. GPs who employed a PA did not express much preference regarding previous professional experience and preliminary training. The majority of GPs employing an NP considered a nursing education required to treat the broad spectrum of complaints in primary care. Moreover, they often considered nursing experience in several clinical hospital departments to be favourable.

In many cases curiosity played a role in the decision to employ a PA/NP and preparation of the implementation was often lacking. Most GPs did not have a clear insight in the role of PAs/NPs in other primary care practices or in the exact curriculum of the training. A clear long-term vision about the role of the PA/NP in their practice was often not expressed.

> *"I should really revisit the differences between a PA and an NP, because for me those definitions somewhat overlap. So, no, we didn't really discuss or look at which professional we would employ."*
>
> *(GP group practice, employing an NP)*

> *"We started without good preparation or a detailed plan about what we exactly wanted to achieve in the long term. How do we want to shape our practice? We weren't sufficiently aware about how the profession in general practices works."*
>
> *(GP group practice, employing an NP)*

> *"The single-handed GP like it used to be is something that is slowly changing and completely disappearing. Now you are building a team within general practices. Maybe it should be called primary care team, in which many professionals collaborate in one centre, with the common goal of improving healthcare in the broadest sense. The GP has a role, just as NPs do. It's the team that puts it together."*
>
> *(GP group practice, employing an NP)*

In contrast to GPs, GPCs made more informed decisions regarding the employment of a PA or an NP. This was often based on the curriculum of the training or preferences of the GPs in their region. They often formulated a long-term vision of the PA's/NP's role within their organisation.

Insecurities regarding the PA/NP profession

GPs without prior experience working with PAs/NPs expressed uncertainties about their own profession, in particular that an actual decrease in their workload is not guaranteed. Almost all GPs expressed uncertainties about the future in terms of the financial reimbursement of primary care and about political decisions regarding legislation and scope of practice of PAs/NPs.

Both GPs and GPCs felt that political and financial uncertainties made it difficult to formulate long-term organisation planning. Moreover, investments in the training and employment of a PA/NP cause uncertainties because there is no guarantee that these will be paid back.

> *"Rules keep on changing during the play. Planning ahead and ensuring a financial base is difficult as there are no certainties in general practice."*
>
> *(GP duo practice, employing an NP)*

Theme III. PAs'/NPs' tasks and responsibilities

Direct patient care

Most GPs had not formulated an exact role description including the scope of PA's/NP's practice and GPs differed considerably in their ideas about the task of the PA/NP within their practice. Some GPs wanted the PA/NP to serve certain target populations, while others wanted the PA/NP to serve a broad range of patient complaints.

Different views were expressed as to whether or not PAs/NPs should treat chronic patients, acute problems, palliative care, gynaecology complaints and care for elderly or young children. In general, there were some complaints that all GPs agreed were suitable for PA/NP practice. These minor ailments included: dermatology, ear nose and throat complaints, musculoskeletal system and influenza. In addition, preventive tasks like social home visits and postoperative consultations were considered suitable. GPs considered complaints to be suitable when they are not life threatening and if there is a low impact when something goes wrong. The role description was based on the curriculum of PA's/NP's training, experience of the PA/NP, the number of patients having those complaints, and being straightforward for triage.

> *"We wanted a professional who could take over parts of our job. For example, we were thinking about ear complaints, children with fever, abdominal pain, urological infections, et cetera. So, well defined areas that are straightforward for triage."*
>
> *(GP duo practice, employing a PA)*

> *"In palliative care, a lot of tasks are not medical based, but rather nurse based. We intend the NP to be responsible for organising everything at home when a patient is discharged from the hospital; keeping everyone informed about agreements and having insight in expected complications."*
>
> *(GP group practice, employing an NP)*

In contrast to the general practices, the GPCs formulated a role description for the PA/NP for the shifts at the GPC. This role description included a number of complaints that were excluded from PA/NP care, all other complaints were considered within PAs'/NPs' scope of practice. At most GPCs those complaints were: abdominal pain, cardiological, neurological and psychiatric complaints and children younger than 1 year old. GPs who trained the PAs/NPs who were employed by the GPC, were free to make decisions on PAs'/NPs' tasks within their practices during office hours. In practice, they usually used the same role description as the GPC.

Indirect or non-patient related tasks

In general, both GPs and GPCs had not considered indirect or non-patient related tasks much. They wanted the PA/NP to focus on direct patient care first. Indirect or non-patient related tasks were likely to be considered when the PA/NP would be more experienced. Tasks considered suitable were: meetings with other primary care professionals, coordination of elderly care, developing protocols and training support staff.

> *"Of course the PA can participate in projects like quality improvement, practice accreditation, but we don't really know exactly yet, we'll just see."*
>
> *(GP group practice, employing a PA)*

Discussion

Employing PAs/NPs in general practices requires role revision. The literature describes two conceptually different approaches to role revision. The first is to employ PAs/NPs as substitutes for GPs, the second as supplements [3]. The GPCs in the current study primarily aim at substitution of GPs within teams offering out-of-hours care. That means PAs/NPs provide the same services as GPs in order to decrease GPs' caseload or increase service capacity as a reaction to the increased workload due to the opening of ECAPs. General practices on the other hand, do not just aim at substitution but also at supplementing GPs. The aim of supplementing is to improve quality of care and extend the range of services to patients. By extending the range of services GPs are able to meet the increase in tasks and patient groups in primary care [3]. An extension in services is also considered a quality improvement. In addition, GPs consider the added value of PAs/NPs as a quality improvement. The services provided by PAs/NPs are considered less medically focussed and instead, often based on their orientation in the nursing discipline, have a more holistic focus [22]. Both GPCs and GPs consider care for patients with minor ailments to be within a broad spectrum suitable for PA/NP care. Some GPs also employ PAs/NPs for certain target populations either as substitute or supplementary to GPs. A study about PAs as case managers for geriatric conditions, suggests that incorporating PAs in supplemental roles for target populations can increase quality of care for previously underdiagnosed and undertreated conditions [2].

According to Contandriopoulos et al. [29] several themes are important for an effective model for integrating new roles in primary healthcare teams. These themes include planning, role definition, practice model, collaboration and team support. The GPCs in the current study put a lot of effort into advance planning. They developed a comprehensive plan and formalised the role of the PA/NP in writing. Moreover, they expressed a clear vision on how the practice model of PAs/NPs in teams together with GPs provides out-of-hours care. In larger organisations like GPCs this clear role formalisation is especially important [29]. Although GPCs put a lot of effort into creating support among their members, due to the large number of members, not all members were supportive about implementing PAs/NPs. As a result, GPCs experience uncertainties about their financial investment in PAs/NPs because GPCs highly depend on general practices to provide the PAs/NPs employment during office hours. Influencing factors, also shown in the literature, for the negative viewpoint among GPs are the lack of support from GPs' professional associations or not being convinced of the added value of PAs/NPs in primary care [30–32].

The implementation process in general practices differs from GPCs. International studies have shown that inadequate planning is very common for general practices [33, 34]. General practices are understood as complex responsive processes of humans relating to each other. GPs do not usually develop a blueprint for the change that comes with the PA/NP role in their practice. However decisions are not simply random either [35]. As Contandriopoulos et al. [29] describe *"integrating NPs into primary care teams is likely to be a dynamic, complex, and messy process"*. Decisions emerge in the interplay of intentions, communicative gestures and responses, power-relating and values-based choices and actions of the partners, practice staff and policy makers in a range of areas [35]. In the current study the determining factors to employ a PA/NP were often: 1. an employee who wanted to start the PA or NP master's programme, or 2. GPs wanting to support the GPC by providing employment and training to the PA/NP during office hours. Just as in previous studies, most GPs expressed that their willingness to employ a PA/NP was influenced by prior knowledge or working experience with PAs/NPs [4, 30, 36]. However, knowledge about the PA/NP profession, legislation and role definitions in general practice is often lacking. Just as in other studies there are preconceived notions about PAs'/NPs' roles and training and the difference between a PA and an NP is not clear [30, 37, 38]. GPs from practices without prior experience working with PAs/NPs felt hesitant about the changes in caseload and whether their workload actually decreases when they employ a PA/NP. Their hesitance can be supported by literature showing that employing PAs/NPs does not always result in a reduced workload, especially when the GP continues to provide the care that has been substituted. Moreover, with the employment of PAs/NPs the complexity of patients for GPs increases [2, 4, 39]. The development of the practice model is, as previously observed in other studies, often emerging through trial and error. GPs base their vision on the needs of their patient population and the experience and preferences of themselves and the PAs/NPs [2, 29]. In addition, the roles of the PAs/NPs are often not well defined. Although many studies indicate an inappropriate and incoherent definition of the PA/NP scope of practice as a big obstacle for PA/NP integration, this does not necessarily mean that roles should be formalised in writing (which is especially the case for small practices). Instead role formalisation should preferably be flexible and allow team members' practices to evolve [29]. Lastly, GPs rarely expressed problems in collaboration and creating team support regarding the employment of a PA/NP.

As there is a lack of international defined role standards and clarity, each organisation formulates its own scope of practice. International standardisation of PA/NP roles can resolve some of the confusion perceived by other professionals and would enable PAs/NPs to practice to their potential [12, 30, 40]. Moreover, like the GPs in the current study indicate, it is important that political decisions and finances regarding the PA/NP profession in the future are clear and transparent [23, 41].

Strengths and limitations

The current study has several limitations. First, only GPs and GPCs who had already decided to train and employ PAs/NPs were included in the study. Therefore a comprehensive overview in barriers perceived by GPs and GPCs who decide not to employ PAs/NPs cannot be given. Moreover, the role of the PA/NP in primary care is still at a pioneering stage in the Netherlands and the implementation might be different when PAs/NPs are more widespread. However, the stage of PA/NP implementation differs a lot between countries and so the current study gives a broad overview about implementation by the early adaptors in the field.

Not all findings were found across all practices or participants. The main variation was found between GPCs and general practices. We did not find variation between practices employing a PA or an NP, confirming that PAs and NPs are often regarded as interchangeable in primary care [18, 19]. Some outcomes, such as how a change in caseload for GPs was perceived, differed considerably between individuals. Lastly, there were few practices that had prior experience with a PA/NP within their practice. As most outcomes did not differ for practices without prior experience then these practices were not treated as a separate subgroup.

A strength of the current study is the large number of interviews. Participants were from a broad geographical area and the variation in type of practices reflects the distribution of practices in the Netherlands [42]. Second, interviews were conducted in a semi-structured manner with open coding, which allowed researchers to preserve all information. A potential limitation might be that the setting of interviews was not identical. The majority of the interviews were conducted by telephone, which allowed the researchers to include practices across the entire country. We did not experience differences between the face-to-face and telephone interviews that could have caused data loss or distortion and this is supported by literature on qualitative research interviews [43].

It should be noted that the current study indicates several themes that influenced implementation of the PA/NP in Dutch general practice. It is difficult to translate these to county-specific characteristics due to differences in PA/NP autonomy, PAs'/NPs' level of education and differences in healthcare systems [17, 31, 44]. Moreover, there is a lack of international and national role standardisation and the implementation of PAs/NPs differs between and within countries [9–12]. In contrast to countries like the United Kingdom, United States, Canada and Australia, the PA/NP role in primary care is relatively new in many countries (including the Netherlands) or non-existent [22, 44]. However, countries with large numbers of PAs/NPs in primary care also struggle with role clarifications and authorities [22]. Further research is therefore needed about the roles and the implementation of PAs/NPs from different countries [5, 11].

Conclusion

The current study considerably improves our understanding of the factors influencing the decision to employ PAs/NPs in primary care. GPCs intended substitution of care of minor ailments and formulated long-term planning and role definitions. They experienced difficulties with creating team support. In general practices, GPs indented both substitution and supplementation of GPs for minor ailments and/or target populations. The decision-making in general practices was a dynamic process with less planning and role definition. Although roles should be able to evolve over time, a comprehensive long-term practice planning is advisable. Role standardisations, long-term political planning and support from professional associations are needed to support policy makers in implementing PAs/NPs in primary care.

Abbreviations

GP: General practitioner; GPC: General practitioners cooperative; NP: Nurse practitioner; PA: Physician assistant

Acknowledgements

We would like to thank the GPs, managers and research assistant (IM) for their invaluable contribution to this paper.

Funding

This study was funded by the Dutch Ministry of Health, Welfare and Sport. The funding body was not involved in the design of the study and collection, analysis and interpretation of data, or in writing the paper.

Authors' contributions

ML, ED and MB conceived and designed the study. MB and ML did the data analysis. MB, ED, MW, ML interpreted the results. MB wrote the first draft of the manuscript. ED, MW and ML revised the manuscript with important intellectual contributions. All authors read and approved the final manuscript.

Authors' information

MB, MSc, PhD student; ED, project coordinator; MW, PhD professor of health services research and implementation science; ML, PhD, professor organisation of healthcare and services.

Competing interests

The authors declare that they have no competing interests.

Consent for publication

Not applicable.

Author details

[1]Radboud university medical center, Radboud Institute for Health Sciences, IQ healthcare, Scientific Center for Quality of Healthcare, P.O. Box 910, Nijmegen 6500 HB, The Netherlands. [2]Foundation for Development of Quality Care in General Practice, Tilburgseweg-West 100, Eindhoven 5652 NP, The Netherlands. [3]Department of General Practice and Health Services Research, Heidelberg University, INF- Marsilius Arkaden, Im Neuenheimer Feld 130.3, Heidelberg 69120, Germany. [4]HAN University of Applied Sciences, Faculty of Health and Social Studies, P.O. Box 6960, Nijmegen 6503 GL, The Netherlands.

References

1. Martinez-Gonzalez NA, Djalali S, Tandjung R, Huber-Geismann F, Markun S, Wensing M, et al. Substitution of physicians by nurses in primary care: a systematic review and meta-analysis. BMC Health Serv Res. 2014. doi:10.1186/1472-6963-14-214.
2. Hooker RS, Everett CM. The contributions of physician assistants in primary care systems. Health Soc Care Commun. 2012. doi:10.1111/j.1365-2524.2011.01021.x.
3. Laurant M, Harmsen M, Wollersheim H, Grol R, Faber M, Sibbald B. The impact of nonphysician clinicians: do they improve the quality and cost-effectiveness of health care services? Med Care Res Rev. 2009. doi:10.1177/1077558709346277.
4. Halter M, Drennan V, Chattopadhyay K, Carneiro W, Yiallouros J, de Lusignan S, et al. The contribution of physician assistants in primary care: a systematic review. BMC Health Serv Res. 2013. doi:10.1186/1472-6963-13-223.
5. Vrijhoef HJ. Nurse practitioners. In: The Wiley Blackwell encyclopedia of health, illness, behavior, and society. 2014.
6. Swan M, Ferguson S, Chang A, Larson E, Smaldone A. Quality of primary care by advanced practice nurses: a systematic review. Int J Qual Health Care. 2015. doi:10.1093/intqhc/mzv054.
7. Dierick- van Daele ATM, Steuten LMG, Romeijn A, Derckx EWCC, Vrijhoef HJM. Is it economically viable to employ the nurse practitioner in general practice? J Clin Nurs. 2010; doi.10.1111/j.1365-2702.2010.03492.x.
8. Sustaita A, Zeigler VL, Brogan MM. Hiring a nurse practitioner: What's in it for the physician? Nurse Pract. 2013. doi:10.1097/01.NPR.0000435783.63014.1c.
9. Pulcini J, Jelic M, Gul R, Loke AY. An international survey on advanced practice nursing education, practice, and regulation. J Nurs Scholarsh. 2010. doi:10.1111/j.1547-5069.2009.01322.x.
10. Freund T, Everett C, Griffiths P, Hudon C, Naccarella L, Laurant M. Skill mix, roles and remuneration in the primary care workforce: who are the healthcare professionals in the primary care teams across the world? Int J Nurs Stud. 2015. doi:10.1016/j.ijnurstu.2014.11.014.
11. Hooker RS, Hogan K, Leeker E. The Globalization of the Physician Assistant Profession. J Physician Assist Educ. 2007. doi:10.1097/01367895-200718030-00011.
12. Lowe G, Plummer V, O'Brien AP, Boyd L. Time to clarify–the value of advanced practice nursing roles in health care. J Adv Nurs. 2012. doi:10.1111/j.1365-2648.2011.05790.x.
13. Timmermans MJ, van Vught AJ, Wensing M, Laurant MG. The effectiveness of substitution of hospital ward care from medical doctors to physician assistants: a study protocol. BMC Health Serv Res. 2014. doi:10.1186/1472-6963-14-43.
14. Dierick-van Daele AT, Metsemakers JF, Derckx EW, Spreeuwenberg C, Vrijhoef HJ. Nurse practitioners substituting for general practitioners: randomized controlled trial. J Adv Nurs. 2009. doi:10.1111/j.1365-2648.2008.04888.x.

15. van der Burgt MR, van Roij R, Derckx EWCC, Meulepas MA. Eindrapport praktijkvoorbeelden: De physician assistant in de eerste lijn. Eindhoven: Stichting KOH; 2015.
16. van der Burgt R, van Roij J, Derckx E, Meulepas M. Eindrapport praktijkvoorbeelden: De verpleegkundig specialist in de eerste lijn. Eindhoven: Stichting KOH; 2015.
17. Hooker RS, Kuilman L. Physician assistant education: five countries. J Physician Assist Educ. 2011. doi:10.1097/01367895-201122010-00010.
18. Sibbald B, Laurant M, Scott A. Changing task profiles. In: Saltman RB, Rico A, Boerma W, editors. Primary care in the driver's seat. New York: Open University Press; 2006. p. 149–64.
19. Ponte PR, O'Neill K. Hiring into advanced practice positions: the nurse practitioner versus physician assistants debate. J Nurs Adm. 2013. doi:10.1097/NNA.0b013e3182942c73.
20. Hass V. Physician assistants and nurse practitioners are not interchangeable. JAAPA. 2016. doi:10.1097/01.JAA.0000481408.81044.4e.
21. De Bruijn-Geraets DP, Van Eijk-Hustings YJ, Vrijhoef HJ. Evaluating newly acquired authority of nurse practitioners and physician assistants for reserved medical procedures in the Netherlands: a study protocol. J Adv Nurs. 2014. doi:10.1111/jan.12396.
22. Kooienga SA, Carryer JB. Globalization and advancing primary health care nurse practitioner practice. J Nurse Pract. 2015. doi:10.1016/j.nurpra.2015.06.012.
23. Naylor MD, Kurtzman ET. The role of nurse practitioners in reinventing primary care. Health Aff (Millwood). 2010. doi:10.1377/hlthaff.2010.0440.
24. van Loenen T, van den Berg MJ, Heinemann S, Baker R, Faber MJ, Westert GP. Trends towards stronger primary care in three western European countries; 2006–2012. BMC Fam Pract. 2016. doi:10.1186/s12875-016-0458-3.
25. van Hassel DTP, Kasteleijn A, Kenens RJ. Cijfers uit de registratie van huisartsen peiling 2015. Utrecht: NIVEL; 2016.
26. Wijers N, Schoonhoven L, Giesen P, Vrijhoef H, van der Burgt R, Mintjes J, et al. The effectiveness of nurse practitioners working at a GP cooperative: a study protocol. BMC Fam Pract. 2012. doi:10.1186/1471-2296-13-75.
27. Giesen P, Smits M, Huibers L, Grol R, Wensing M. Quality of after-hours primary care in the Netherlands: a narrative review. Ann Intern Med. 2011. doi:10.7326/0003-4819-155-2-201107190-00006.
28. Tong A, Sainsbury P, Craig J. Consolidated criteria for reporting qualitative research (COREQ): a 32-item checklist for interviews and focus groups. Int J Qual Health Care. 2007. doi:10.1093/intqhc/mzm042.
29. Contandriopoulos D, Brousselle A, Dubois C-A, Perroux M, Beaulieu M-D, Brault I, et al. A process-based framework to guide nurse practitioners integration into primary healthcare teams: results from a logic analysis. BMC Health Serv Res. 2015. doi:10.1186/s12913-015-0731-5.
30. Niezen MG, Mathijssen JJ. Reframing professional boundaries in healthcare: a systematic review of facilitators and barriers to task reallocation from the domain of medicine to the nursing domain. Health Policy (New York). 2014; doi.10.1016/j.healthpol.2014.04.016.
31. Buerhaus PI, DesRoches CM, Dittus R, Donelan K. Practice characteristics of primary care nurse practitioners and physicians. Nurs Outlook. 2015. doi:10.1016/j.outlook.2014.08.008.
32. Morqan P, Himmerick KA, Leach B, Dieter P, Everett C. Scarcity of primary care positions May divert physician assistants into specialty practice. Med Care Res Rev. 2016. doi:10.1177/1077558715627555.
33. Sangster-Gormley E, Martin-Misener R, Downe-Wamboldt B, Dicenso A. Factors affecting nurse practitioner role implementation in Canadian practice settings: an integrative review. J Adv Nurs. 2011. doi:10.1111/j.1365-2648.2010.05571.x.
34. Sullivan-Bentz M, Humbert J, Cragg B, Legault F, Laflamme C, Bailey PH, et al. Supporting primary health care nurse practitioners' transition to practice. Can Fam Physician. 2010;56:1176–82.
35. Booth BJ, Zwar N, Harris MF. Healthcare improvement as planned system change or complex responsive processes? a longitudinal case study in general practice. BMC Fam Pract. 2013. doi:10.1186/1471-2296-14-51.
36. Sangster-Gormley E, Martin-Misener R, Burge F. A case study of nurse practitioner role implementation in primary care: what happens when new roles are introduced? BMC Nurs. 2013. doi:10.1186/1472-6955-12-1.
37. Hevesy M, Aitchison R, Ruiz A, Bednar S. Nurse practitioners and physician assistants in primary care: An update of changes since 2008. Dis Mon. 2016. doi:10.1016/j.disamonth.2016.01.002.
38. Bailey P, Jones L, Way D. Family physician/nurse practitioner: stories of collaboration. J Adv Nurs. 2006. doi:10.1111/j.1365-2648.2006.03734.x.
39. Laurant M, Reeves D, Hermens R, Braspenning J, Grol R, Sibbald B. Substitution of doctors by nurses in primary care. Cochrane Database Syst Rev. 2005. doi:10.1002/14651858.CD001271.pub2.
40. Buchan J, O'May F, Ball J. New role, new country: introducing US physician assistants to Scotland. Hum Resour Health. 2007. doi:10.1186/1478-4491-5-13.
41. Zwijnenberg NC, Bours GJ. Nurse practitioners and physician assistants in Dutch hospitals: their role, extent of substitution and facilitators and barriers experienced in the reallocation of tasks. J Adv Nurs. 2012. doi:10.1111/j.1365-2648.2011.05823.x.
42. van Hassel DTP, Kenens RJ. Cijfers uit de registratie van huisartsen; peiling 2012. Utrecht: Netherlands institute for health services research (NIVEL); 2013.
43. Novick G. Is there a bias against telephone interviews in qualitative research? Res Nurs Health. 2008. doi:10.1002/nur.20259.
44. Groenewegen P, Heinemann S, Gress S, Schafer W. Primary care practice composition in 34 countries. Health Policy (New York). 2015; doi.10.1016/j.healthpol.2015.08.005.
45. Dutch government: Wet medisch-wetenschappelijk onderzoek met mensen. 2015.
46. Association of Universities in the Netherlands (VSNU). The netherlands code of conduct for academic practice. The Hague: Association of Universities in the Netherlands (VSNU); 2014.

8

Who is on the primary care team? Professionals' perceptions of the conceptualization of teams and the underlying factors

Kirti D. Doekhie[1*], Martina Buljac-Samardzic[1], Mathilde M. H. Strating[1] and Jaap Paauwe[1,2,3]

Abstract

Background: Due to the growing prevalence of elderly patients with multi-morbidity living at home, there is an increasing need for primary care professionals from different disciplinary backgrounds to collaborate as primary care teams. However, it is unclear how primary care professionals conceptualize teams and what underlying factors influence their perception of being part of a team. Our research question is: *What are primary care professionals' perceptions of teams and team membership among primary care disciplines and what factors influence their perceptions?*

Methods: We conducted a mixed-methods study in the Dutch primary care setting. First, a survey study of 152 professionals representing 12 primary care disciplines was conducted, focusing on their perceptions of which disciplines are part of the team and the degree of relational coordination between professionals from different disciplinary backgrounds. Subsequently, we conducted semi-structured interviews with 32 professionals representing 5 primary care disciplines to gain a deeper understanding of the underlying factors influencing their perceptions and the (mis)alignment between these perceptions.

Results: Misalignments were found between perceptions regarding which disciplines are members of the team and the relational coordination between disciplines. For example, general practitioners were viewed as part of the team by helping assistants, (district) nurses, occupational therapists and geriatric specialized practice nurses, whereas the general practitioners themselves only considered geriatric specialized practice nurses to be part of their team. Professionals perceive multidisciplinary primary care teams as having multiple inner and outer layers. Three factors influence their perception of being part of a team and acting accordingly: a) knowing the people you work with, b) the necessity for knowledge exchange and c) sharing a holistic view of caregiving.

Conclusion: Research and practice should take into account the misalignment between primary care professionals' perceptions of primary care teams, as our study notes variations in the conceptualization of primary care teams. To enhance teamwork between professionals from different disciplinary backgrounds, professionals acknowledge the importance of three underlying conditions: team familiarity, regular and structured knowledge exchange between all professionals involved in the care process and realizing and believing in the added value for patients of working as a team.

Keywords: Primary care, Primary care professionals, Primary care teams, Teamwork, Team fluidity, Relational coordination, Mixed-methods

* Correspondence: doekhie@eshpm.eur.nl
[1]Erasmus School of Health Policy and Management (ESHPM), Erasmus University Rotterdam, PO Box 1738, Rotterdam 3000, DR, The Netherlands
Full list of author information is available at the end of the article

Background

The number of elderly patients aged 65 years or older with multiple chronic conditions living at home is rapidly rising [1, 2]. Research shows different high prevalence rates of elderly with multiple chronic conditions worldwide, ranging between 55% and 98% [3]. Because of their high and complex needs, care for these patients is delivered by multiple primary care professionals from different disciplinary backgrounds [1, 4]. Strong collaboration between these professionals is important [5], as it can lead to better patient outcomes in terms of patient-centred, high quality care and can improve not only patient satisfaction with care [6, 7], but also work satisfaction of professionals [8].

In research, the concept of collaboration is often used as a general term to describe a range of collaborative structures [9–12]. For example, a collaboration could consist of professionals with minimal interaction and no shared goal [10, 11]. Members of these type of collaborations are more task focused and often feel little necessity for interpersonal contact [10]. This type of collaboration is often defined as a 'group' or 'network' [10, 11]. A collaboration could also exist of members with a shared common goal, well defined tasks, task interdependency and stable membership [13]. Historically, this type of collaboration is defined as a 'team' [10, 11, 13].

In primary care, collaborations are often defined as 'primary care teams' [14–16]. Professionals from different disciplinary backgrounds can collaborate in formal structures, for example within the same organization, in which primary care teams are purposefully established, a common and shared care goal is set and professionals fulfil designated roles within the team. In such teams, accountability and procedural structures are embedded in the team, and the team membership of primary care professionals is clear [10, 17].

However, in recent years, teams have tended to become more fluidly structured, operating within loose boundaries and accordingly leading to dynamic team membership [7, 13, 17–21]. Present-day teams are expected to continuously and rapidly adapt to changes and issues in their environment, for example to changing patient expectations and demands [13, 22]. Team membership has a dynamic nature [13]; therefore, professionals can be members of multiple teams at the same time (i.e., multiple team membership) [13, 23]. Such teams are conceptualized as fluid entities in which membership is based more on task interdependency than formal structures [10, 13, 17]. Fluid teams are often described as having an ad hoc or multi-layered structure [13, 17]. In ad hoc teams, a team is built of members with diverse expertise to address specific needs, after which the team is dissolved and a new team is built [13, 20]. Teams with multi-layered structures consist of multiple inner and outer layers. The inner layer is formed by members who have a central and permanent role in the team, whereas the outer layers consist of team members who are members for a limited time period during which their specific expertise is required [13, 24].

Research on team fluidity shows both positive and negative effects of having dynamic team membership. By increasing the diversity of knowledge, team creativity and the opportunity for open discussions can be enhanced, which ultimately positively affects team performance [25, 26]. However, dynamic team membership can also lead to less coordination and team familiarity, as team members have less shared work experience [19, 21]. According to Mortensen [21], dynamic team membership can lead to a misalignment of team members' perceptions regarding who is considered part of the team, which is referred to as the membership divergence phenomenon.

Although one could argue that the membership divergence phenomenon [21] may be an issue in the primary care setting due to the variety of conceptualizations of primary care teams, little research has focused on primary care professionals' perceptions of team membership [27]. Therefore, the basic questions regarding how primary care professionals conceptualize teams and whether they perceive themselves as working as a team with professionals from other disciplinary backgrounds remain unanswered. Due to the changing and more fluid structure of present-day teams, is it debatable whether the term 'team' is still the appropriate term to describe these type of collaborations [17]. Regardless of the structures or perceptions of the type of collaborations between primary care professionals, collaborations are frequently labelled as teams merely on the assumption that teamwork will lead to superior outcomes [14, 15]. This phenomenon is discussed by Allen and Hecht [28] as the 'romance of teams'. However, if primary care professionals do not perceive themselves as working as a team, it may not result in superior outcomes and is more likely to negatively affect their collaboration and ultimately the quality of care [10, 29].

Research suggests different underlying factors that could influence professionals' perceptions of which disciplines they consider to be part of a team [8, 21–31]. These factors revolve around the presence of formal work processes within teams (e.g., communication, clearly defined goals and regular feedback loops to improve team performance [7, 8, 30, 32]) and informal social processes (e.g., mutual respect, trust and understanding of each other's roles) [7, 29, 31, 32].

The interrelation between formal and social processes in teams is described in the 'relational coordination' theory [33, 34] and is defined as *"a mutually reinforcing process of interaction between communication and relationships carried out for the purpose of task integration*" [33]. This theory identifies key concepts regarding the communication and relationship ties between team members that underpin effective teamwork [34]. The quality of communication consists of four dimensions: frequency, timeliness, accuracy and a focus on problem solving rather than blaming [35]. The quality of relationships consists of three dimensions: the extent to which team members have shared goals, shared knowledge and mutual respect [35]. Although the relational coordination theory often focuses on the ties between core team members, Gittell [36] pleas for an extension of the theory beyond the inner layer and to include relational coordination with non-core participants (i.e., the outer layers), as these participants may also play an important role in the work process [13]. This approach emphasizes the importance of including a broad range of team structures and taking team fluidity into account.

Research on relational coordination suggests an interaction and mutually reinforcing effect between the degree of relational coordination and professionals' perceptions of team membership. On the one hand, relational coordination can positively affect the perception of team membership [37]. Research shows that for primary care delivery, specifically disease-management programmes for chronically ill patients, higher degrees of relational coordination exist between professionals from different disciplinary backgrounds compared to professionals from the same disciplinary background [38]. This could be explained by the emphasis of disease-management programmes on multidisciplinary interactions, as the effectiveness of chronic care delivery is dependent on the communication and relationships between professionals [38]. Following this line of reasoning, we could say that professionals from different disciplinary backgrounds who share high degrees of relational coordination are more likely to perceive each other as members of the same team and to collaborate as a team. On the other hand, the degree of relational coordination between professionals could be enhanced by facilitating interactions between professionals in multidisciplinary meetings [39]. This suggests that when professionals from different disciplinary backgrounds get the opportunity to meet each other, they are more likely to perceive each other as part of the same team, which could result in higher degrees of relational coordination.

In this study, the perceptions of primary care professionals from different disciplinary backgrounds are our central focus. We aim to provide more insight into the concept of primary care teams and the functioning of these teams from the perspective of primary care professionals themselves. Our research question is the following: *What are primary care professionals' perceptions of teams and team membership among primary care disciplines and what factors influence their perceptions?*

Methods

In this paper, a sequential mixed-methods approach was used. First, a questionnaire survey study was conducted focusing on the perceived team membership and relational coordination between professionals from different backgrounds. The quantitative results showed a misalignment of the perceptions of professionals from different disciplinary backgrounds regarding which disciplines were part of the team. This analysis will be discussed in more depth in the results and discussion sections. Subsequently, semi-structured interviews with professionals representing different primary care disciplines were conducted to gain a deeper understanding of the misalignment and insight into the influencing factors.

Setting and participants

This study was performed in the primary care setting in the Netherlands. The Netherlands, comparable to other European countries such as the United Kingdom and Denmark, has been identified as having a strong primary care system with high access to primary care [40, 41]. Similar to systems in Italy, Norway, Sweden and Estonia, primary care in the Netherlands is characterized by a referral system to secondary care and a gatekeeping position of general practitioners [41, 42]. Although different professionals are considered to be primary care professionals, such as physiotherapists and pharmacists, general practitioners are seen as the central care providers and first contact persons in care for patients [41]. These professionals deal with a large range of health problems and diseases and patients need to obtain their referral to medical specialist care. Moreover, practice nurses play a more central role in care in countries such as the Netherlands, Poland and Sweden [41]. In the Netherlands, these nurses often provide health programs such as dietary programs to elderly and sometimes focus on a specific patient groups like diabetic patients [41].

In light of the growing aging population, many European countries such as the Netherlands, France and Germany emphasize 'ageing in place': treating patients at home for as long as possible [43]. From this viewpoint, these countries have restructured their health system with a decentralization of government responsibilities at local (municipality) level, focusing on strengthening the primary care system [43, 44]. With this decentralization, patients need to live independently at home for as long as possible and rely on their informal care network before applying for professional care provision [43].

In this paper, we solely focus on the perceptions of primary care professionals and exclude social care and informal caregivers. Prior to the data collection for the questionnaire, the researchers composed a list of common primary care disciplines involved in care for chronically ill elderly patients based on existing research on primary care (Table 1) [45]. Convenience sampling was used to select participants. Managers of multiple types of primary care practices, for example primary care centres and monodisciplinary centres such as general practitioner centres, were approached by telephone or email.

The questionnaires were filled out anonymously. Informed consent was assumed by completion of the questionnaire. Participants were given two weeks to complete the questionnaire. After one week, a reminder was sent to all participants. The total sample consisted of 152 primary care professionals from 37 different primary care organisations (response rate of 38%). The participant characteristics can be found in Table 2.

For the interviews, professionals from five main primary care disciplines were approached. In order to determine these five disciplines, we analysed our quantitative results and organized meetings with stakeholders in primary care. This approach resulted in the inclusion of the following disciplines: general practitioners, physiotherapists, occupational therapists and (district) nurses. During the interviews, multiple participants emphasized the importance of geriatric specialized practice nurses in elderly primary care. This discipline was therefore included as well. Convenience sampling and a snowball method were used to select participants. We conducted interviews until no new perspectives or underlying factors were being offered (i.e., saturation strategy), which finally resulted in 32 interviews. During the recruitment process of the participants as well as at the start of the interviews, all participants were repeatedly informed on the aims and purpose of the study. Informed consent was assumed by agreeing and completion of the interviews. Moreover, participants were repeatedly informed about the recording the interviews. At the start of each interview, the participants were explicitly asked for verbal consent for recording of the interviews. At all times, participants were allowed to withdraw their consent and end the interview. The participant characteristics can be found in Table 3.

Table 1 List of common primary care disciplines

1. General Practitioners	7. (District) Nurses
2. General Practitioner Assistants	8. Helping Assistants
3. Physiotherapists	9. Primary Care Psychologists
4. Remedial Therapists	10. Geriatric Specialized Practice Nurses
5. Pharmacists	11. Occupational Therapists
6. Dieticians	12. Speech Therapists

Table 2 Quantitative survey: Participants characteristics (n = 152)

Characteristic	*n*	%	
Sex			
Male	33	21.7	
Female	119	78.3	
Education level completed			
Secondary school	13	8.6	
Secondary vocational	35	23	
Bachelor degree	89	58.6	
Master degree	14	9.2	
Other	1	0.7	
Discipline			
Physiotherapist	36	23.7	
Helping Assistant	31	20.4	
Remedial Therapist	22	14.5	
(District) Nurse	19	12.5	
General Practitioner Assistant	12	7.9	
General Practitioner	9	5.9	
Primary Care Dermatologist	6	3.9	
Geriatric Specialized Practice Nurse	5	3.3	
Dietician	5	3.3	
Occupational Therapist	2	1.3	
Speech Therapist	2	1.3	
Primary Care Psychologist	2	1.3	
Other	1	0.7	
	Mean	SD	Range
Team tenure	6	7.2	1–35
Age (years)	40	12.1	21–64
Team size	9.9	5.4	2–40
Team diversity	.46	.30	0–.93

Note. SD = Standard deviation

Quantitative questionnaire

The questionnaire was divided into two sections. The first section contained two questions on primary care professionals' perceptions regarding team membership, focusing on their perceived team size ("How many team members are on your team?") and team diversity ("Which of the following disciplines do you consider part of your team?"). The latter question was based on Table 1. Participants were asked to answer openly, without reference to their specific work setting or structure. For example, the general practitioners were asked to indicate which other primary care disciplines (as presented in Table 1) they considered part of their team. In the second section, the degree of relational coordination was assessed using a seven-item relational coordination scale. This scale was originally developed to measure airline

Table 3 Qualitative interviews: Participants characteristics ($n = 32$)

Variable	General Practitioner ($n = 6$)	Physio- therapist ($n = 7$)	Occupational therapist ($n = 7$)	(District) Nurse ($n = 9$)	Geriatric specialized practice nurse ($n = 3$)
Gender					
Male	2	2	0	1	0
Female	4	5	7	8	3
Age in years					
< 30	0	2	2	3	0
30–50	5	3	4	2	2
> 50	1	2	1	4	1
Work setting					
Home care organization	0	0	0	9	0
General practitioner centre	2	0	0	0	2[a]
Physiotherapy centre	0	3	0	0	0
Occupational therapy centre	0	0	5	0	0
Primary health care centre	4	4	2	0	1
Number of years practicing					
< 15	2	3	3	5	1
15–30	1	2	3	1	2
> 30	3	2	1	3	0

[a]In the Netherlands, geriatric specialized practice nurses often work within general practitioner centres

operations [46] but has also been applied in health care settings [34]. Sample questions include "How frequently do you communicate with each of these disciplines about a patient?" and "To what degree do people in these disciplines share your goals for the care of your patients?" A five-point Likert scale ranging from 1 ("never") to 5 ("always") was used. Participants were asked to answer the questions with respect to the other disciplines. For example, the physiotherapists were asked to score how frequently they communicated with the helping assistants about a patient. The used questionnaire can be found in Additional file 1. Principal component analyses revealed that the seven items loaded onto two factors with eigenvalues of 3.53 and 1.48, which explained 71.61% of the variance.

Qualitative interviews

The topic list for the semi-structured interviews was developed by the primary researcher and revised based on input from the full research team. The design of the topic list allowed an in-depth investigation of the underlying dimensions of the misalignment on team membership among professionals. Participants were first asked how they would define 'teams' and if they felt to be members of a team. Example questions include "What elements of teamwork could make you feel more like a member of a team?" and "What is important to you when collaborating with other disciplines?" The interview guide can be found in Additional file 2.

Quantitative analysis

The data were analysed using IBM SPSS 22.0. Descriptive statistics were used to analyse the sample characteristics, the perceived team size, and the relational coordination between disciplines. Each discipline's perceived team diversity was analysed using Blau's index for diversity [47]. The index ranges between zero (completely homogeneous teams) and one (completely heterogeneous teams). To explore the different perceptions among disciplines regarding who is a member of the team, UCINET Software for Social Network Analysis was used to create a social network figure of the different disciplines. To analyse the relationship between perceptions regarding who is part of the team and the degree of relational coordination between disciplines, correlation analysis was performed.

Qualitative analysis

The interviews were audiotaped, transcribed verbatim and analysed using Atlas TI (version 7). Data analysis was a combination of inductive coding and deductive framework analysis and included several steps. First, the primary researcher read the transcripts multiple times to gain a preliminary understanding of the experiences of the participants. Then, the primary researcher initiated an open coding of all the data. Next, the full research team compared the codes to derived insights from literature on teams and team membership. Specific attention was paid to participants' conceptualization of primary care teams and factors that participants mentioned that could increase their perception of being part of a primary care team. During this process, the codes found from the open coding process were grouped into subthemes, which were then grouped into major themes. For example, the codes 'flying in and out' and 'loose boundaries' were grouped into the subtheme 'team versus loose network', which was then included under the major theme 'conceptualization of teams'. To ensure reliability, the themes were discussed among the full research team until consensus was reached, which was the case after five meetings with the full research team.

Results

Quantitative results

Who is part of the team

The average indicated team size was 9.9 members and the average diversity in disciplines in the team was .46. When specifying team size per discipline (Additional file 3), primary care dermatologists reported the largest team size (15 members), and primary care psychologists reported the smallest team size (7 members). Regarding team diversity, occupational therapists reported the highest diversity (.79), and remedial therapists reported the lowest diversity (.09).

Alignments and misalignments between the perceptions of professionals from different disciplinary backgrounds were found, as illustrated in Fig. 1. Notably, most arrows point towards physiotherapists, general practitioners, dieticians, helping assistants and (district) nurses, which indicates that these disciplines were most often considered to be part of the team. Helping assistants and (district) nurses consider each other to be part of their team; 89.5% of the helping assistants consider a (district) nurse to be part of their team and 81.1% vice versa. There is a maximum alignment of perceptions between general practitioners and geriatric specialized practice nurses, as both disciplines considered each other to be part of their team at a level of 100%. Although general practitioners only considered geriatric specialized practice nurses to be part of their team, they were considered part of the team by three additional disciplines: helping assistants (45.2%), (district) nurses (42.1%) and occupational therapists (50%), indicating a misalignment in perceptions between general practitioners and these disciplines. Physiotherapists were considered to be part of the team by the remedial therapists (77.3%), speech therapists (100%), occupational therapists (100%) and (district) nurses (47.4%), whereas less than 40% of the physiotherapists considered any of these disciplines to be part of their team. Moreover, no arrows are present between physiotherapists and general practitioners or between general practitioners and dieticians, indicating that less than 40% of these disciplines considered one another to be part of their team.

Relational coordination

A (mis)alignment of perceptions was also found with regard to the perceived degrees of relational coordination.

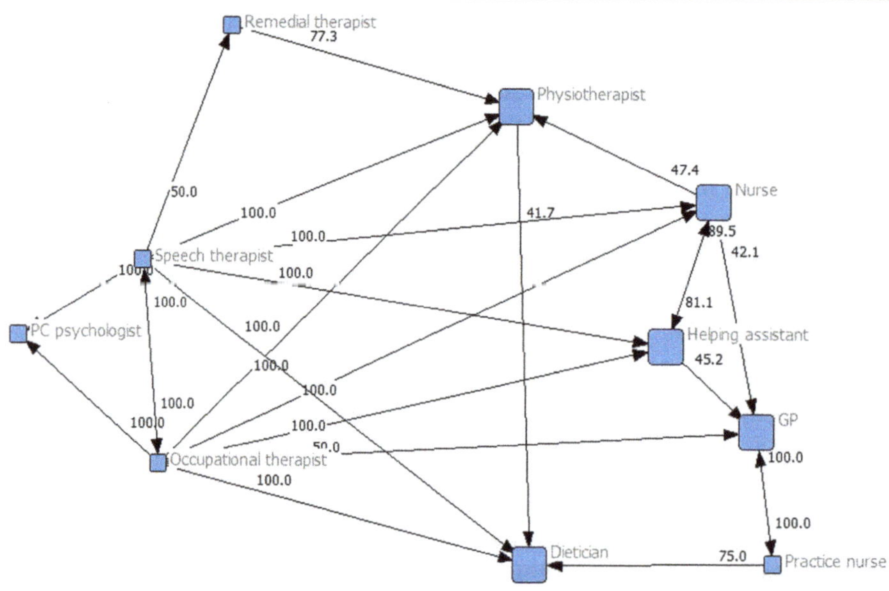

Fig. 1 Social network figure on professionals' perceptions on team membership. The social network figure illustrates participants' perceptions of which disciplines are part of their team. The arrows and percentages show which disciplines and how many participants from a specific disciplinary background consider another discipline to be part of the team. The arrows represent percentages higher than 40%. The absence of an arrow implies a percentage lower than 40%. All percentages, also lower than 40%, are provided in Additional file 3. For example, Fig. 1 shows that 77.3% of the remedial therapists considered a physiotherapist to be part of the team

On a scale of one to five, Additional file 4 shows the average degree of relational coordination between professionals from different disciplinary backgrounds, subdivided into the communication and relationship dimensions. Overall, the means scores on the communication dimensions are lower than those on the relationship dimensions.

Helping assistants and (district) nurses not only often perceive each other's discipline to be part of the team (Fig. 1), but also share roughly similar degrees of relational coordination on both dimensions. From the perspective of (district) nurses, the perceived degree of relational coordination on the communication dimensions with helping assistants was 4.54, and the perceived degree of relational coordination on the relationship dimensions was 4.49. Vice versa, the perceived degree of relational coordination on the communication dimensions was 4.74 and on the relationship dimensions 4.78. Misalignments in the degrees of relational coordination were found for general practitioners. For example, from the perspective of (district) nurses, the perceived degree of relational coordination with general practitioners on the communication dimensions was 3.43 and on the relationship dimensions 3.64, while vice versa, the perceived degrees of relational coordination were 2.44 and 2.48, respectively.

Additional file 5 shows the correlation matrix between a specific discipline perceived to be part of the team and the perceived degree of relational coordination with that discipline, subdivided into the communication and relationship dimensions of the relational coordination theory. Overall, higher correlations were found between being perceived as part of the team and the communication dimensions of relational coordination (i.e., frequency, timeliness, accuracy and a focus on problem solving rather than blaming), but the overall mean scores for the relationship dimensions were higher. Following the identified misalignment in perceptions as illustrated in Fig. 1 and Additional file 4, the correlation matrix shows ambiguous relationships between a specific discipline considered to be part of the team and the perceived degree of relational coordination (i.e., communication and relationship) with that discipline. For general practitioners, there are relatively low correlations between perceiving that discipline to be part of the team and both the communication dimensions and the relationship dimensions ($r = .35$ and $r = .17$ respectively), although 40.9% of the participants considered general practitioners to be part of their team. Conversely, high correlations were found for primary care psychologists on both the communication dimensions and the relationship dimensions ($r = .65$ and $r = .56$ respectively), although only 18.8% of the participants considered this discipline to be part of their team. The (district) nurses and helping assistants showed high correlations on both the communication ($r = .76$ and $r = .67$ respectively) and relationship ($r = .76$ and $r = .68$ respectively) dimensions.

Qualitative results

The aim of the interviews was to investigate the reasoning for the identified misalignment of the perceptions of primary care professionals regarding which other disciplines they consider to be part of their team. Analyses of these interviews showed two lines of reasoning. The first theme, 'conceptualization of teams', focuses on the different perspectives of the participants regarding the concept of primary care teams. Second, our analysis identified three factors that could minimize the misalignment of perceptions: 'knowing the people you work with', 'the necessity for knowledge exchange' and 'sharing a holistic perspective of caregiving'. These three factors are combined in the theme 'factors influencing the perception of working as a team'. Specific quotes are included under each (sub) theme to provide meaning and context to the participants' perspectives.

Conceptualization of teams

The first theme involved the meaning of the concept of teams. Most participants mentioned that teams consist of multiple layers. According to most of the general practitioners, the inner layer is formed by the general practitioners themselves, geriatric specialized practice nurses and (district) nurses, as these three disciplines are considered to have central tasks in caregiving and are involved for a long period of time. This contrasts the questionnaire results, in which less than 40% of the general practitioners considered the (district) nurse part of the team. The outer circles are formed by professionals whose expertise is needed for a limited period of time. According to the general practitioners, these professionals are often physiotherapists and occupational therapists.

> *"A team to me is when together you provide high quality care for a patient. A network is more like loose grains of sand. A real team is often the general practitioners, the home care organization and the practice nurses. And occasionally, other people [KD: disciplines] are flown in like a physiotherapist or an occupational therapist. But the core of the team really is the general practitioner and the home care organization." (General practitioner 1)*

> *"For example, an occupational therapist can arrange walkers for patients with Parkinson's. But long-term care, they don't provide that. They are more or less flown in, do their business and fly out again. And it could very well be that you need them again later, but not structurally." (General practitioner 2)*

However, most occupational therapists and physiotherapists felt that in the eyes of patients, they do belong to the core of the team around a patient, as their fields of expertise focus more on helping a patient with daily activities than treating their medical condition. According to the occupational therapists, knowing how to manage daily life and how to remain independent are important goals for patients.

Which disciplines are considered by a professional to be part of the inner layer and the outer layer seem to be related to the extent to which professionals from different disciplinary backgrounds are familiar with each other and the frequency of contact. Some participants felt a lower "team familiarity" with professional who they do not meet or speak to on a regular basis. The importance of knowing the people you work with in relation to perceiving to work as a team is described more in depth in the second theme.

> *"Well, a social worker might be involved whom I have never spoken to or whose patient goals I might not know. That person will have a lower team familiarity towards me than the physiotherapist whom I regularly speak with regarding a client's condition. That may be via phone or email, that's not important to me. So in that sense there are multiple layers." (Occupational therapist 1)*

The extent to which participants felt that they were part of a team was divided and seemed to be related to the type of work structure (i.e., working within the same building or not). Professionals working within the same building often referred to each other as members of the same team. However, for professionals who work in a monodisciplinary centre, the team concept applies to professionals from the same disciplinary background.

> *"The centre I am currently working in does feel like a team, but actually, my team members are merely my fellow general practitioners." (General practitioner 3)*

With regard to teamwork with professionals from other disciplinary backgrounds outside a formal structure or the same building, participants did not perceive to work as a team. These multidisciplinary collaborations were often described as "loose networks" around a single patient. The participants did not refer to these collaborations as teams because of the perceived incidental structure of the collaboration. Professionals who do not structurally work together for the same patient group are not perceived as a team.

> *"It [KD: collaboration with different disciplines] doesn't feel like a team because it's usually a one-time collaboration around a patient. And perhaps you meet the same people around another patient, but that doesn't make it a team. It's more an incidental collaboration around a patient. So it's more like a network." (Occupational therapist 4)*

Although most participants felt that all professionals ultimately want the best care for their patients, the participants felt that professionals work individually with few mutual connections.

> *"When I look at the care for the elderly that we give, I feel that the older person is at the centre and we as professionals stand around the patient. And everybody does their own thing. But it would be very nice if all of those professionals had connections with each other." (General practitioner 5)*

Factors influencing the perception of working as team

The three most mentioned factors that could influence the perception of working as a team are described below.

Knowing the people you work with Having met the other professionals in person and knowing who that person is could positively influence communication and coordination by increasing the levels of familiarity and trust. Professionals know what to expect from each other, know their mutual responsibilities and can hold each other accountable for their actions. The occupational therapists, physiotherapists and geriatric specialized practice nurses particularly emphasized the importance of knowing the other professionals involved in the care for the same patient.

> *"Well, there's a difference between knowing each other in the sense of 'I know the other person's name' and knowing in the sense of 'I've seen his or her face'. If you recognize each other's faces, the collaboration will be ten times better because usually right after five minutes you'll know things like, 'Oh, everything will be all right with that physiotherapist,' or 'Oh, that general practitioner is very involved'." (Occupational therapist 2)*

> *"It does help a lot if you know each other. For example, the geriatric specialized nurse doesn't work in this building, but since you know each other, you've already seen each other, and together you've invested time in knowing each other's roles and expertise. You know what you can and can't expect from each other. Or you can sometimes think along with another professional. That works really well, and I also think it's important in elderly care." (Physiotherapist 1)*

The general practitioners also acknowledged the positive effects of knowing the other professionals, but mentioned a lack of time as a hindering factor. Additionally, the fact that multiple professionals represent the same discipline in care for the same patient was viewed as a barrier to getting to know each other. This was especially the case for (district) nurses working in the same home care organization, where multiple (district) nurses can be involved in the care for a single patient.

Knowing each other could not only benefit the professionals but also the patients. Participants felt that patient satisfaction and patients' trust in the care delivery could be increased if all of the professionals involved know each other and collaborate.

> *"What I notice with the elderly people whom I visit is that they like it very much when everyone involved in their care knows each other. For example, when I visit a patient, and they say "Yeah, my physiotherapist is M!", then I would say "Oh, I know her. I just saw her at another patient's home". "Oh that's great!" So you can see that they like it when they know that you know the other professionals." (Occupational therapist 6)*

THE NECESSITY FOR KNOWLEDGE EXCHANGE

Some participants expressed their desire for regular multidisciplinary team meetings to discuss patient cases. However, a lack of time often hinders the organization of these meetings. Communication therefore usually takes place via email or phone.

Both the frequency and the content of communication seem to be related to the degree of (task) interdependency between professionals and the patient's medical condition. Regarding the frequency of communication, all participants acknowledged that communication mostly occurs when the coordination of tasks is necessary regarding a patient's condition. When a patient is stable, communication is considered to be less necessary and thus less present. In that sense, communication is considered to be more incidental than structural.

> *"I think that everyone [KD: primary care professionals] is highly involved in the care for patients with multimorbidity, so there's no real necessity to have contact in any way. Look, as far as I'm concerned, when things go really wrong, then there's a need to deliberate." (General practitioner 1)*

As a side note, compared to the other disciplines, occupational therapists and physiotherapists found it more important to update the other disciplines on their tasks on a weekly basis, especially the general practitioners. These disciplines found it particularly important to keep the other disciplines informed, as they highly valued providing holistic care to patients. However, communication is often felt to be one-directional; the general practitioners rarely respond to their emails.

Regarding the content of communication, participants found that information sharing solely focuses on a patient's medical condition; the professionals rarely communicate for personal (social) reasons. Some participants, particularly the occupational therapists and physiotherapists, expressed a desire for more proactive communication between disciplines to prevent further deterioration of a patient's condition. Instead of solely reacting to a patient's – deteriorating – condition, professionals should more proactively communicate with other disciplines when their expertise could be helpful. Some occupational therapists expressed a desire for professionals to focus on multidisciplinary patient goals and not solely focusing on patient goals within their own field of expertise.

> *"To me, it's important that other professionals know how to find me if they have any questions regarding my treatment of a patient. For example, that they inform me when they see a patient goal related to occupational therapy. And that they share important developments in their own fields of expertise with me. I currently feel that I share what I am doing more often, that as an occupational therapist, I see patient goals within the field of expertise of other disciplines and make these disciplines aware of these goals than the other way around. That happens sometimes." (Occupational therapist 4)*

SHARING A HOLISTIC VIEW OF CAREGIVING

Most participants felt that one of the core steps in enhancing teamwork is that each professional should have a holistic view of caregiving, meaning that professionals should not work individually and solely focus on the patient's needs within their own field of expertise, but should collectively try to address all of the patient's needs. Professionals should truly believe in the added value of working as a team around a patient instead of as distant individual professionals. As a result, they would actually want to work as a team. However, when professionals share little task interdependency, it can be difficult to see the added value of collaborating as a team, and they are therefore less likely to invest in teamwork.

> *"It really also depends on your own perspective, whether you see each other as complementary and see each other's added value, or if you rather like to keep things to yourself." (Physiotherapist 7)*

Some (district) nurses expressed a desire for more teamwork with general practitioners, but they felt that the general practitioners often prefer to work solo. The results from the general practitioners on this matter were mixed. Some expressed a wish for more teamwork between different disciplines on a regular and structured basis, while others felt that teamwork is only necessary on an incidental basis when a patient's condition is unstable.

> *"General practitioners always say "we are so busy". Nobody else in the world is busy, but they are. If we work with a general practitioner, he visits a patient on his own time. He doesn't adapt to my schedule. It doesn't matter if I'm there or not. It makes me sad because sometimes the patient needs a bandage and he [KD: general practitioner] won't do it. We [KD: (district) nurses] are like a necessary evil. Nothing comes from the general practitioners that says that they're willing to collaborate. The love always needs to come from the other side." ((District) nurse 2)*

Discussion

Our study explored the perceptions of primary care professionals from different disciplinary backgrounds regarding the conceptualization of teams and which disciplines they consider to be part of their team.

Conceptualization of teams

Building further on the membership model divergence phenomenon of Mortensen [21], our study first shows that for the complex primary care setting professionals from multiple disciplinary backgrounds have different perceptions of which disciplines are part of a primary care team. For example, (district) nurses frequently consider general practitioners to be part of the team, but the latter often do not consider (district) nurses to be part of their team.

This misalignment can be linked to how primary care professionals conceptualize teams. In line with the team fluidity literature [13, 17], our study shows that primary care teams are perceived to have a fluid nature and consist of multiple inner and outer layers. Primary care teams have an inner layer consisting of disciplines with long-term involvement in care and outer layers of disciplines who are only team members when necessary. However, primary care professionals perceive which disciplines are part of the inner or outer layers differently. To illustrate, our interview results show that general practitioners do not consider occupational therapists as part of their team, because they help patients with specific problems and are only involved for a limited amount of time. However, the occupational therapists felt that they are part of the inner layer, giving their field of expertise to help patients with daily life activities.

Task interdependency is frequently mentioned as a core characteristic of teams [14, 48–50] and has been shown to positively affect team processes and effectiveness [8]. This study emphasizes the importance of task interdependency in primary care teams and suggests that the extent to which professionals perceive other disciplines to be part of the inner or outer layers of the team is dependent on task interdependency. When task interdependency is low, the perceived need for professionals to communicate and interact with other professionals in order to achieve their goals is also low. Consequently, these professionals are more likely to consider each other as members of the outer layer of a team. Vice versa, when task interdependency is high, professionals are more likely to consider each other part of the inner layer of the team, and the perceived need for communication and knowledge exchange will be higher.

In addition, this study emphasize the importance of the perceived goal interdependency, which refers to the interconnection among team members implied by the type of goal (individual or team) that guides their performance [51]. Professionals who perceive patient care as a holistic process and acknowledge that achieving patient goals from their own discipline is dependent on patient goals from other disciplines, will be more likely to want to collaborate as a team and consider each other as team members.

Underlying factors

For certain combinations of professionals from different disciplinary backgrounds, the (mis)alignment of perceptions regarding which disciplines are part of the team seems to be related to the perceived degree of relational coordination. For example, (district) nurses and helping assistants not only frequently consider each other to be part of the team but also share high degrees of relational coordination. This result suggests that (district) nurses and helping assistants often perceive each other to be part of the inner layer of a team and likely share equal expectations regarding, for example, their roles and responsibilities, shared goals and the frequency of their communication. When focusing on general practitioners in relation to the other disciplines, the expectations do not always align. For example, general practitioners are perceived to be part of the team by both (district) nurses and helping assistants, who also perceive relatively high degrees of relational coordination with general practitioners on both dimensions. However, vice versa, only a small percentage of the general practitioners consider these two disciplines to be part of the team, and their perceived degrees of relational coordination with (district) nurses and helping assistants are relatively low.

In practice, general practitioners are often considered to have a central role in the caregiving process [52]. Our study suggests that most primary care professionals acknowledge this central role of general practitioners, but that general practitioners do not always acknowledge the central role that other disciplines could play in the caregiving process. By having a highly medicalised focus on patient needs, some general practitioners tend to not perceive disciplines with a less medicalised contribution to patient care as part of the inner layer. However, these disciplines (e.g. occupational therapists) are crucial for patients' quality of life as they focus on daily life activities. Our study also indicates a lack of or little communication between general practitioners and other disciplines. Communication was often a one way road towards general practitioners as they fail to respond to emails or phone calls. The misalignment in perceptions and lack of communication between general practitioners and other disciplines also suggests power differentials between the former and latter. Research shows that power can negatively affect team effectiveness [8] and affects the strategic choices of care professionals whether to collaborate, with whom and to what level [53]. Research by Rieck [54] on the relationship between general practitioners and pharmacists shows that power distances exist between these disciplines and is based on knowledge and expertise differences. General practitioners had little trust in the expertise of the pharmacists and felt to perform tasks better independently than as a team with the pharmacists. Following this line of reasoning, we could say that in our study, power differentials between general practitioners and other disciplines exist. General practitioners felt little necessity to function as a team with especially disciplines with a less medicalised contribution to care. This lack of communication and teamwork could negatively influence the quality of delivered care [55].

Our study suggests three underlying factors of the misalignment in perceptions: 1) knowing the people you work with, 2) the necessity of knowledge exchange, and 3) sharing a holistic view of caregiving. These factors are related to the communication and relationships between primary care professionals and could contribute to enhancing their perception of being part of a team.

In line with other studies such as that of Gucciardi and colleagues [32], our study emphasizes the importance of investing in communication and relationships between all professionals involved in the care for a single patient. Research has shown that high levels of trust, mutual respect and mutual understanding of each other's roles are important characteristics of effective teamwork [7, 29, 32]. Building further on other research [32], the responses of our participants suggest that familiarity could increase mutual levels of trust, respect and understanding between professionals. By enabling primary care professionals from different disciplinary backgrounds to meet and get to know each other, trust, respect and understanding are nurtured. Furthermore, this study suggests that getting to know each other could also positively affect the quality of communication between professionals, as the professionals will be more familiar with each other.

Practice and research implications

To provide patient-centred holistic care to chronically ill elderly patients, all of the primary care professionals involved need to work together as one team, regardless of whether they perceive task interdependency. The importance of holistic care has often been emphasized in health policy, and our study shows that primary care professionals themselves acknowledge the need for a holistic view of caregiving. To provide holistic care, our study underscores the importance of strengthening the communication and relationships between professionals involved in the care for the same patient, as the professionals may have different expectations of each other.

In line with other research [32, 56], we suggest that to improve team functioning, all professionals involved in the care for the same patient could benefit from meetings in which they have the opportunity to get to know each other and discuss their mutual roles, responsibilities and expectations. Research stresses the importance of informal contact between team members to enhance role clarification and social processes within the team [30, 32, 57]. By organizing these meetings, professionals can build on their mutual levels of trust, respect and understanding, and role conflict can be minimized. However, it is crucial that hindering factors such as a lack of time, motivation and the perceived added value of informal contact and engaging with each other are taken into account. This could for example be realised by not organizing specific meetings focused on informal contact, role clarification and engagement, but to integrate these elements into multidisciplinary team meetings in which critical incidents are discussed. For example, informal contact, role clarification and engagement could be integrated into simulation-based trainings at the workplace for professionals who already work together or need to communicate and coordinate their activities [58]. Within these simulation trainings, professionals have the opportunity to re-enact a real life case to stimulate and improve their teamwork around a patient [58]. Research has shown that simulation training improves technical skills as well as non-technical skills of professionals [59–61]. Further research is needed to gain more knowledge of underlying conditions that are necessary for these meetings to succeed.

Moreover, different researchers [14–16, 28] have debated the definition of teams and have shown that the label "team" is often applied to a collaboration in the belief that teamwork leads to superior outcomes. Some research argues that in reality, many of these so-called teams consist of professionals who work individually, rarely communicate or do not share a common goal [14, 15]. Adding to this debate, this study shows that although a collaboration is frequently labelled as a primary care team, professionals from different disciplinary backgrounds often do not perceive themselves as part of a team and have different perceptions regarding which disciplines are part of the team. Rather, some primary care professionals may perceive that they work on a team, while others may perceive that they work in a network. However, as our study shows that these networks are multi-layered, the actual structure and formal and social processes within networks may vary in different contexts. This also implies that researched primary care teams or primary care networks may vary in their actual structure and membership, making it difficult for example to compare primary care team effectiveness across studies. Thus, policy-makers, managers and researchers should carefully consider the specific context in which teamwork takes place and the perceptions of professionals on team membership and the conceptualization of teams and networks. Our study shows that professionals may have different perceptions on team membership and task interdependency, frequency and content of communication between professionals varies. Therefore, when using the terms 'primary care team' or 'primary care network', it is important to specify who the members are and what their task interdependency and communication is.

Our study shows a misalignment in perceptions of primary care professionals and suggests different underlying factors influencing their perception. Further research is needed to more in depth explore this misalignment, for example by focusing on factors on a patient level. The extent to which professionals see each other as part of the inner or outer layer could be influenced by patient characteristics, such as complexity of patient condition, intensity of treatment and patient involvement.

Moreover, research on self-management and health care consultations underscores the importance of patient involvement and indicates that patients fulfil different roles, from passive recipients of care to active participants or co-producers of their care [62]. Therefore, future research on primary care teams should focus on the different roles of patients in the self-management of their diseases and on patients' team membership in primary care teams. In addition, because of the growing prevalence of informal caregivers and their unique role as semi-patients and semi-professionals [63], future research should also focus on informal caregivers' team membership.

Limitations

When interpreting our results, careful consideration must be paid to the following. First, due to our cross-sectional design, we cannot draw any conclusions regarding causality between the extent to which professionals perceive specific disciplines as part of their team and their perceived degree of relational coordination. At the same time, due to our mixed-methods design, our study does suggest that these concepts are related and that investing in communication and relationships between professionals is important for teamwork. Second, the quantitative component of our study included a moderate sample size and had an unequal distribution of participants per discipline. However, our sample included a large variety of primary care professionals from different disciplinary backgrounds, reflecting the diversity of primary care services for chronically ill elderly patients.

Third, in both the quantitative and well as the qualitative component of our study we did not include all primary care disciplines from the same primary care practice, such as all members of one community care team, because we aimed to openly explore the relationships between professionals from different disciplinary backgrounds. We therefore cannot draw any conclusions on (mis)alignments of perceptions between professionals involved in the care for a specific patient. Future research could focus on exploring teams and networks around a specific patient and the perceptions of the professionals within these structures.

Conclusion

Our study shows that from the perspective of primary care professionals, the concept of primary care teams is ambiguous and misalignments exist regarding how these teams are conceptualized and which disciplines are perceived as part of the team. To create more alignment and to enhance professionals' perceptions of being part of a team, professionals emphasize the importance of knowing the people you work with, exchanging knowledge with all professionals involved and sharing a holistic view of caregiving. By focusing on these underlying conditions of teamwork, professionals are not only more likely to perceive themselves and professionals from other disciplines as team members but are also more likely to collaborate as a team.

Additional files

Additional file 1: Questionnaire survey data. The questionnaire used for quantitative data collection on collaboration and relational coordination between primary care professionals.

Additional file 2: Interview guide. The interview guide used for qualitative data collection on collaboration and teams.

Additional file 3: Team size, diversity and part of the team. The table indicates the average team size and diversity and which primary care disciplines are considered as part of the team by professionals from other disciplinary backgrounds

Additional file 4: Mutual degrees of relational coordination, subdivided into communication and relationship dimensions. The table indicates the degrees of relational coordination between primary care professionals from different disciplinary backgrounds as perceived by the professionals themselves.

Additional file 5: Descriptives and correlations between perceived as part of the team and the degree of relational coordination. The table indicates the correlation between the perceptions of all participants on the team membership of professionals from a specific disciplinary background in the team and the perceived degrees of relational coordination with these professionals

Aknowledgements
We would like to thank all participants of this study.

Funding
No funding was obtained for this study.

Authors' contributions
All authors (KD, MBS, MS and JP) designed the study. KD, MBS and MS collected the data and KD initiated the analysis of the data. All authors frequently discussed the appropriate methods for analysis and results of the analysis. Regarding the qualitative data specifically, KD in interaction with MBS, MS and JP came to a final set of codes and themes. KD drafted the first version of the manuscript and based on input and reformulations of sentences of MBS, MS and JP, KD revised the manuscript. All authors read and approved the definitive version of the manuscript and agree to be accountable for all aspects of the study.

Consent for publication
Not applicable.

Competing interests
The authors declare that they have no competing interests.

Author details
[1]Erasmus School of Health Policy and Management (ESHPM), Erasmus University Rotterdam, PO Box 1738, Rotterdam 3000, DR, The Netherlands. [2]Department of Applied Economics, Erasmus University Rotterdam , PO Box 1738, Rotterdam 3000, DR, The Netherlands. [3]Department of Human Resource Studies, Tilburg University, PO Box 90153, Tilburg 5000, LE, The Netherlands.

References

1. van Dongen, Jerôme Jean Jacques, van Bokhoven MA, Daniëls R, van der Weijden T, Emonts, Wencke Wilhelmina Gerarda Petronella, Beurskens A. Developing interprofessional care plans in chronic care: a scoping review. BMC Fam Pract. 2016;17(1):137.
2. Scherer M, Hansen H, Gensichen J, Mergenthal K, Riedel-Heller S, Weyerer S, et al. Association between multimorbidity patterns and chronic pain in elderly primary care patients: a cross-sectional observational study. BMC Fam Pract. 2016;17(1):1.
3. Marengoni A, Angleman S, Melis R, Mangialasche F, Karp A, Garmen A, et al. Aging with multimorbidity: a systematic review of the literature. Ageing Research Rev. 2011;10(4):430–9.
4. Bähler C, Huber CA, Brüngger B, Reich O. Multimorbidity, health care utilization and costs in an elderly community-dwelling population: a claims data based observational study. BMC Health Serv Res. 2015;15(23):1–12.
5. Loeb DF, Bayliss EA, Candrian C, Binswanger IA. Primary care providers' experiences caring for complex patients in primary care: a qualitative study. BMC Fam Pract. 2016;17(1):1.
6. Trivedi D, Goodman C, Gage H, Baron N, Scheibl F, Iliffe S, et al. The effectiveness of inter-professional working for older people living in the community: a systematic review. Health & Social Care in the Community. 2013;21(2):113–28.
7. Mulvale G, Embrett M, Razavi SD. 'Gearing up' to improve interprofessional collaboration in primary care: a systematic review and conceptual framework. BMC Fam Pract. 2016;17(1):83.
8. Lemieux-Charles L, McGuire WL. What do we know about health care team effectiveness? A review of the literature. Med Care Res Rev. 2006;63(3):263–300.
9. D'Amour D, Ferrada-Videla M, San Martin Rodriguez L, Beaulieu M. The conceptual basis for interprofessional collaboration: core concepts and theoretical frameworks. Journal of interprofessional care. 2005;19(S1):116–31.
10. Saltman DC, O'Dea NA, Farmer J, Veitch C, Rosen G, Kidd MR. Groups or teams in health care: finding the best fit. J Eval Clin Pract. 2007;13(1):55–60.
11. Gilley A, Kerno SJ. Groups, teams, and communities of practice: a comparison. Adv Dev Hum Resour. 2010;12(1):46–60.
12. Grumbach K, Bodenheimer T. Can health care teams improve primary care practice? JAMA. 2004;291(10):1246–51.
13. Tannenbaum SI, Mathieu JE, Salas E, Cohen D. Teams are changing: are research and practice evolving fast enough? Ind Organ Psychol. 2012;5(1):2–24.
14. West MA, Lyubovnikova J. Illusions of team working in health care. Journal of Health Organization and Management. 2013;27(1):134–42.
15. Lyubovnikova J, West MA, Dawson JF, Carter MR. 24-karat or fool's gold? Consequences of real team and co-acting group membership in healthcare organizations. European Journal of Work and Organizational Psychology. 2014;24(5):1–22.
16. West MA, Lyubovnikova J. Real teams or pseudo teams? The changing landscape needs a better map. Ind Organ Psychol. 2012;5(1):25–8.
17. Wageman R, Gardner H, Mortensen M. The changing ecology of teams: new directions for teams research. J Organ Behav. 2012;33(3):301–15.
18. Bushe GR, Chu A. Fluid teams: solutions to the problems of unstable team membership. Organ Dyn. 2011;40(3):181–8.
19. Summers JK, Humphrey SE, Ferris GR. Team member change, flux in coordination, and performance: effects of strategic core roles, information transfer, and cognitive ability. Acad Manag J. 2012;55(2):314–38.
20. Huckman RS, Staats BR. Fluid tasks and fluid teams: the impact of diversity in experience and team familiarity on team performance. Manufacturing & Service Operations Management. 2011;13(3):310–28.
21. Mortensen M. Constructing the team: the antecedents and effects of membership model divergence. Organ Sci. 2014;25(3):909–31.
22. Mickan S, Rodger S. The organisational context for teamwork: comparing health care and business literature. Aust Health Rev. 2000;23(1):179–92.
23. O'leary MB, Mortensen M, Woolley AW. Multiple team membership: a theoretical model of its effects on productivity and learning for individuals and teams. Acad Manag Rev. 2011;36(3):461–78.
24. Humphrey SE, Morgeson FP, Mannor MJ. Developing a theory of the strategic core of teams: a role composition model of team performance. J Appl Psychol. 2009;94(1):48.
25. Choi H, Thompson L. Old wine in a new bottle: impact of membership change on group creativity. Organ Behav Hum Decis Process. 2005;98(2):121–32.
26. Hirst G. Effects of membership change on open discussion and team performance: the moderating role of team tenure. European Journal of Work and Organizational Psychology. 2009;18(2):231–49.
27. Jaruseviciene L, Liseckiene I, Valius L, Kontrimiene A, Jarusevicius G, Lapão LV. Teamwork in primary care: perspectives of general practitioners and community nurses in Lithuania. BMC Fam Pract. 2013;14(1):1.
28. Allen NJ, Hecht TD. The 'romance of teams': toward an understanding of its psychological underpinnings and implications. J Occup Organ Psychol. 2004;77(4):439–61.
29. Sargeant J, Loney E, Murphy G. Effective interprofessional teams:"contact is not enough" to build a team. J Contin Educ Heal Prof. 2008;28(4):228–34.
30. Xyrichis A, Lowton K. What fosters or prevents interprofessional teamworking in primary and community care? A literature review. Int J Nurs Stud. 2008;45(1):140–53.
31. Sheard A, Kakabadse A. From loose groups to effective teams: the nine key factors of the team landscape. Journal of Management Development. 2002; 21(2):133–51.
32. Gucciardi E, Espin S, Morganti A, Dorado L. Exploring interprofessional collaboration during the integration of diabetes teams into primary care. BMC Fam Pract. 2016;17(1):1.

33. Hoffer GJ. Coordinating mechanisms in care provider groups: relational coordination as a mediator and input uncertainty as a moderator of performance effects. Manag Sci. 2002;48(11):1408–26.
34. Gittell JH, Weinberg D, Pfefferle S, Bishop C. Impact of relational coordination on job satisfaction and quality outcomes: a study of nursing homes. Hum Resour Manag J. 2008;18(2):154–70.
35. Gittell JH. Relational coordination: coordinating work through relationships of shared goals, shared knowledge and mutual respect. In: Kyriakidou O, Özbilgin M, editors. Relational perspectives in organizational studies. A research companion Cheltenham, UK: Edward Elgar Publishers; 2006. p. 74-94.
36. Gittell JH. New directions for relational coordination theory. In: Cameron K, Spreitzer G, editors. The Oxford handbook of positive organizational scholarship. New York: Oxford University Press; 2011. p. 400–11.
37. Cramm JM, Nieboer AP. In the Netherlands, rich interaction among professionals conducting disease management led to better chronic care. Health Aff (Millwood). 2012;31(11):2493–500. https://doi.org/10.1377/hlthaff.2011.1304.
38. Cramm JM, Nieboer AP. Relational coordination promotes quality of chronic care delivery in Dutch disease-management programs. Health Care Manag Rev. 2012;37(4):301–9.
39. Hartgerink JM, Cramm JM, Bakker TJEM, Eijsden AM, Mackenbach JP, Nieboer AP. The importance of multidisciplinary teamwork and team climate for relational coordination among teams delivering care to older patients. J Adv Nurs. 2014;70(4):791–9.
40. Kringos DS, Boerma WGW, Hutchinson A, Saltman RB, (Eds.). Building primary care in a changing Europe. European observatory on health systems and policies, Observatory studies series, vol. 38 (2015).
41. Kringos D, Boerma W, Bourgueil Y, Cartier T, Dedeu T, Hasvold T, et al. The strength of primary care in Europe: an international comparative study. Br J Gen Pract. 2013;63(616):e742–50. https://doi.org/10.3399/bjgp13X674422.
42. Kringos DS, Boerma WG, Hutchinson A, van der Zee J, Groenewegen PP. The breadth of primary care: a systematic literature review of its core dimensions. BMC Health Serv Res. 2010;10:65. https://doi.org/10.1186/1472-6963-10-65.
43. Triantafillou J, Naiditch M, Repkova K, Stiehr K, Carretero S, Emilsson T, et al. Informal care in the long-term care system European overview paper. 2010.
44. Pavolini E, Ranci C. Restructuring the welfare state: reforms in long-term care in western European countries. Journal of European Social Policy. 2008; 18(3):246–59. https://doi.org/10.1177/0958928708091058.
45. Wiegers T, Hopman P, Kringos D, Bakker Dd. NIVEL Overzichtstudies: de eerste lijn. 2011.
46. Gittell JH. Supervisory span, relational coordination and flight departure performance: a reassessment of postbureaucracy theory. Organ Sci. 2001; 12(4):468–83.
47. Blau PM. Inequality and heterogeneity. New York: Free Press; 1977.
48. Kvarnström S. Difficulties in collaboration: a critical incident study of interprofessional healthcare teamwork. Journal of Interprofessional Care. 2008;22(2):191–203.
49. Wageman R, Hackman JR, Lehman E. Team diagnostic survey: development of an instrument. J Appl Behav Sci. 2005;41(4):373–98.
50. Thylefors I, Persson O, Hellström D. Team types, perceived efficiency and team climate in Swedish cross-professional teamwork. Journal of Interprofessional Care. 2005;19(2):102–14.
51. Saavedra R, Earley PC, Van Dyne L. Complex interdependence in task-performing groups. J Appl Psychol. 1993;78(1):61.
52. Weenink J, van Lieshout J, Jung HP, Wensing M. Patient care teams in treatment of diabetes and chronic heart failure in primary care: an observational networks study. Implement Sci. 2011;6(6):66.
53. McDonald J, Jayasuriya R, Harris MF. The influence of power dynamics and trust on multidisciplinary collaboration: a qualitative case study of type 2 diabetes mellitus. BMC Health Serv Res. 2012;12(1):63.
54. Rieck AM. Exploring the nature of power distance on general practitioner and community pharmacist relations in a chronic disease management context. Journal of interprofessional care. 2014;28(5):440–6.
55. Hartgerink JM, Cramm JM, Bakker TJEM, Eijsden RAM, Mackenbach JP, Nieboer AP. The importance of relational coordination for integrated care delivery to older patients in the hospital. J Nurs Manag. 2014;22(2):248–56.
56. Gittell JH. Transforming relationships for high performance. Palo Alto: Stanford University Press; 2015.
57. King N, Ross A. Professional identities and interprofessional relations: evaluation of collaborative community schemes. Soc Work Health Care. 2004;38(2):51–72.
58. Buljac-Samardzic M, Dekker-van Doorn CM, van Wijngaarden JD, van Wijk KP. Interventions to improve team effectiveness: a systematic review. Health Policy. 2010;94(3):183–95.
59. Doumouras AG, Keshet I, Nathens AB, Ahmed N, Hicks CM. A crisis of faith? A review of simulation in teaching team-based, crisis management skills to surgical trainees. Journal of surgical education. 2012;69(3):274–81.
60. Murphy M, Curtis K, McCloughen A. What is the impact of multidisciplinary team simulation training on team performance and efficiency of patient care? An integrative review. Australas Emerg Nurs J. 2016;19(1):44–53.
61. Tan SB, Pena G, Altree M, Maddern GJ. Multidisciplinary team simulation for the operating theatre: a review of the literature. ANZ J Surg. 2014;84(7–8):515–22.
62. Thompson AG. The meaning of patient involvement and participation in health care consultations: a taxonomy. Soc Sci Med. 2007;64(6):1297–310.
63. Weinberg DB, Lusenhop RW, Gittell JH, Kautz CM. Coordination between formal providers and informal caregivers. Health Care Manag Rev. 2007; 32(2):140–9. https://doi.org/10.1097/01.HMR.0000267790.24933.4c.
64. Dutch Government. Wet medisch-wetenschappelijk onderzoek met mensen. 2016.

9

Experiences of adult patients using primary care services in Poland – a cross-sectional study in QUALICOPC study framework

Marek Oleszczyk[1*], Anna Krztoń-Królewiecka[1], Willemijn L. A. Schäfer[2], Wienke G. W. Boerma[2] and Adam Windak[1]

Abstract

Background: Patients as real healthcare system users are important observers of primary care and are able to provide reliable information about the quality of care. The aim of this study was to explore the patients' experiences and their level of satisfaction with the process and outcomes of care provided by primary care physicians in Poland and to identify the characteristics of the patients, their physicians, and facilities associated with patient satisfaction.

Methods: The study is based on data from the Polish part of the Quality and Costs of Primary Care in Europe (QUALICOPC) cross-sectional, questionnaire-based study. In Poland, a nationally representative sample of 220 PC physicians and 1980 of their patients were recruited to take part in the study. As a study tool we used 3 out of 4 QUALICOPC questionnaires: "Patient Experience", "PC Physician" and "Fieldworker" questionnaires.

Results: The areas of the best quality perceived by Polish PC patients are: equity, accessibility of care and quality of service. Coordination and comprehensiveness of care are evaluated relatively worse. The patients' and their physicians' characteristics have a limited influence on patient satisfaction and experiences with Polish primary care.

Conclusions: Primary health care in Poland is of good overall quality as perceived by the patients. Study participants were at most satisfied with accessibility and equity of care and less satisfied with coordination and comprehensiveness of care. Longer patient-doctor relationship and older age of patients were found as the most influential determinants of higher satisfaction. However, variables used in this study poorly explain the overall level of satisfaction. Further research is needed to identify the other determinants of patient satisfaction in the Polish population. Rural practices deserve additional attention due to highest proportions of both extremely satisfied and dissatisfied patients.

Keywords: Primary health care, Quality of health care, Family medicine, Patient satisfaction, Poland

Background

Primary health care (PHC) in Poland was shaped mostly by the 1999 health care reform introducing the health insurance system. Important changes in PHC were initiated in the early 1990s, stimulated by worsening economic effectiveness of the health care system (HCS) based on the multi-specialists model (Shemashko's model of polyclinics). PHC in Poland in this era was associated with difficult access to health services, the low reputation of physicians, continuously declining patients' satisfaction and their instrumental treatment [1]. A new model of PHC was developed mostly based on family medicine – a medical specialty with a wide range of competencies, similar to the solutions found in countries with strong PHC (such as the United Kingdom, Netherlands, Australia, Canada, Scandinavian countries) [2]. Physicians already acting in PHC were given transition time to get trained in family medicine. Their services financed by general health insurance were standardized according to the decree of the Ministry of Health [3].

Adaptation and approximation to European Union standards also required strengthening of the position of patients in the health care system [4]. The 1999 HCS reform allowed patients to freely choose the place to use medical

* Correspondence: marek.oleszczyk@uj.edu.pl
[1]Department of Family Medicine, Chair of Internal Medicine and Gerontology, Jagiellonian University Medical College, 4 Bochenska St., 31-061, Krakow, Poland
Full list of author information is available at the end of the article

services, including free choice of PHC physician. Patients' rights were gathered in one bill in 2008. New legal regulations, strengthening the patients' position have been added in following years.

The issues of quality of care received a much higher level of attention in the new model. One of its important dimensions is patients' opinions and satisfaction with the quality of care [5]. The classical approach according to A. Donabedian allows for the evaluation and description of complex and multi-dimensional quality in HCS in a three-level model: Structure-Process-Outcome [6]. Within this model, 10 core dimensions to evaluate primary health care were identified: "Governance", "Economic conditions", "Workforce" at "Structure level"; "Accessibility", "Comprehensiveness", "Continuity", "Coordination" at "Process" level; and "Quality of care", "Efficiency" and "Equity" at "Outcome" level [7]. This approach was developed within the Primary Health Care Monitor in Europe (PHAMEU) study in 2007–2010, which results showed an association between PHC structure and overall performance. The methodology of this study, based on the analysis of existing published data (gray-literature review as well as experts' and key-informants' opinions) left gaps in numerous areas. The researchers were unable to track in detail the links between structure, process, and outcomes, yet the study gave a conceptual and organizational foundation for future research [8, 9].

Studies on patient satisfaction in PHC have been performed in Poland since the early 1990s. The results show an overall high level of satisfaction [10–15]. However, it is difficult to generalize the results due to the fact that they have been performed in few practices or at small regional level. The diversity of methodologies used in the above-mentioned studies do not allow to compare the results with the data from other countries.

The aim of this study was to explore the experiences of real users of primary care in Poland. The study was designed to answer the following questions:

1. What is the level of patient satisfaction with the process and outcomes of care, provided by Polish PC physicians?
2. Are patients' personal characteristics related to their satisfaction?
3. Do professional characteristics of the PC physicians and their practices influence the patient satisfaction with the received care?

Methods

Design of the study

The study is based on data from the Polish part of the Quality and Costs of Primary Care in Europe (QUALICOPC) cross-sectional, questionnaire-based study, aiming to compare the quality of PHC in 34 countries. The detailed protocol for the QUALICOPC study has already been published and is available elsewhere [16, 17].

According to the international protocol of the QUALICOPC study, participating patients were approached through their general practitioners. A nationally representative sample of 220 primary care physicians was selected from the database of the Polish National Health Fund (statutory health insurance company in Poland) by a stratified random sampling procedure. The detailed description of the physicians' recruitment has been already published [18]. The participating physicians agreed that a trained fieldworker would distribute questionnaires to patients who have consulted them. On a set date, the fieldworker visited the participating PC practice, obtained written consent from the general practitioner and handed her/him the "PC Physician" questionnaire. Then, in the waiting-hall, the fieldworker consecutively invited 10 adult patients of the selected physicians, who were eligible and agreed to participate in the study. The first nine of them filled out the "Patient Experiences" questionnaire, the tenth – "Patient Values". Participants completed the questionnaires in the PC practice, just after the consultation with their GP. Each study participant returned the questionnaire in a sealed envelope to the fieldworker. The detailed scheme of the study track is shown in Fig. 1.

The study was approved by the Jagiellonian University Bioethics Committee (approval number KBET/104/B/2011).

Study participants

According to the international framework of QualicoPC study, we aimed to recruit 1980 participants. To gather this number of participants, the fieldworkers had to invite 4663 patients to take part in the study, and thus the response rate was 47%. One patient was excluded from the data analysis, because of incompleteness and high inconsistency of the answers to the survey questions. We checked the representativeness of the participating patients by comparing them with regard to age, gender, education and employment status to national statistics. Our study group included more women and more patients with secondary and higher level education than the general population.

Study tool

The QUALICOPC coordinator from the Netherlands Institute for Health Services Research (NIVEL) Consortium developed a survey set, which included four questionnaires: (1) one for general practitioners ("PC Physician" questionnaire) focused on the structural aspects and process of care; (2) one for patients about their experiences with one specific GP consultation ("Patient Experience" questionnaire) focused on the care processes and outcomes, (3) another for patients about the values of PHC they consider important ("Patient Values" questionnaire), and (4) a practice questionnaire about the structure of the PHC setting ("Fieldworker"

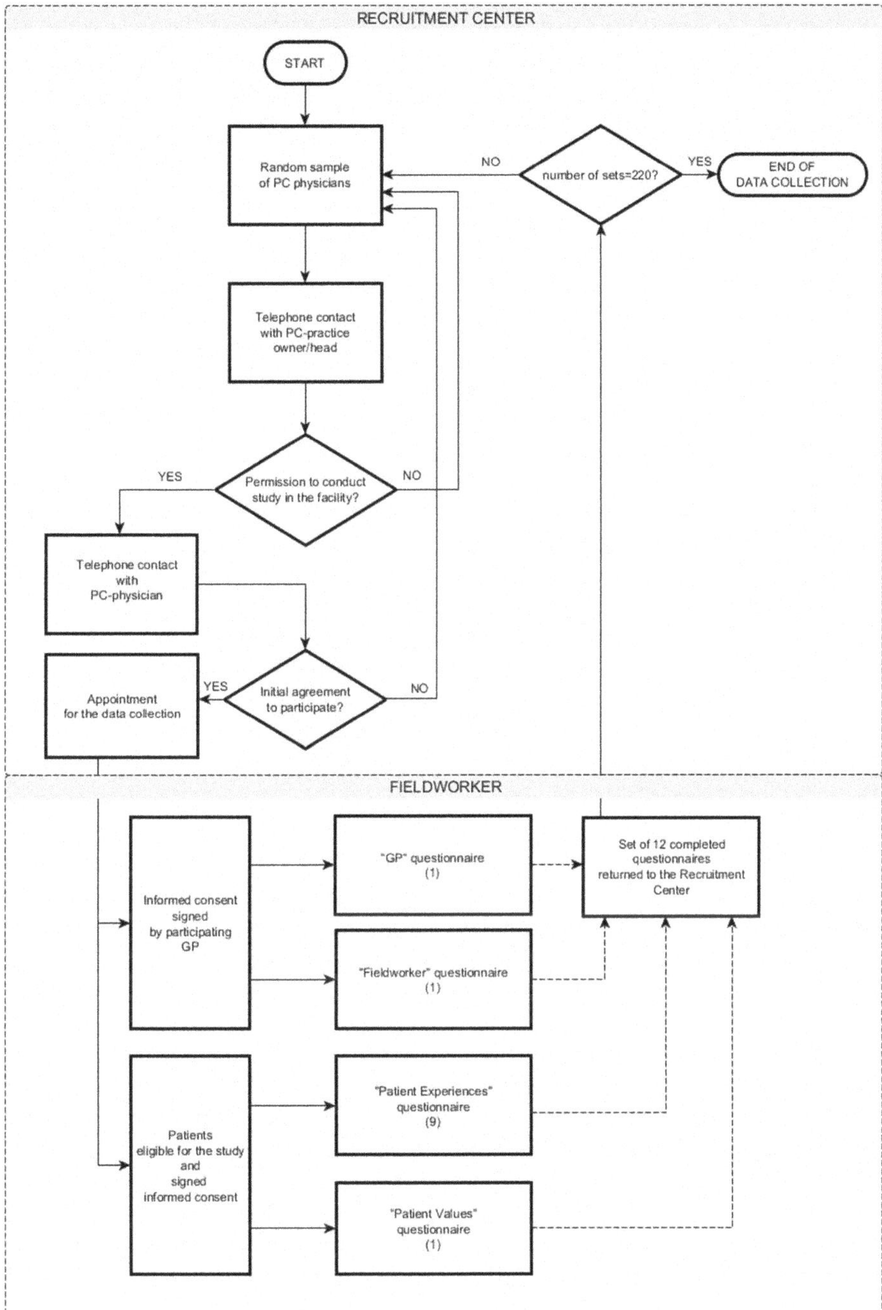

Fig. 1 Recruitment Center

questionnaire). The original questionnaires in English have been already published elsewhere [16]. The Polish version was translated and culturally adjusted in a formal process, common for all participating countries and included the controlled process of back-translation and validation. A detailed description of the conducted cross-cultural adaptation procedure is available in Additional file 1 [see Additional file 1]. In our study we used items from 3 out of 4 QUALICOPC questionnaires: "Patient Experience", "PC Physician" and "Fieldworker" questionnaires.

Dependent variables

To describe patients experiences we developed a satisfaction index (SI) for all seven studied PC areas: "Accessibility" (ACCS), "Continuity" (CONT), "Comprehensiveness" (COMP), "Coordination" (COOR), "Quality of care" (QUAL),

"Equity" (EQ), and "Efficiency" (EFF). All the variables (questionnaire items) from the "Patient Experience" questionnaire were assigned to areas of care, according to the key provided by the international study coordinator of QUALICOPC [16]. We rescaled all variables to a uniform scale ranging from −1 (extremely negative) to +1 (extremely positive). We assigned positive values to good experiences and negative values to poor experiences. In case of dichotomous variables and two possible answers (Yes/No), the values (+1) or (−1) were assigned respectively. For variables measured on ordinal scale, for questions with more than two answers, values from (−1) (for extremely negative) to (+1) (extremely positive) were given, the other were given intermediate values (−0.5), (0), (+0.5). The satisfaction indexes were calculated as an arithmetic mean (μ) of variables representing particular PC areas.

In the final analysis, we used three approaches to the satisfaction indexes. First, we analyzed them as interval dependent variables ranging from −1 to +1. Second, we categorized the interval variables in 5 categories: "extremely negative experience" when the SI equaled −1, "negative experience" for the SI (−1, −0.2), "neutral experience" for the SI [−0.2, 0.2], "positive experience" for the SI (0.2, 1) and "extremely positive experience" when SI equaled 1. Third, from the interval variables we derived dichotomous variables: "negative experience", for the SI below 0 and "positive experience", for SI 0 to +1.

Independent variables

As independent variables, we used 9 socio-demographic characteristics of patients from the "Patient Experience" questionnaire, including age, gender, education, employment status, the presence of children in the household, the presence of other adults in the household, declared income, self-estimated health status, and presence of chronic medical conditions. The PC physicians' characteristics were obtained from the "PC physician" questionnaire. The following 7 independent variables were used: age, gender, medical specialties, years of work in PC, physicians' involvement in pre and postgraduate medical education, PC practice location, declared the average time of consultation. Additionally, the analysis employed 8 variables, retrieved from "the Fieldworker" questionnaire, characterizing the infrastructure of the facility: handicap adjustment (parking place, physical barriers in the access to the practice building, location of the practice on the ground floor or presence of an elevator, accessible toilet); reception and waiting room confidentiality; information about opening hours and out-of-hours PHC services.

Statistical analysis

For statistical analysis, we used Statistica 10 software package (Statsoft Inc.). To illustrate respondents' characteristics and SI in all studied areas of PHC, we calculated descriptive stats as distributions for categorical data and means, medians, and ranges for numerical data.

Multivariate analyses were conducted to estimate the influence of patients' socio-demographic characteristics and the corresponding GPs' and practices' characteristics on satisfaction index in individual areas. As we included 24 independent variables in the analysis, we used backward stepwise regression to determine the models with the most variance explained using the fewest explanatory variables. When analyzing SIs as interval dependent variables, step-down linear regression was performed. We employed step-down logistic regression models for SI analyzed as binary independent variables. An alpha level of $p = 0.05$ was accepted as tests of statistical significance.

Results

Characteristics of respondents

In total 1980 patients took part in the study. Mean age of respondents was 48.2 (SD ±16.6, min. 18, max. 87 years). Their detailed sociodemographic characteristics are presented in Table 1.

The study participants were the patients of PC physicians of mean age 49.7 (SD ±8.7 years). The youngest and the oldest physician were 30 and 82, respectively. Most of the doctors were women (64%). Almost half (46%) of the physicians had been working in PC setting for more than 15 years. Those with PC experience shorter than 5 years represented 5%. Three-fourths had specialty training in family medicine. Almost half (47%) was in different ways involved in pre- or postgraduate medical education. More detailed information on participating physicians has been already published [18].

The primary care practices, in which the respondents visited their PC physician, were located mainly in an urban area (city: 30%, town: 30%, suburbs 7%), 27% were situated in rural areas, and 11% on the border between small towns and rural areas. In a clear majority of practices, there was readable information on opening hours and availability of out-of-hours care (96% and 80%, respectively). Almost all (95%) practices were located on the ground floor or had an elevator. In 84% of facilities, there was a handicap adjusted toilet and almost half (46%) had special parking places. Serious barriers for people using wheelchairs or parents with strollers existed in every eleventh practice. 64% practices had conditions to protect the privacy of conversation at the reception desk, and only in 7% of them could hear or see what was happening in the office during the consultation.

Satisfaction indexes

In the studied primary care areas, the mean values of the satisfaction index were as follows: "Accessibility" 0.64 (SD = 0.33); "Continuity" 0.60 (SD = 0.52); "Comprehensiveness" 0.30 (SD = 0.40); "Coordination" 0.44 (SD = 0.48); "Quality"

Table 1 Socio-demographic characteristics of study participants

Item	%	National statistics*
Gender		
Women	60.6	52.4
Born in Poland		
Participant	98.7	99.9
Participant's mother	97.8	N/A
Occupation/employment status		
Employed	38.9	34.1
Self-employed or family business	8.6	6.9
Student	6.9	5.8
Jobseeker/ unemployed	8.1	12.3
Unable to work due to illness or disability	5.3	5.3
Retired	27.4	18.0
Mainly homemaker (incl. Caring for children)	8.9	5.3
Education		
No qualifications/primary/vocational	32	29.2
Secondary	43.3	43.5
Higher	24.7	27.4
Skills in the Polish language		
Fluent/native speaker	96.5	96.2
Sufficient	2.8	2.0
Moderate/poor/not at all	0.7	0.5
Declared household income		
Below average	39.9	N/A
Around average	48.5	N/A
Above average	11.6	N/A
Self-evaluated health status		
Very good	11.3	18.9
Good	41.4	36.6
Fair	29.8	31.5
Poor	17.5	13.0
Chronic disease/condition	51.8	57.2

*Data derived from national statistics of Central Statistical Office: Demographic database, Statistical Yearbook of the Republic of Poland 2013, Healthcare in Households 2013; Employment in national economy in 2012 (www.stat.gov.pl)

0.77 (SD = 0,.9); "Equity" 0.8 (SD = 0.34); and "Efficiency" 0.55 (SD = 0.29). Figure 2 presents distributions of satisfaction indexes in particular areas of primary care.

Experience with primary care

The percentage of "positive experiences" (SI ranging from 0 to +1) in particular primary care area was for "Accessibility" 94%; "Continuity" 95%; "Comprehensiveness" 95%; "Coordination" 82%; "Quality of care" 81%; "Equity" 84%; and "Efficiency" 92% .

Figure 3 shows the detailed data about patients' experiences in each area of care categorized in 5 categories from "extremely negative" to "extremely positive" experience. The highest ratio of "extremely positive" experiences was noted in "Equity" (54%), the lowest in "Accessibility" (4%). The highest ratio of neutral scores was noted in "Quality of care" (27%). The percentage of "negative" and "extremely negative" experiences in particular areas ranged from 1% for "Continuity" to 14% for "Coordination". "Extremely negative" experiences were absent in three areas of care: "Accessibility", "Comprehensiveness" and "Efficiency".

Predictors of satisfaction

Table 2 shows a summary of step-down linear regression models evaluating the associations between satisfaction indexes and patients' and their corresponding GPs' and practices' characteristics.

The strongest determinants of patient satisfaction in the studied primary care areas were as follows: for "Accessibility" – very good self-estimated health status in comparison to poor health status ($p < 0.001$); for "Continuity" and "Quality of care" – 5-10 years of physician's experience in PC in comparison to shorter experience ($p < 0.001$); for "Comprehensiveness" and "Coordination" – PC practice setting in a rural area in comparison to a city ($p < 0.001$ and $p < 0.01$ respectively); for "Equity" - the duration of consultation ($p < 0.001$); for "Efficiency" the presence of children in household ($p < 0.001$).

Predictors of negative experiences

The determinants of patients' negative experiences with a particular PC area were analyzed in logistic regression are presented in Figs. 4, 5, 6, 7, 8, 9, 10.

The strongest predictors of negative experience with primary care were: location of the practice (town vs. city) in the area of "Accessibility of care" ($p < 0.01$); diagnosis of a chronic condition in the area of "Continuity of care" ($p < 0.01$); location of the practice in rural area in comparison to the location in a city in the area of "Comprehensiveness of care", "Coordination of care" and "Efficiency of care" ($p = 0.001$, $p < 0.001$ and $p < 0,.5$ respectively); declared household incomes above average in comparison to below average in the area "Quality of services" and "Equity of care" ($p < 0.05$ and $p < 0.05$, respectively).

Discussion

Summary of key findings

The Polish patients reported explicitly positive experiences with primary health care. The satisfaction index was positive in all studied areas. Quality of service, equity of care (where personal contact and communication skills of GPs and their staff were evaluated) and accessibility scored the best. Relatively lower (but still positive) satisfaction with comprehensiveness and coordination was found. Where the patients faced formal regulation and limitations of health care system e.g. few

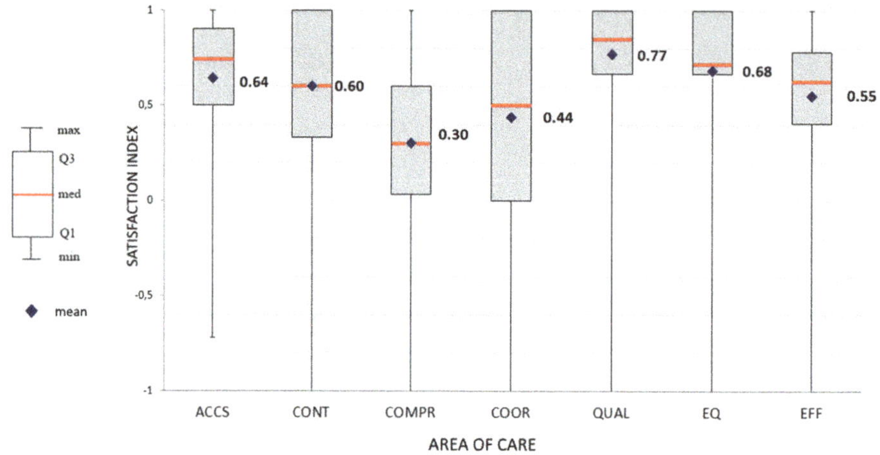

Q1 - the first quartile, Q3 - the third quartile, min - the minimum, max - the maximum;
ACCS – accessibility; CONT – continuity; COMP – comprehensiveness; COOR – coordination; EQ: equity;
QUAL – quality of services; EFF – effectiveness

Fig. 2 Satisfaction indexes in areas of primary care

invasive procedures performed in PHC (e.g. small surgery) or direct access to some specialist in secondary care (e.g. gynecologist or ophthalmologist). Lack of efficient information flow (amongst GPs and between primary and secondary care) could be another explanation of worse evaluation of coordination of care. We found that only a small part of the variability in patients' satisfaction can be explained by socio-demographic characteristics of patients and their PHC physicians. Primary care was better perceived by older patients, with chronic medical conditions, loneliness, inactivity in the labor market, and lower declared incomes. The higher satisfaction of PC services was reported by patients from rural areas and those treated by physicians with long professional experience in primary care. Specialty training in family medicine of the PC physician seemed to be

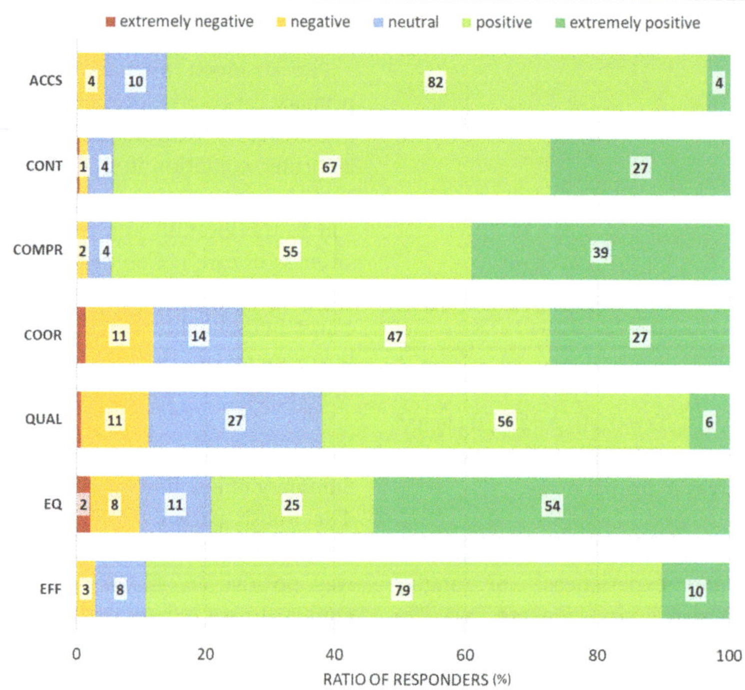

ACCS – accesibility; CONT – continuity; COMPR – comprehensiveness; COOR – coordination; QUAL – quality of services; EQ – equity; EFF – effectiveness

Fig. 3 Patients' experiences in the areas of primary care

Table 2 Step-down linear regression models: predictors of patient satisfaction in particular primary care areas in Poland

In cells: b and (95% CI)

Area of care Variable		ACCS	CONT	COMP	COOR	QUAL	EQ	EFF
Patient's age		0.002644 (0.001693; 0.003595)	0.005609 (0.004081; 0.007137)	0.004994 (0.003957; 0.006031)	0.004368 (0.002917; 0.005819)	0.002169 (0.001408; 0.002930)		0.003841 (0.002960; 0.004722)
Patient's gender male			−0.088791 (−0.132572; −0.045010)		0.080721 (0.037485; 0.123957)			−0.068408 (−0.098400; −0.038416)
Self-estimated health status	very good	0.10684 (0.055496; 0.158184)	−0.143814 (−0.216872; −0.070756)					
	good	0.054535 (0.022178; 0.086892)						
Diagnosis of chronic condition			0.166293 (0.114663; 0.217923)		0.115596 (0.066976; 0.164216)			
Children in household								−0.095592 (−0.149626; −0.041558)
Practice setting	rural	0.133077 (0.098952; 0.167202)	0.15093 (0.099386; 0.202474)	0.123771 (0.080141; 0.167401)	0.146834 (0.096665; 0.197003)	0.117116 (0.085533; 0.148699)		
	town							−0.077099 (−0.109392; −0.044806)
Duration of consultation		−0.013498 (−0.016463; −0.010533)				−0.006800 (−0.009503; −0.004097)	−0.007314 (−0.010018; −0.004610)	
Physician's age				0.004046 (0.001997; 0.006095)		−0.002980 (−0.004745; −0.001215)		
Specialty of - physician	family medicine (only)	−0.075238 (−0.107313; −0.043163)				−0.057494 (−0.087416; −0.027572)		
	family medicine (and other)				0.081966 (0.040626; 0.123306)			
Physician's experience in PC setting	5–10 years		0.235482 (0.122157; 0.348807)			0.146124 (0.077975; 0.214273)		
	10–15 years		0.253207 (0.145450; 0.360964)			0.191715 (0.126441; 0.256989)		0.114692 (0.074341; 0.155043)
	>15 years		0.356765 (0.250963; 0.462567)			0.201085 (0.135023; 0.267147)		0.104759 (0.066685; 0.142833)
Physician's involvement in medical education				0.062629 (0.026822; 0.098436)				
R^2		0.1	0.16	0.07	0.07	0.08	0.08	0.08
Area of care		ACCS	CONT	COMP	COOR	QUAL	EQ	EFF

ACCS – accessibility; CONT – continuity; COMPR – comprehensiveness; COOR – coordination; QUAL – quality of service; EQ – equity; EFF – effectiveness; PC – primary care; b – beta coefficient; CI – confidential interval; R^2 – proportion of variation explained

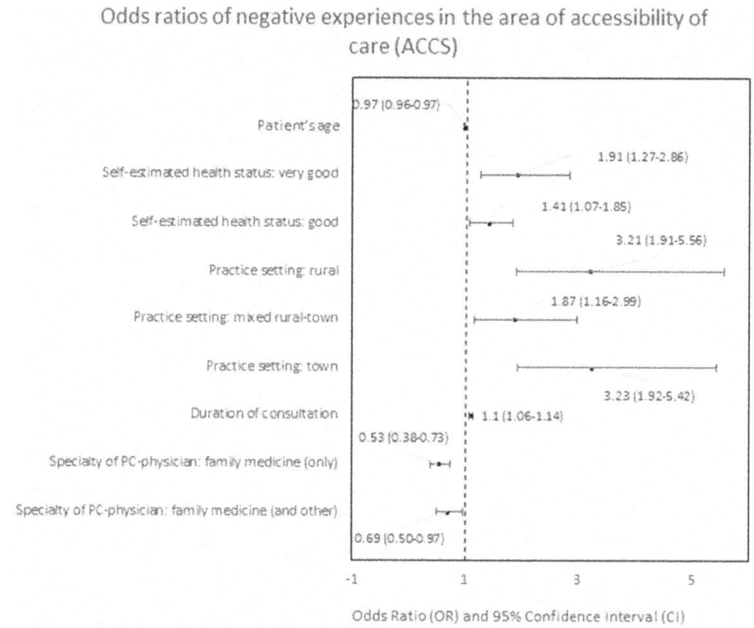

Fig. 4 Odds ratios of negative experiences in the area of accessibility

important, but not a sufficient condition of satisfactory care. Our study did not reveal any correlations between practice infrastructure and patients' experiences.

Strengths and limitations

The strength of our study was a large sample size, representing all adult primary care patients in Poland. To check the representativeness, the socio-demographic characteristics of study participants were compared to those of the general population. This comparison showed that the study group included more women and more patients with secondary and higher level education than the general population, which could be expected, as female gender and education level are proved to be

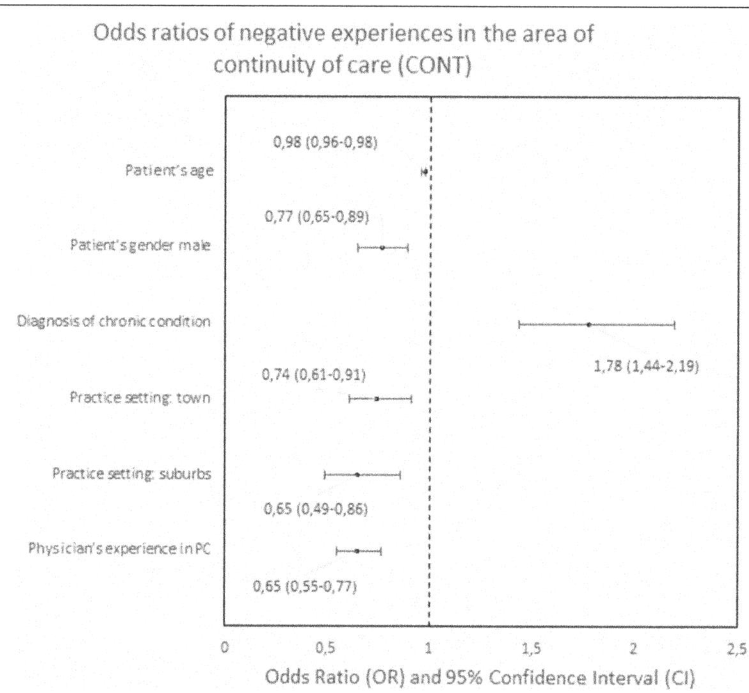

Fig. 5 Odds ratios of negative experiences in the area of continuity

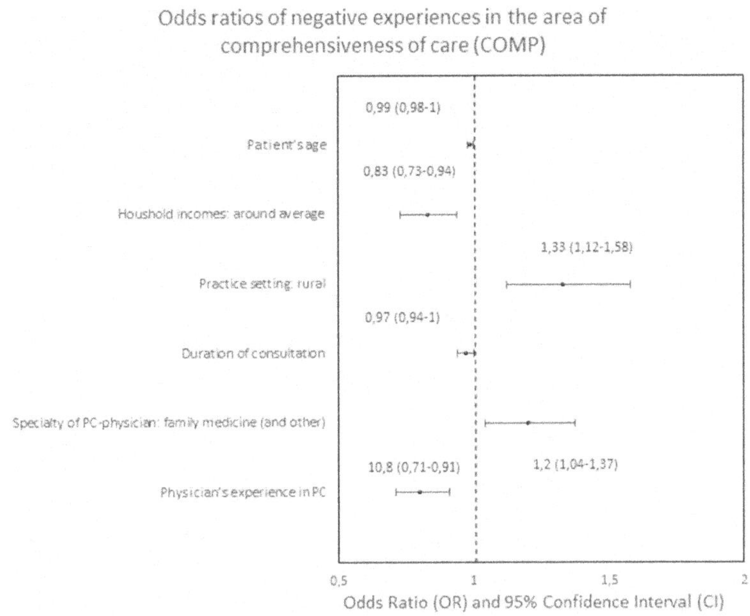

Fig. 6 Odds ratios of negative experiences in the area of comprehensiveness

important determinants of health care seeking behaviors [19].

The international, uniform methodology of the QUALICOPC study allowed for direct comparisons between countries. However, the national data from particular countries could be limited, as the in-country specific conditions were not taken into consideration when developing the study tool. Another limitation of the study is the use of self-reported questionnaires to gather data, which is linked to response bias caused by misunderstanding, underreport, exaggeration, etc.

As a limitation, we wanted to point out the fact that in our multiple regression analyses R-squared values were low, which is common in health services research in which outcomes are harder to predict [20]. However, it indicates the existence of other predictors of patient satisfaction, which were not included in our study. Another limitation is relatively low response rate and potential bias

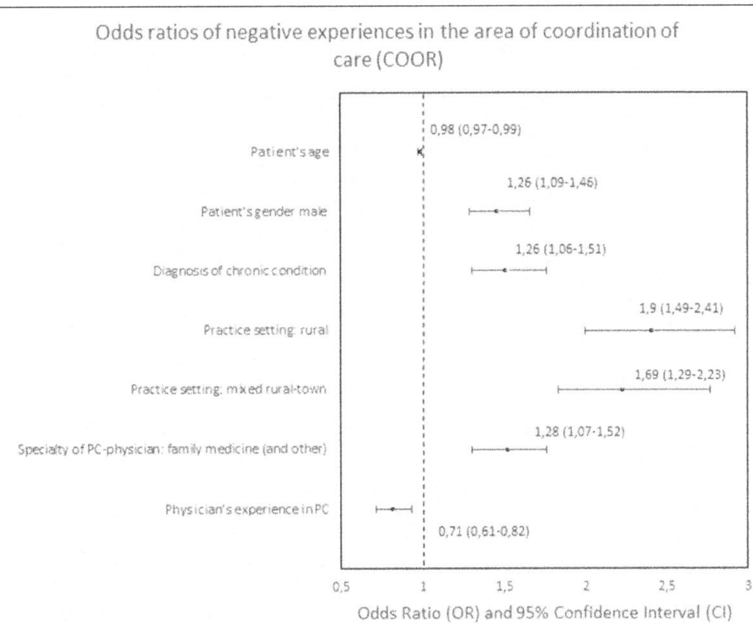

Fig. 7 Odds ratios of negative experiences in the area of coordination of care

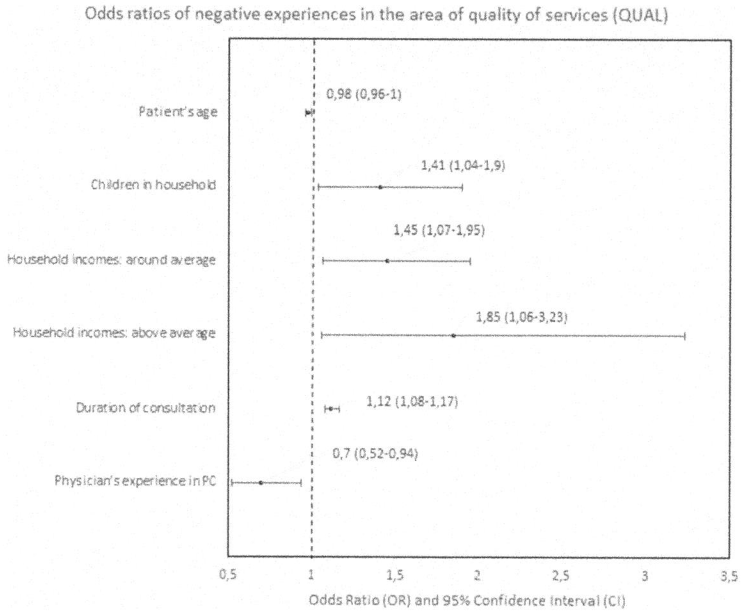

Fig. 8 Odds ratios of negative experiences in the area of quality of services

caused by this fact. We suppose that this is the result of a "real life" design and data collection system – there were no special invitations and incentives for participants and the recruitment was performed by an anonymous field-worker. Another limitation and a potential source of bias were that the GPs were contacted before and they were aware of the day of patient's recruitment; and that the questionnaires were filled by the participants in the waiting hall of PC facility, directly after seeing their GP.

Findings in light of other studies

In the PHAMEU study, Poland was classified as a country with medium PHC strength, characterized by good accessibility and coordination and poorly developed comprehensiveness [9]. The QUALICOPC survey conducted among primary care physicians in Poland showed that doctors were very critical of the areas of care in process and outcomes of PHC services. Coordination, quality of care and equity were evaluated negatively by

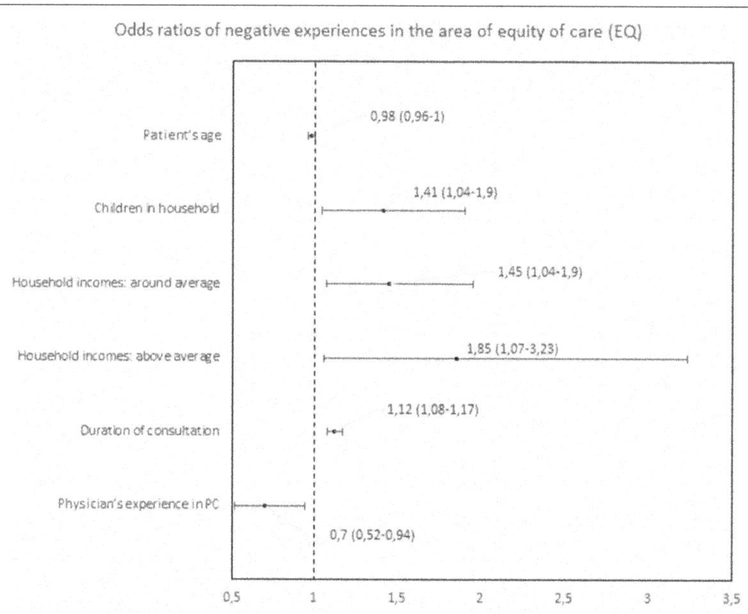

Fig. 9 Odds ratios of negative experiences in the area of equity

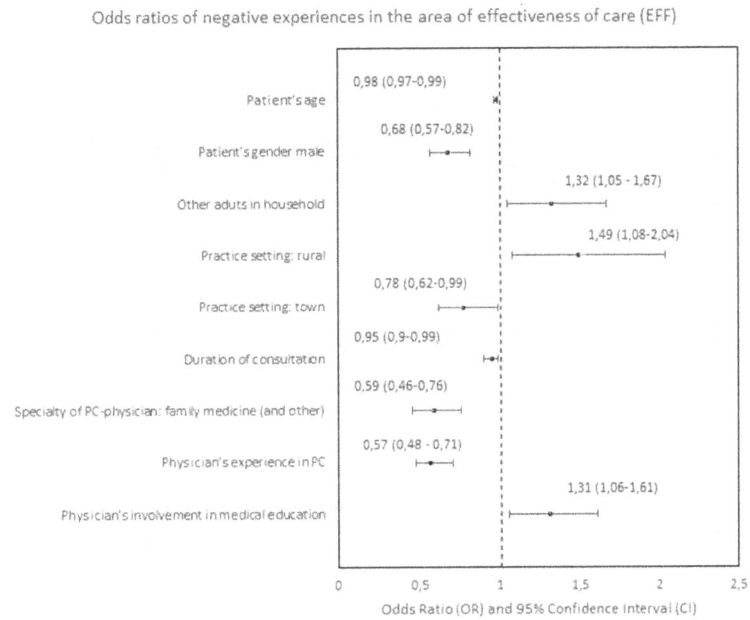

Fig. 10 Odd ratios of negative experiences in the area of efficiency

PC physicians, while accessibility, continuity, and comprehensiveness received neutral scores [18]. Contrary to poor evaluations of PC on the system level, patients (users of PC services) in our study had predominantly positive experiences with primary care in Poland. These findings are consistent with several previously published Polish studies on patient satisfaction with primary care. Marcinowicz et al. reported high satisfaction with communication skills of GPs (with scores around 4.5 on 1 to 5 scale) and length of consultation (88% satisfied) [11]. Kurpas et al. conclude in their paper on satisfaction with PHC of chronically ill patients, that they were at most satisfied with GP consultation (interview and physical examination) and their empathetic attitude, kindness and willingness to help [21]. In another national survey on patient's satisfaction, 78% of participants evaluated positively accessibility of PHC with mean satisfaction value +0.32 (range:-1.0 to 1.0), which was the highest score of all areas of care. [22]. In our study, we found that the length of a doctor's professional experience was a noticeable predictor of positive PC evaluation. The years of physician's experience in primary care may be associated with the duration of the relationship and shared experiences with patients and their physician. Although the therapeutic alliance and the long-term patient-doctor relationship are important and beneficial for both of them, it seems to be essential for the patient's satisfaction. According to Noyes et al., having a primary care physician and duration of that relationship is a key element determining the quality of care perceived by family medicine patients [23]. Interpersonal continuity with a regular provider is the most important predictor of patient satisfaction, as reported in Balkan populations by Gajovic et al. and in the USA by Nutting et al. [24, 25]. The findings of Mainous et al. showed that the patients place value on continuity with their regular physician [26]. According to Plomodon et al., PHC providers turnover was associated with worse patient satisfaction of care [27].

The difference between patients' (overall good) and physicians' (overall skeptical) evaluation of PHC was very likely to be linked to the negative evaluation of economic conditions and the structure of PHC in Poland by physicians. On the other hand, GPs might be more aware of their limitations or diagnostic uncertainty and less optimistic in the evaluation of their abilities to help patients [18, 28].

Exploring the positive PC experience predictors, we found a positive relationship between increasing age and patient satisfaction in all studied primary care areas. These results are compatible with other literature on patient evaluations of care [21, 29–31]. Kontopantelis et al. suggested that differences in satisfaction by age group could be due to differences in actual care received or to different response tendencies of individual population groups [31].

Our findings indicate that specialty training in family medicine is one of the desired PC physicians' characteristics associated with higher patient satisfaction, especially if the physician has more than one specialty. The introduction of family medicine into the primary health care system in Turkey resulted in an increase of patient satisfaction [32]. Similar observations were found in studies by Gavran et al. [33]. However, the study conducted by Chu-Weiniger et al. showed that giving patients the possibility of free choice of physician is more important than the doctor's specialty.

The free choice of PC provider helped to establish a trusting relationship [34].

The American research by Ly and Glied showed that patient satisfaction is not influenced by the number of PC physicians per inhabitant. Unexpectedly, longer waiting times for appointment were observed in practices with a higher physician-to-population ratio [35]. It may explain at least partially the observed discrepancies in satisfaction between patients from rural PC practices and those visiting PC physicians in big cities. In a national patient survey in Sweden, the higher satisfaction of care was observed among patients from smaller practices and practices where a high proportion of all visits were with a doctor [36]. According to Tung et al., the doctor's technical skill was the most important determinant of satisfaction, followed by the doctor's interpersonal skill. Staff care, access and providing patient education during the visit on prevention and prophylaxis were associated with improved patient satisfaction [37].

In our study, the infrastructure of facilities did not influence quality assessment. The literature review by Rozenblum et al. reported that the expansion of health information technologies did not significantly improve patient satisfaction [38]. These results may indicate that investments only in infrastructure and new technologies do not necessarily increase satisfaction.

Conclusions

PHC in Poland is of good overall quality as perceived by the patients. The areas of best quality are equity of care, accessibility of care and quality of service. Coordination and comprehensiveness of care are evaluated relatively worse. Organizational obstacles, like poor information flow, limited range of procedures in primary care and direct access to some services in secondary care might be responsible for lower satisfaction with coordination and comprehensiveness of care. The patients' and their physicians' characteristics have a limited influence on patient satisfaction and experiences with Polish primary care. Further research (including qualitative studies) is needed to identify other determinants of patient satisfaction. Because of the homogeneity of our study population, other studies are needed to explore experiences of ethnic minorities and other vulnerable groups of patients with their use of PHC. Similarly, other studies analyzing the quality of PHC in the rural setting are suggested, where best scoring in satisfaction was accompanied with the highest chance for negative experiences in this subpopulation of patients. Our findings suggest that creating a stable and sustainable environment to support long-lasting interpersonal patient-doctor relationship might be one of the most important factors to maintain and improve PHC patient's satisfaction.

Abbreviations

ACCS: Accessibility; COMP: Comprehensiveness; CONT: Continuity;; COOR: Coordination; EFF: Effectiveness; EQ: Equity; NIVEL: Netherlands Institute for Health Services Research; PC: Primary care; PHAMEU: Primary Health Care Activity Monitor in Europe; PHC: Primary health care; QUAL: Quality; QUALICOPC: Quality and Costs of Primary Care in Europe; SD: Standard deviation; SI: Satisfaction index

Acknowledgements

The study is a Polish arm of the QUALICOPC (Quality and Costs of Primary Care in Europe) project, co-funded by the European Commission under the Seventh Framework Programme. We would like to thank the primary care physicians and their patients for participation in the study, Ewa Wójtowicz MSc for her contribution to data analysis and Francis Ball MD for his contribution in the revision of the English manuscript.

Funding

The study is part of the QUALICOPC (Quality and Costs of Primary Care in Europe) project, co-funded by the European Commission under the Seventh Framework Programme (FP7/2007–2013) under grant agreement 242,141.

Authors' contributions

MO was involved in conceptual work, study design, data collection, and analysis, drafting and revising of the manuscript. AKK had a contribution in conception and design of the study, data collection, data analysis, drafting and revising of the manuscript. WLAS contributed to conceptual work, study design, drafting and revising of the manuscript. WGWB had a contribution in conception and design of the study, drafting and revising of the manuscript. AW was involved in conceptual work, study design, data collection, and analysis, drafting and revising of the manuscript. All co-authors have approved the final version of the article, including the authorship list. All authors read and approved the final manuscript.

Consent for publication

Not applicable.

Competing interests

The authors declare that they have no competing interests.

Author details

[1]Department of Family Medicine, Chair of Internal Medicine and Gerontology, Jagiellonian University Medical College, 4 Bochenska St., 31-061, Krakow, Poland. [2]NIVEL, Netherlands Institute for Health Services Research, PO Box 1568, 3500, BN, Utrecht, the Netherlands.

References

1. Figueras J, McKee M, Cain J, Lessof S, editors. Health systems in transition: learning from experience. Copenhagen: European Observatory on Health Systems and Policies; 2004. http://www.euro.who.int/__data/assets/pdf_file/0007/98395/E83108.pdf?ua=1. Accessed 29 Aug 2017.
2. Rechel B, McKee M. Health reform in central and eastern Europe and the former soviet union. Lancet. 2009;374:1186–95.
3. Windak A. The return of old family doctors in the new Europe. Eur J Gen Pract. 1998;4:168–70.
4. Together For Health: A Strategic Approach for the EU 2008–2013. White Paper. Brussels;2007; https://ec.europa.eu/health/ph_overview/Documents/strategy_wp_en.pdf. Accessed 29 Aug 2017.
5. Grol R, Baker R, Wensing M, Jacobs A. Quality assurance in general practice: the state of the art in Europe. Fam Pract. 1994;11:460–7.

6. Donabedian A. The quality of care. JAMA. 1988;260:1743.
7. Kringos DS, Boerma WG, Hutchinson A, van der Zee J, Groenewegen PP. The breadth of primary care: a systematic literature review of its core dimensions. BMC Health Serv Res. 2010;10:65.
8. Kringos DS, Boerma WG, Bourgueil Y, Cartier T, Hasvold T, Hutchinson A, et al. The European primary care monitor: structure, process and outcome indicators. BMC Fam Pract. 2010;11:81.
9. Kringos DS, Boerma WGW, Bourgueil Y, Cartier T, Dedeu T, Hasvold T, et al. The strength of primary care in Europe: an international comparative study. Br J Gen Pract. 2013;63:742–50.
10. Marcinowicz L, Chlabicz S. Improvement in the accessibility and organization of services of family physicians in a small town in Poland: a comparison of patient opinions between 1998 and 2002. Adv Med Sci. 2006;51:226–31.
11. Marcinowicz L, Konstantynowicz J, Chlabicz S. The patient's view of the acceptability of the primary care in Poland. Int J Qual Heal Care. 2008;20: 277–83.
12. Marcinowicz L, Rybaczuk M, Grebowski R, Chlabicz S. A short questionnaire for measuring the quality of patient visits to family practices. Int J Qual Heal Care. 2010;22:294–301.
13. Windak A, Gryglewska B, Tomasik T, Narkiewicz K, Grodzicki T. General practitioners ignore high normal blood pressure. Blood Press. 2008;17:42–9.
14. Parnicka A, Wizner B, Fedyk-Łukasik M, Windak A, Grodzicki T. Knowledge about heart failure in primary care: need for strengthening of continuing medical education. Cardiol J. 2013;20:356–63.
15. Marcinowicz L, Grebowski R, Chlabicz S. Exploring negative evaluations of health care by polish patients: an attempt at cross-cultural comparison. Health Soc Care Community. 2009;17:187–93.
16. Schäfer WL a, Boerma WGW, Kringos DS, De Ryck E, Greß S, Heinemann S, et al. Measures of quality, costs and equity in primary health care instruments developed to analyse and compare primary care in 35 countries. Qual Prim Care 2013;21:67–79.
17. Schäfer WLA, Boerma WGW, Kringos DS, De Maeseneer J, Gress S, Heinemann S, et al. QUALICOPC, a multi-country study evaluating quality, costs and equity in primary care. BMC Fam Pract. 2011;12:115.
18. Krztoń-Królewiecka A, Oleszczyk M, Schäfer WLA, Boerma WG, Windak A, Starfield B, et al. Quality of primary health care in Poland from the perspective of the physicians providing it. BMC Fam Pract. 2016;17:151.
19. MacKian S. A review of health seeking behaviour: problems and prospects. Manchester: University of Manchester; 2003. http://citeseerx.ist.psu.edu/viewdoc/download?doi=10.1.1.473.8350&rep=rep1&type=pdf. Accessed 29 Aug 2017.
20. Hamilton DF, Ghert M, Simpson AHRW. Interpreting regression models in clinical outcome studies. Bone Joint Res. 2015;4:152–3.
21. Kurpas D, Church J, Mroczek B, Hans-Wytrychowska A, Nitsch-Osuch A, Kassolik K, et al. The quality of primary health care for chronically ill patients - a cross-sectional study. Adv Clin Exp Med. 2013;22:501–11.
22. [Opinions on the function of the health care system A.D. 2014] [Polish with summary in English]. Komunikat z badań CBOS. Warszawa; 2014;http://cbos.pl/SPISKOM.POL/2012/K_034_12.PDF. Accessed 29 Aug 2017.
23. Noyes R, Kukoyi OA, Longley SL, Langbehn DR, Stuart SP. Effects of continuity of care and patient dispositional factors on the physician-patient relationship. Ann Clin Psychiatry. 2011;23:180–5.
24. Gajovic G, Kocic S, Radovanovic S, Ilic B, Milosavljevic M, Radevic S, et al. Satisfaction of users in primary health care. HealthMED. 2012;6:4185–93.
25. Nutting P, Goodwin M, Flocke S, Zyzanski SJ, Stange KC. Continuity of primary care: to whom does it matter and when? Ann Fam Med. 2003;1:149–55.
26. Mainous AG III, Goodwin MA, Stange KC. Patient-physician shared experiences and value patients place on continuity of care. Ann Fam Med. 2004;2:452–4.
27. Plomondon ME, Magid DJ, Steiner JF, MaWhinney S, Gifford BD, Shih SC, et al. Primary care provider turnover and quality in managed care organizations. Am J Manag Care. 2007;13:465–72.
28. Alam R, Cheraghi-Sohi S, Panagioti M, Esmail A, Campbell S, Panagopoulou E. Managing diagnostic uncertainty in primary care: a systematic critical review. BMC Fam Pract. 2017;18:79.
29. Sánchez-Piedra CA, Prado-Galbarro FJ, García-Pérez S, Santamera AS. Factors associated with patient satisfaction with primary care in Europe: results from the EUprimecare project. Qual Prim Care. 2014;22:147–55.
30. Campbell JL, Ramsay J, Green J. Age, gender, socioeconomic, and ethnic differences in patients' assessments of primary health care. Qual Health Care. 2001;10:90–5.
31. Kontopantelis E, Roland M, Reeves D. Patient experience of access to primary care: identification of predictors in a national patient survey. BMC Fam Pract. 2010;11:61.
32. Baltaci D, Celesun T, Eroz R, Saritas A, Celer A, Musulu C, et al. Evaluation of patient satisfaction with family physicians after implementation of family medicine in Turkey. HealthMED. 2012;6:469–75.
33. Gavran L, Jašarević E, Hasanica N. Patient satisfaction with primary care: are there differences between the approaches in family and general medicine? Med. Glas. (Zenica). 2013;10:379–84.
34. Chu-Weininger MYL, Balkrishnan R. Consumer satisfaction with primary care provider choice and associated trust. BMC Health Serv. Res. 2006;6:139.
35. Ly DP, Glied SA. Variations in the service quality of medical practices. Am J Manag Care. 2013;19:e378–85.
36. Glenngård AH. Is patient satisfaction in primary care dependent on structural and organizational characteristics among providers? Findings based on data from the national patient survey in Sweden. Heal Econ Policy Law. 2013;8:317–33.
37. Tung Y-C, Chang G-M. Patient satisfaction with and recommendation of a primary care provider: associations of perceived quality and patient education. Int J Qual Heal Care. 2009;21:206–13.
38. Rozenblum R, Donze J, Hockey PM, Guzdar E, Labuzetta MA, Zimlichman E, et al. The impact of medical informatics on patient satisfaction: a USA-based literature review. Int J Med Inform. 2013;82:141–58.

10

Recognition of depression by primary care clinicians in rural Ethiopia

Abebaw Fekadu[1,2,3*], Girmay Medhin[4], Medhin Selamu[2], Tedla W. Giorgis[5], Crick Lund[6], Atalay Alem[2], Martin Prince[7] and Charlotte Hanlon[2,7]

Abstract

Background: Depression is a common health condition affecting up to a third of patients attending primary care, where most of the care for people with depression is provided. Adequate recognition of depression is the critical step in the path to effective care, particularly in low income countries. As part of the Programme for Improving Mental healthcare (PRIME), a project supporting the implementation of integrated mental healthcare in primary care, we evaluated the level of recognition of depression by clinicians working in primary care in rural Ethiopia prior to in service training. We hypothesised that the detection rate of depression will be under 10% and that detection would be affected by gender, education and severity of depression.

Methods: Cross-sectional survey in eight health centres serving a population of over 160,000 people. A validated version of the 9-item patient health questionnaire (PHQ-9) was administered as an indicator of probable depression. In addition, primary care clinicians completed a clinician encounter form. Participants were consecutive primary care attendees aged 18 years and above.

Results: A total of 1014 participants were assessed. Primary care clinicians diagnosed 13 attendees (1.3%) with depression. The PHQ9 prevalence of depression at a cut-off score of ten was 11.5% ($n = 117$), of whom 5% ($n = 6/117$) had received a diagnosis of depression by primary care clinicians. Attendees with higher PHQ scores and suicidality were significantly more likely to receive a diagnosis of depression by clinicians. Women ($n = 9/13$) and participants with higher educational attainment were more likely to be diagnosed with depression, albeit non-significantly. All cases diagnosed with depression by the clinicians had presented with psychological symptoms.

Conclusion: Although not based on a gold standard diagnosis, over 98% of cases with PHQ-9 depression were undetected. Failure of recognition of depression may pose a serious threat to the scale up of mental healthcare in low income countries. Addressing this threat should be an urgent priority, and requires a better understanding of the nature of depression and its presentation in rural low-income primary care settings.

Keywords: Detection of depression, Developing country, Ethiopia, Integrated mental healthcare, Primary care

Background

Depression is established as a major public health problem because of its relatively high prevalence, globally affecting 10–20% of the population [1–9], and associated disability. Depression is particularly high in primary care settings [5, 10]. In the largest study of primary care patients, which involved 14 countries, mental disorders, mostly depression, were detected, on average, in 24% of attendees [6]. The few studies from Africa suggest comparable figures [11]. Depression is the second leading cause of years of life lived with disability [12] and accounts for 11 million suicide Disability Adjusted Life Years (DALYs) and for about four million DALYS of Ischaemic Heart Disease [13]. It is often co-morbid with other medical conditions with adverse outcomes [14–16]. Depression also increases risk of mortality in high [17, 18] and low income countries alike [7, 8], even when subthreshold [19]. Although depression is treatable [20, 21], most patients with

* Correspondence: abe.wassie@kcl.ac.uk
[1]Center for Innovative Drug Development and Therapeutic Trials for Africa (CDT-Africa), Addis Ababa University, College of Health Sciences, PO Box 9086, Addis Ababa, Ethiopia
[2]Department of Psychiatry, Addis Ababa University, College of Health Sciences, School of Medicine, Addis Ababa, Ethiopia
Full list of author information is available at the end of the article

depression, particularly those from low and middle income countries (LMIC), are untreated [22, 23]. In the world mental health survey, the treatment gap for "serious cases" in "less developed" countries was 76.3–85.4% [23]. The higher treatment gap in LMIC is unlikely to be explained by scarcity of specialists alone [24]; most patients with depression in high income countries are treated by primary care doctors and not by specialists [5]. Indeed, it is estimated that up to 90% of episodes of depression are managed in primary care [25].

Integrated care, i.e., task-shifted care provided at the primary care level by non-specialists, has been the key strategy proposed to address the treatment gap in LMIC [26]. For example, the mental health gap action programme intervention guide (mhGAP-IG) of the World Health Organization (WHO) provides a set of evidence-based clinical algorithms for the assessment and management of mental disorders specifically designed for use by non-specialist health workers [26]. Yet, the primary care setting in LMIC is very different to high income settings. The most important differences are: (1) care is provided by non-physicians with lower level of training; (2) the health facility to population ratio is extremely low and therefore there is a higher level of patient flow per clinician; (3) the chronic care model in which patients have the opportunity to engage with a single physician and be monitored regularly is almost unheard of in many LMICs; (4) the profile of patients in terms of education, awareness about mental health and socio-economic status differs substantially from those in high income settings. These factors, individually and in combination, conspire against service use or detection of depression in many LMICs. Thus, whereas on average about 50% of cases with depression attending primary care in high income countries may go undetected [6, 27], studies from Africa have reported detection rates close to 0% [28, 29], which do not improve significantly with brief [29, 30] or more intensive training [28]. In the WHO supported mhGAP programme in Ethiopia, the detection of depression in the 20 pilot health centres over a 6 month period was extremely low (available at: http://www.who.int/mental_health/mhgap/mhgap_ethiopia_proof_of_concept_2013.pdf; accessed 12/02/2014). Although detection does not ensure good quality care, it is a critical step in the pathway to quality care. Poor detection will also have serious downstream impacts on efforts to scale up integrated care, including loss of political commitment. Understanding the factors that impact on detection of depression by primary care staff is of crucial importance. As part of the PRogramme for Improving Mental health carE (PRIME), which aims to support integration of mental healthcare in five low and middle income countries [31], we conducted a study to determine the detection rate of depression in the eight primary care facilities that provide care to a population of over 160,000 people [32, 33]. We hypothesised that the detection rate would be low, under 10%, and that higher education level, female gender and increased severity of depression would be associated with improved detection.

Methods

The study was a facility-based, cross-sectional survey.

Setting

The study was conducted in Sodo district, Gurage Zone, Southern Nations, Nationalities and Peoples Region (SNNPR), a predominantly rural district located about 100 km south of the capital city, Addis Ababa. The population of the district at the start of the project was 161,952 (79,356 men; 82,596 women) living in 58 subdistricts (*kebeles*) [32, 33]. The largest ethnic group in the district is Sodo Gurage (85.3%) followed by Oromo (11.6%) and Amhara (1.5%) and Amharic is the official language. The majority of the population is Orthodox Christian (97%), with Muslims making up 2.3%. The district has eight health centers, five rural and three urban, in addition to the health posts (total $n = 58$) found in each sub-district. The health centers are staffed by nurses and health officers (clinicians with 3–4 years of training). Health officers run outpatient clinics. Each health post is staffed by a pair of health extension workers, female high school graduates with 1 year of training in health, focusing on prevention. At the time of the study, there were no mental health services in the district other than those initiated with the support of the PRIME project. Sodo is a relatively typical rural district for Ethiopia, and is located close to the research infrastructure of the Butajira research project of severe mental disorders [8, 34] and the Butajira Demographic Surveillance Site [11, 12]. The site is also within 30–50 km distance from specialist mental health services.

Assessment of depression and risk factors

We used the 9-item patient health questionnaire (PHQ-9) [35] to screen for depression. The PHQ was validated in the primary healthcare settings of the neighbouring district of Butajira (Meskan and Mareko) [36], as well as a general hospital setting in Ethiopia [37]. In the general hospital study, the PHQ-9 showed very good internal consistency and test-retest reliability, and at a cut-off point of 10, showed good sensitivity and specificity. However, in the primary care study, the optimum cut-off was determined to be five, with lower sensitivity and specificity. The disability item (10th item) of the PHQ that enquires about impairment in day to day functioning among those who responded positively to any of the preceding nine items was also included. This item specifically asks "how difficult have these problems made it for you to do your work, take care of things at home or get along with other people?"

The response options are "Not difficult at all, somewhat difficult, very difficult, extremely difficult".

Demographic factors hypothesised to be relevant for detection (gender, education) were assessed using a structured questionnaire developed for this purpose. Severity indicators were PHQ9 score (higher score indicating more severe illness) and suicidality. Suicidality was assessed using the suicide items included in the Composite International Diagnostic Interview (CIDI) [38]. The questions in the CIDI refer to suicidal ideation, suicide plan and suicide attempt. The CIDI has good face validity, feasibility and reliability [39] and has been used previously in community based studies in Ethiopia [40, 41]. Data collectors were high school graduates with 5 years experience of data collection. They were trained for 4 days on the instruments and the instruments were then pretested on 25 adults before the conduct of the actual study.

Clinicians (health officers) working at the primary care completed a clinical encounter form. The form was a simple, custom made tool that allowed the clinician to record the presenting complaint, history of the presenting illness, any pertinent past history, findings of the physical examination, diagnosis, any investigations requested and treatment provided. In our study, all nine health officers working at the eight health centres participated. All the health officers were men. Most were aged 25 and above and had been practicing at the centres for more than 1 year. They were trained in mental health as part of their undergraduate education.

Participants

Participants were selected through systematic random sampling of adults attending primary care facilities in all eight health centres (primary care facilities) of the Sodo district. To be included in the study, attendees had to be aged 18 years and above, be residents of the Sodo district, as evidenced by residence of 6 months or more in the district, and speak the local official language, Amharic, as the language of interview was Amharic. In estimating the sample size, we assumed a 5% detection rate at baseline (in the current study) and a 15% improvement in detection (to 20% detection) after training through the PRIME project. Assuming 80% power at 95% confidence, and 20% non-response, 978 participants were required. The eventual sample size ($n = 1014$), would enable us to estimate a detection rate by primary care clinicians of 5.0% with a margin of error of 1.3%. and a level of confidence of 95%. The number of participants for each health centre was allocated based on the number of sub-districts (anticipated population size) covered by each health centre. To obtain the number to be allocated to each health centre, the number of kebeles (nk) was divided by the total number of kebeles (NK) and multiplied by the total sample size (SS): [((nk/NK) × SS)].

Data management and analysis

Data were entered in Epidata v3.0 (http://www.epidata.dk/) and exported into STATA for Windows (version 13) for further analysis. PHQ-9 cut-off scores of five and ten were used to distinguish severity grades of depression. Other secondary depression criteria were the PHQ-2, in which those who score 3 or more were considered to have depression [42]. The PHQ-9 was also converted into DSM-5 criteria for major depressive disorder [43]. A proportion of patients who responded positively to the PHQ items were also asked about their feelings towards discussions about stress and emotional difficulties. Furthermore, we used data from a neighbouring district, in which PHQ was validated against a gold standard diagnosis by psychiatric nurses [36], to generate weights that were then used to determine the weighted prevalence of depression. Probability of being "clinically" depressed was derived from probability weights of the Butajira PHQ validation data. In this validation study, psychiatric nurses used the Mini International Neuropsychiatric Interview with additional open clinical questions to confirm clinical depression [36]. From these validation data, the probability of receiving "valid" diagnosis of depression within a range of PHQ score categories and disability from depressive symptoms were computed. These probabilities were then used as a weight in establishing a more conservative prevalence of depression in Sodo. Analyses were primarily descriptive in nature because of the low number of participants with clinically detected depression.

Results

Demographic characteristics

All consecutive participants who were approached ($n = 1014$) agreed to participate and were interviewed, with complete information available for 1009 participants. Most participants were from the Gurage ethnic group (89.6%), married (63.0%) and followers of Orthodox Christian religion (Table 1). Just over half (54.1%) were women. The mean age of participants was 35.5 years (SD = 15.7) with 11.3% aged 60 or above. Nearly half of the participants had formal education (49.5%).

The prevalence of depression

The prevalence of depression varied depending on the cut-off score of the PHQ used to define depression (Table 2). At a PHQ9 cut-off score of 10, 11.6% of the participants had potential depression. At the lower cut-off score of five, which was the optimum cut-off in primary care settings of the region [36], the prevalence of depression was much higher, 42.8%. However, weighting back against the gold standard diagnosis from primary care data

Table 1 Socio-demographic characteristics of participants (n = 1014)

Characteristics		Number(%)
Sex	Male	465(45.9)
	Female	549(54.1)
Age categories (years) (n = 1008)	18–24	282(28.0)
	25–34	286(28.4)
	35–44	181(18.0)
	45–59	145(14.4)
	60+	114(11.3)
Age (years) (=1008)	Mean(SD)	35.5(15.7)
Marital status	Married	639(63.0)
	Never married	269(26.5)
	Formerly married	106(10.5)
Ethnicity	Gurage	908(89.6)
	Others	206(10.4)
Religion	Orthodox Christian	876(86.4)
	Protestant	105(10.4)
	Others	33(3.3)
Education	Non-literate	399(39.4)
	Literate but no formal education	113(11.1)
	Formal Education	502(49.5)
Occupation (n = 1012)	Civil servant	105(10.4)
	Employed in private sector	21(2.1)
	Self employed	356(35.2)
	Voluntary work	5(0.5)
	Housewife	258(25.5)
	Jobless	24(2.4)
	Student	83(8.2)
	Pensioner	20(2.0)
	Other	140(13.8)
Number of children	No child	352(34.7)
	1–4 children	346(34.1)
	More than 4 children	31.6(31.2)

for validating the PHQ in the neighbouring district of Butajira [36], the prevalence was 7.1%.

In terms of impairment in day to day functioning, nearly 80% (79.4%) of those with PHQ9 score of five and above and over 85% of those with score of ten and above reported at least some degree of impairment.

Clinician diagnosis of depression

In total, 38 participants (4.0%) were diagnosed by clinicians as having either depression (n = 13; 1.3%) or other psychiatric conditions (n = 25; 2.5%) (Table 3). All clinician-diagnosed cases of depression had a PHQ9 score of five and above. Most diagnosed with other psychiatric conditions (82%) also had PHQ score of at least five. Suicidality and symptom severity were associated significantly with receiving a diagnosis of depression (Table 3). Although more women and those with formal education received a diagnosis of depression, these were not statistically significant. Those receiving a PHQ2 diagnosis of depression, although not a DSM-5 diagnosis of depression, were more likely to receive a clinician diagnosis of depression ($P = 0.007$ for PHQ2).

The sensitivity of clinician diagnosis of depression against the PHQ9 was between 2.8 and 5.1% (Table 4). This also translates into low positive and negative predictive values.

Clinical encounter

"Stress" and "headache" were the leading presenting complaints in clinically diagnosed cases of depression, occurring in 53.8% ($n = 7/13$) and 30.8% ($n = 4/13$) (Table 5), respectively. Cases with clinical diagnosis of depression had PHQ score of five and above (Table 5). "Distress" was also the most common diagnosis among attendees with a diagnosis of a psychiatric condition other than depression (Table 6). Headache was the leading presenting complaint among those with other psychiatric conditions, occurring in 57% ($n = 16/28$). Stress, dizziness and sleep problems occurred in two cases each while palpitations, chest pain, eye pain, pain during micturition, paralysis and suicidality were each presenting complaints for one case. No laboratory investigations were ordered for any of the cases diagnosed with depression. In terms of medication, eight were prescribed analgesics, two were counselled and another two were referred for further psychiatric assessment and treatment. Follow-up arrangements were made for ten of the cases. However, only five cases reported discussing about depression with the clinician. Those who discussed depression reported that they found their discussion useful (somewhat useful (n = 1) or very much useful (n = 4)).

Discussion

Depressive symptoms are prevalent in this sample of primary care attendees. While nearly half of the participants had depressive symptoms above the optimum cut-off point of five, about 11% had symptom severity compatible with a diagnosis of major depressive disorder (PHQ score of 10 and above). Yet, the detection rate of depression by primary care clinicians was extremely low, with over 95% of patients presenting to primary care with potential depression not receiving a clinical diagnosis of depression. This level of non-detection is much higher than reported in high income countries where about 50% of cases with depression may be unrecognised [44]. With ongoing engagement for a

Table 2 Diagnostic categories versus clinician diagnosis of study participants

Characteristics	Total n(%)	Depression n(%)	Other psychiatric morbidity (%)	Depression and other psychiatric morbidity n(%)	Epilepsy n(%)	Other health problems
PHQ9 total score						
5+	432(42.8)	13(3.0)	21(4.9)	34(7.9)	3(0.7)	395(91.4)
< 5	578(57.2)	0(0.0)	4(0.7)	4(0.7)	3(0.5)	571(98.8)
10+	117(11.6)	7(6.0)	7(6.0)	14(12.0)	2(1.7)	101(86.3)
< 10	893(88.4)	6(0.7)	18(2.0)	24(2.7)	4(0.5)	865(96.9)
PHQ2 score						
3+	116(11.5)	6(5.2)	2(1.7)	8(6.9)	3(2.6)	105(90.5)
< 3	894(88.5)	7(0.8)	23(2.6)	30(3.4)	3(0.3)	861(96.3)
DSM5 criteria						
Depressed	34(3.4)	1(2.9)	2(5.9)	3(8.8)	2(5.9)	29(85.3)
Non-depressed	976(96.6)	12(1.2)	23(2.4)	35(3.6)	4(0.4)	937(96.0)

period of 6 months, the proportion with unrecognized depression goes down to 20% [45]. However, such an alarmingly low rate of detection is not unique for these rural Ethiopian facilities with the limited evidence from sub-Saharan Africa indicating a detection rate of depression in primary care close to 0% [11, 28]. The significance of this finding looms large in the context of the current international effort to scale up mental health care in low and middle income countries through services provided by primary care clinicians. It is also very important because most patients with depression, whether in low income or high income country settings, are bound to receive treatment in primary care. Thus the low detection represents a major threat as well as opportunity to address an important public health challenge.

Although further work is required, the apparent low detection of depression is unlikely to be due to low rates of depression. In a validation study in primary care facilities of the adjoining rural districts of Meskan and Mareko, the prevalence of depression based on mental health professional diagnosis was 5% [36]. In the current study, nearly half of the participants had depressive symptoms with a PHQ score of five and above while about one in ten had a PHQ score of ten and above. Although not all those with high levels of PHQ depressive

Table 3 Clinician diagnosis of depression as a function of selected clinical and demographic characteristics of study participants

Characteristics	Total n(%)	Depression n(%)	Other psychiatric morbidity n(%)	Depression and other psychiatric morbidity n(%)
Severity measured with PHQ9 score				
< 5	578(57.2)	0 (0.0)	4(0.7)	4(0.7)
5–9	315 (31.2)	6(1.9)	14(4.4)	20(6.3)
10 + [a]	117(11.6)	7(6.0)	7(6.0)	14(12.0)
Suicidality				
Yes[a]	100(9.9)	6 (6.0)	8(8.0)	14(14.0)
No	910(90.1)	7(0.8)	17(1.9)	24(2.6)
Sex				
Male	461(45.6)	4(0.9)	16(3.5)	20(4.3)
Female	549(54.4)	9(1.6)	9(1.6)	18(3.3)
Education				
Non-literate	398(39.4)	4(1.0)	7(1.8)	11(2.8)
Literate but no formal education	124(12.3)	0(0.0)	3(2.4)	3(2.4)
Formal Education	488(48.3)	9(1.8)	15(3.1)	24(4.9)

[a]Differences statistically significant [Fisher's exact p <0.001]

Table 4 Clinician diagnosis of depression and the PHQ diagnosis of depression at varied thresholds of diagnosis

Target parameter	Point estimate and confidence Interval	Detection criteria			
		PHQ9 (5+)	PHQ9 (10+)	PHQ2 (3+)	DSM 5
Prevalence	%	42.6	11.5	11.4	3.4
	95% CI	39.6, 45.7	9.6, 13.5	9.5, 13.4	2.2, 4.7
Sensitivity	%	3.0	6.0	5.2	2.9
	95% CI	1.4, 4.6	1.6, 10.3	1.1, 9.3	−3.0, 8.9
Specificity	%	100.0	99.3	99.2	98.8
	95% CI	99.4, 100.0	98.5, 99.8	98.4, 99.7	97.9, 99.4
PPV	%	100.0	53.8	46.2	7.7
	95% CI	75.3, 100.0	25.1, 80.8	19.2, 74.9	0.2, 36.0
NPV	%	58.0	89.0	89.0	96.7
	95% CI	54.8, 61.1	86.9, 90.8	86.9, 90.8	95.4, 97.7

PHQ Patient Health Questionnaire

symptoms are likely to have major depressive disorder, it appears that these symptoms might not have been trivial in that the majority of participants who reported depressive symptoms also reported at least some degree of impairment in their day to day functioning. Suicidal ideation was also increased among those reporting depressive symptoms in the PHQ rating. These provide indirect evidence for the clinical relevance of the depressive symptoms recorded. Although studies from high income countries suggest that those with undetected depression have mild illness and benefit of treatment may be uncertain [41], the extremely low detection rate in the current study and in the few studies from Sub-Saharan African countries mean that a proportion of the missed cases are likely to have more severe illness and to benefit from treatment.

The reasons for the low detection are likely to be multifaceted and related to health system features, and patient and clinician factors [46–49]. The health system in many low and middle income countries, particularly in sub-Saharan African countries, is geared towards acute care. Although, ongoing contact with a service increases the chances of detection, patients in these settings are rarely seen more than once and clinicians and patients rarely form ongoing therapeutic relations. Explanatory models of illness regarding mental illness, which tend to be shared by clinician and patient with mental disorders, are likely to influence both clinician and patient. Social attributions, emotional burden and concern about dealing with social issues that might have led to the depression in the first place have been reported as important barriers [48]. The expectation of patients, and how symptoms are presented and communicated influence the ability of the clinician to detect depression. Family members are also important in influencing decisions of diagnosis and treatment and their

Table 5 Presenting complaints and selected demographic characteristics of clinician detected cases

Age	Gender	First presenting complaint	Second presenting complaint	PHQ scores
19	F	Stress	Lack of sleep	15
19	M	Stress	————	8
20	F	Headache	Fever	10
20	F	Stress	————	7
20	F	Stress	————	5
20	F	Headache	Depression	14
23	M	Suicide attempt	Sleep problem	10
25	F	Headache	Hearing difficulty	16
25	M	Stress	Lack of sleep	6
38	M	Depression	Headache	12
40	F	Fever/Headache	Ear discharge	9
41	F	Stress	————————	5
44	F	Stress	Headache	10

Table 6 Psychiatric diagnosis other than depression made by primary care clinicians

Specific diagnosis	Number	Percent
Schizophrenia	1	3.6
Anxiety disorder	4	0.4
Distress	12	1.2
Insomnia	2	0.2
Mental and behavioural disorder	5	0.5
Worry ("Thinking")	1	0.1
Suicidality	1	0.1
Total	26	2.6

explanatory model is likely to have a role. Clinicians and patients are also likely to share similar attitude towards mental illness as the community they live in. Negative attitude towards mental illness is thus likely to influence the diagnosis of depression. The low level of knowledge and skill of clinicians have important impact on diagnosis. Recognition of depression may be affected by a number of illness related features. Presentation with mood symptoms, past history of illness, more severe depressive symptoms and reporting suicidal tendencies increase the chance of detection [50]. In the current study, clinician detection of depression relied on direct report by patients of psychological symptoms; however, in primary care settings, most patients present with somatic rather than psychological symptoms [5]. Improving detection of depression in routine care requires interventions that address the system level needs, and the needs of the clinician as well as addressing patient and family/community level barriers.

Detection does not always lead to care. For example, a series of studies conducted in high income countries have indicated that only a quarter to one third of those detected receive appropriate intervention [51–53]. Therefore, intervention to improve detection should also address this "detection-intervention" gap. Addressing this gap will require changes at all the levels that are relevant for detection. The health system need to adopt the chronic care approach, which has the potential not only to improve depression care but also cost [54]; clinicians have to be equipped with the necessary knowledge and skill; the attitude of clinicians, patients and the public at large needs to encourage detection and treatment.

The results of this study should be interpreted with some important limitations in mind. The proportion with detected depression was too small to make generalizable conclusions regarding the implication of the detected depression. The report is also primarily descriptive because of the apparent risk of unstable estimation. However, although this is an important limitation, we believe the descriptive nature of the paper should not detract from the clear relevance of its content. First, the paper fills an important knowledge gap regarding the detection of depression in LMICs given the dearth of evidence in LMIC settings. Secondly, as we have indicated, our report comes in the context of the concerted effort to scale up mental healthcare in LMICs. In this regard, the report shows a crucial challenge for scaling up care and has the potential to spur researchers and clinicians to develop interventions to improve detection of depression. Detection is an unresolved conundrum that awaits concerted multidisciplinary effort, particularly in LMICs. Thirdly, despite the limited number, we have provided detailed clinical description of the cases, which might be used for training of primary healthcare workers.

Further assessment to understand what the PHQ symptoms mean would have allowed a more accurate interpretation of the ratings. The reasons provided for the under-detection are theoretical and further studies to understand the role of the various proposed mechanisms for the low detection, for example through qualitative studies, need to be explored. The cross-sectional nature of the assessment may introduce bias, particularly recall bias. However, the depressive symptoms were assessed for the preceding 2 weeks and the impact of recall bias should be minimal.

Conclusion

Detection is the rate limiting step in the path to care for people with depression in low and middle income countries. Findings from this study indicate that the level of detection is unacceptably low. Even if it was concluded that only a small proportion of these cases would require treatment, still a major opportunity for intervention has been missed.

However, several issues have to be addressed in order to deal with the detection barrier. First, understanding the question of the nature of depression in these settings is important and should be explored carefully. The second crucial issue is understanding the process of detection. Finally understanding the system level barriers and the organizational or structural requirements of the health system are crucial. Improving detection should be one of the priorities of global mental health studies.

Abbreviations

CIDI: Composite International Diagnostic Interview; DALY: Disability adjusted life year; LMIC: Low and Middle Income Countries; mhGAP: Mental health Gap Action Programme; mhGAP-IG: mhGAP intervention guide; PHQ: Patient Health Questionnaire; PRIME: Programme for Improving Mental Health Care; SNNPR: Southern Nations Nationalities and Peoples Region; WHO: World Health Organization

Acknowledgements

Not applicable.

Funding
The study was funded by the Department for International Development, Government of the UK.

Authors' contributions
AF, GM, MS, TWG, CL, AA, MJP and CH participated in the design of the study. AF, GM, MS, CH contributed to data collection. AF, GM, MP analysed the data. AF drafted the paper. AF, GM, MS, TWG, CL, AA, MJP and CH revised the draft and made critical intellectual contributions and agreed for the submission. All authors read and approved the final manuscript.

Authors' information
Abebaw Fekadu, MD, PhD, MRCPsych: Head, Centre for Innovative Drug Development and Therapeutic Trials for Africa (CDT-Africa) and MRC African Research Leader.
Girmay Medhin, PhD: Associate Professor and epidemiologist, Aklilu Lemma Institute of Pathobiology, Addis Ababa University.
Medhin Selamu, MA: Intervention Coordinator for the PRIME project in Ethiopia and a PhD student at the Department of Psychiatry, Addis Ababa University.
Tedla W Giorgis, PhD: Mental Health Advisor to the Minister, Federal Ministry of Health of Ethiopia.
Crick Lund, PhD: Professor and Head, Alan J Flisher Centre for Public Mental Health, Department of Psychiatry and Mental Health, University of Cape Town
Atalay Alem, MD, PhD: Professor, Department of Psychiatry, Addis Ababa University.
Martin Prince: MD, FRCPsych: Professor, Head, Health Services and Population Research Department, and Co-Director, Center for Global Mental Health, Institute of Psychiatry, Psychology and Neuroscience, King's College London
Charlotte Hanlon, PhD, MRCPsych: Associate Professor, Department of Psychiatry, Addis Ababa University.

Competing interests
All authors declare no conflict of interest. AF is supported by the Medical Research Council and DfID to develop intervention to improve detection of depression through the African Research Leader Scheme.

Consent for publication
Not applicable.

Author details
[1]Center for Innovative Drug Development and Therapeutic Trials for Africa (CDT-Africa), Addis Ababa University, College of Health Sciences, PO Box 9086, Addis Ababa, Ethiopia. [2]Department of Psychiatry, Addis Ababa University, College of Health Sciences, School of Medicine, Addis Ababa, Ethiopia. [3]Department of Psychological Medicine, Centre for Affective Disorders, King's College London, Institute of Psychiatry, Psychology and Neuroscience, London, UK. [4]Aklilu Lemma Institute of Pathobiology, Addis Ababa University, Addis Ababa, Ethiopia. [5]Federal Ministry of Health, Addis Ababa, Ethiopia. [6]Alan J Flisher Centre for Public Mental Health, Department of Psychiatry and Mental Health, University of Cape Town, Cape Town, South Africa. [7]King's College London, Institute of Psychiatry, Psychology and Neuroscience, Health Services and Population Research Department, London, UK.

References

1. Bromet E, Andrade L, Hwang I, Sampson N, Alonso J, de Girolamo G, de Graaf R, Demyttenaere K, Hu C, Iwata N, et al. Cross-national epidemiology of DSM-IV major depressive episode. BMC Med. 2011;9(1):90.
2. Weissman M, Bland R, Canino G, Faravelli C, Greenwald S, Hwu H, Joyce P, Karam E, Lee C, Lellouch J, et al. Cross-national epidemiology of major depression and bipolar disorder. JAMA. 1996;276(4):293–9.
3. Alonso J, Angermeyer MC, Bernert S, Bruffaerts R, Brugha TS, Bryson H, de Girolamo G, Graaf R, Demyttenaere K, Gasquet I, et al. Prevalence of mental disorders in Europe: results from the European Study of the Epidemiology of Mental Disorders (ESEMeD) project. Acta Psychiatr Scand Suppl. 2004;420:21–7.
4. Andrade L, Caraveo-Anduaga JJ, Berglund P, Bijl RV, De Graaf R, Vollebergh W, Dragomirecka E, Kohn R, Keller M, Kessler RC, et al. The epidemiology of major depressive episodes: results from the International Consortium of Psychiatric Epidemiology (ICPE) Surveys. Int J Methods Psychiatr Res. 2003;12(1):3–21.
5. Tylee A, Gandhi P. The importance of somatic symptoms in depression in primary care. Prim Care Companion J Clin Psychiatry. 2005;7:167–76.
6. Ustun TB, Sartorius N. Mental Illness in General Health Care. Chichester: Wiley; 1995.
7. Mogga S, Prince M, Alem A, Kebede D, Stewart R, Glozier N, Hotopf M. Outcome of major depression in Ethiopia: Population-based study. Br J Psychiatry. 2006;189(3):241–6.
8. Fekadu A, Medhin G, Kebede D, Alem A, Cleare AJ, Prince M, Hanlon C, Shibre T. Excess mortality in severe mental disorders: a 10-year population-based cohort study in rural Ethiopia. Br J Psychiatry. 2015;206:289–96.
9. Fekadu A. Studies on Affective Disorders in Rural Ethiopia. Umea: Umea University; 2010.
10. Katon W, Schulberg H. Epidemiology of depression in primary care. Gen Hosp Psychiatry. 1992;14:237–47.
11. Udedi M. The prevalence of depression among patients and its detection by primary health care workers at Matawale Health Centre (Zomba). Malawi Med J. 2014;26(2):34–7.
12. Vos T, Flaxman AD, Naghavi M, Lozano R, Michaud C, Ezzati M, Shibuya K, Salomon JA, Abdalla S, Aboyans V, et al. Years lived with disability (YLDs) for 1160 sequelae of 289 diseases and injuries 1990?2010: a systematic analysis for the Global Burden of Disease Study 2010. Lancet. 2012;380(9859):2163–96.
13. Ferrari AJ, Charlson FJ, Norman RE, Patten SB, Freedman G, Murray CJL, Vos T, Whiteford HA. Burden of Depressive Disorders by Country, Sex, Age, and Year: Findings from the Global Burden of Disease Study 2010. PLoS Med. 2013;10(11):e1001547.
14. Frasure-Smith N, Lespérance F, Talajic M. Depression following myocardial infarction: Impact on 6-month survival. JAMA. 1993;270(15):1819–25.
15. Frasure-Smith N, Lespérance F, Talajic M. Depression and 18-Month Prognosis After Myocardial Infarction. Circulation. 1995;91(4):999–1005.
16. Januzzi Jr JL, Stern TA, Pasternak RC, DeSanctis RW. THe influence of anxiety and depression on outcomes of patients with coronary artery disease. Arch Intern Med. 2000;160(13):1913–21.
17. Cuijpers P, Smit F. Excess mortality in depression: a meta-analysis of community studies. J Affect Disord. 2002;72(3):227–36.
18. Harris EC, Barraclough B. Excess mortality of mental disorder. Br J Psychiatry. 1998;173(1):11–53.
19. Cuijpers P, Vogelzangs N, Twisk J, Kleiboer A, Li J, Penninx BW. Differential mortality rates in major and subthreshold depression: meta-analysis of studies that measured both. Br J Psychiatry. 2013;202(1):22–7.
20. Patel V, Simon G, Chowdhary N, Kaaya S, Araya R. Packages of Care for Depression in Low- and Middle-Income Countries. PLoS Med. 2009;6(10): e1000159. doi:10.1371/journal.pmed.1000159.
21. Sobocki P, Ekman M, ÅGren H, Runeson B, JÖNsson B. The mission is remission: health economic consequences of achieving full remission with antidepressant treatment for depression. Int J Clin Pract. 2006;60(7):791–8.
22. Kohn R, Saxena R, Levav I, Saraceno B. The treatment gap in mental health care. Bull World Health Organ. 2004;82:858–66.
23. The WHO World Mental Health Survey Consortium. Prevalence, Severity, and Unmet Need for Treatment of Mental Disorders in the World Health Organization World Mental Health Surveys. JAMA. 2004;291:2581–90.
24. Jenkins R, Kiima D, Okonji M, Njenga F, Kingora J, Lock S. Integration of mental health into primary care and community health working in Kenya: context, rationale, coverage and sustainability. Ment Health Fam Med. 2010;7(1):37–47.
25. Scott J, Thorne A, Horn P. Effects of a multifaceted approach to detecting and managing depression in primary care. BMJ. 2002;325:951–4.
26. World Health Organization. mhGAP Intervention Guide for mental, neurological and substance use disorders in non-specialized health settings. Geneva: WHO Press; 2010.
27. Mitchell AJ, Rao S, Vaze A. International comparison of clinicians' ability to identify depression in primary care: meta-analysis and meta-regression of predictors, vol. 61. 2011.
28. Jenkins R, Othieno C, Okeyo S, Kaseje D, Aruwa J, Oyugi H, Bassett P, Kauye F. Short structured general mental health in service training programme in Kenya improves patient health and social outcomes but not detection of

mental health problems - a pragmatic cluster randomised controlled trial. Int J Ment Heal Syst. 2013;7(1):25.
29. Udedi M. The Prevalence of depression among patients and its detection by Primary Health Care Workers at Matawale Health Centre (Zomba). Malawi Med J. 2014;26:34–7.
30. Alexander CL, Arnkoff DB, Kaburu AW, Glass CR. Detecting depression in rural primary care clinics in central Kenya: Impact of a brief training intervention. Int Perspect Psychol Res Pract Consultation. 2013;2:14–28.
31. Lund C, Tomlinson M, Silva M, Fekadu A, Shidhaye R, Jordans M, Petersen I, Bhana A, Kigozi F, Prince M. PRIME: a programme to reduce the treatment gap for mental disorders in five low- and middle-income countries. PLoS Med. 2012;9(12):e1001359.
32. Fekadu A, Medhin G, Selamu M, Hailemariam M, Alem A, Giorgis TW, Breuer E, Lund C, Prince M, Hanlon C. Population level mental distress in rural Ethiopia. BMC Psychiatry. 2014;14:194.
33. Hanlon C, Luitel NP, Kathree T, Murhar V, Shrivasta S, Medhin G, Ssebunnya J, Fekadu A, Shidhaye R, Petersen I, et al. Challenges and opportunities for implementing integrated mental health care: a district level situation analysis from five low- and middle-income countries. PLoS ONE. 2014;9(2):e88437.
34. Kebede D, Alem A, Shibre T, Negash A, Fekadu A, Fekadu D, Deyassa N, Jacobsson L, Kullgren G. Onset and clinical course of schizophrenia in Butajira-Ethiopia–a community-based study. Soc Psychiatry Psychiatr Epidemiol. 2003;38(11):625–31.
35. Kroenke K, Spitzer RL, Williams JB. The PHQ-9: validity of a brief depression severity measure. J Gen Intern Med. 2001;16(9):606–13.
36. Hanlon C, Medhin G, Selamu M, Breuer E, Worku B, Hailemariam M, Lund C, Prince M, Fekadu A. Validity of brief screening questionnaires to detect depression in primary care in Ethiopia. J Affect Disord. 2015;186:32–9.
37. Gelaye B, Williams MA, Lemma S, Deyessa N, Bahretibeb Y, Shibre T, Wondimagegn D, Lemenhe A, Fann JR, Vander Stoep A, et al. Validity of the Patient Health Questionnaire-9 for depression screening and diagnosis in East Africa. Psychiatry Res. 2013;210(2):653–61.
38. World Health Organization. Composite International Diagnostic Interview, version 2.1. Geneva: WHO; 1997.
39. Rashid E, Kebede D, Alem A. Evaluation of an Amharic version of the Composite International Diagnostic Interview (CIDI) in Ethiopia. Ethiop J Health Dev. 1996;10:69–77.
40. Fekadu A, Kebede D, Alem A, Fekadu D, Mogga S, Negash A, Medhin G, Beyero T, Shibre T. Clinical outcome in bipolar disorder in a community-based follow-up study in Butajira, Ethiopia. Acta Psychiatr Scand. 2006;114(6):426–34.
41. Fekadu A, O'Donovan MC, Alem A, Kebede D, Church S, Johns L, Medhin G, Prince M, Shibre T. Validity of the concept of minor depression in a developing country setting. J Nerv Ment Dis. 2008;196(1):22–8.
42. Kroenke K, Spitzer RL, Williams JB. The Patient Health Questionnaire-2: validity of a two-item depression screener. Med Care. 2003;41(11):1284–92.
43. American Psychiatric Association. Diagnostic and Statistical Manual of Mental Disorders, 5th Edition: DSM-5. Washington, DC: APA; 2013.
44. Tylee A, Freeling P, Kerry S, Burns T. How does the content of consultations affect the recognition by general practitioners of major depression in women? Br J Gen Pract. 1995;45:575–8.
45. Paykel ES, Priest RG. Recognition and management of depression in general practice: consensus statement. Br Med J. 1992;305(6863):1198–202.
46. Gilbody S, Whitty P, Grimshaw J, Thomas R. Educational and organizational interventions to improve the management of depression in primary care: a systematic review. JAMA. 2003;289(23):3145–51.
47. Gilbody SM, Whitty PM, Grimshaw JM, Thomas RE. Improving the detection and management of depression in primary care. Qual Saf Health Care. 2003;12:149–55.
48. Petersen I. Comprehensive integrated primary mental health care. Pipedream or possibility. Soc Sci Med. 2000;51:321–34.
49. Mendenhall E, De Silva MJ, Hanlon C, Petersen I, Shidhaye R, Jordans M, Luitel N, Ssebunnya J, Fekadu A, Patel V, et al. Acceptability and feasibility of using non-specialist health workers to deliver mental health care: stakeholder perceptions from the PRIME district sites in Ethiopia, India, Nepal, South Africa, and Uganda. Soc Sci Med. 2014;118:33–42.
50. Wittchen HU, Pittrow D. Prevalence, recognition and management of depression in primary care in Germany: the Depression 2000 study. Hum Psychopharmacol. 2002;17 Suppl 1:S1–11.
51. Kessler RC, Zhao S, Katz SJ, Kouzis AC, Frank RG, Edlund M, Leaf P. Past-year use of outpatient services for psychiatric problems in the National Comorbidity Survey. Am J Psychiatry. 1999;156(1):115–23.
52. Wang PS, Berglund P, Kessler RC. Recent care of common mental disorders in the United States. J Gen Intern Med. 2000;15(5):284–92.
53. WHO International Consortium in Psychiatric Epidemiology. Cross-national comparisons of the prevalences and correlates of mental disorders. Bull World Health Organ. 2000;78(4):413–26.
54. Bodenheimer T, Wagner EH, Grubach K. Improving primary care for patients with chronic illness: The chronic care model, Part 2. JAMA. 2000;288:1909–14.

11

Migrants' motives and expectations for contacting out-of-hours primary care

Ellen Keizer[1*], Peter Bakker[1,2], Paul Giesen[1], Michel Wensing[1], Femke Atsma[1], Marleen Smits[1] and Maria van den Muijsenbergh[2,3]

Abstract

Background: Migrants are more likely to use out-of-hours primary care, especially for nonurgent problems. Their motives and expectations for help-seeking are as yet unknown. The objective of this study is to examine the motives and expectations of migrants for contacting out-of-hours primary care.

Methods: We used data from a survey study of 11,483 patients who contacted a General Practitioner (GP) cooperative in the Netherlands between 2009 and 2014 (response rate 45.6%). Logistic regression analysis was used to test differences in motives and expectations between non-western and western migrants and native Dutch patients.

Results: The main motives for contacting a GP cooperative for non-western and western migrants were an urgent need for contact with a GP (54.9%–52.4%), worry (49.3%–43.0%), and a need for medical information (21.3%–26.2%). These were also the most important motives for native Dutch patients. Compared to native Dutch patients, non-western migrants more often perceived an urgent need for a GP (OR 1.65; 99% CI 1.27–2.16), less often needed information (OR 0.59; 99% CI 0.43–0.81), and more often experienced problems contacting their own GP during office hours (OR 1.71; 99% CI 1.21–2.43). Western migrants also reported experiencing problems more often in contacting their own GP (OR 1.38; 99% CI 1.04–1.84).
As well as for natives, most non-western and western migrants expected to see a doctor (46.2%–46.6%) or get advice (39.6%–41.5%). Non-western migrants expected more often to get physical examination (OR 1.53; 99% CI 1.14–2.04), and prescription (OR 1.37; 99% CI 1.00–1.88). We found no differences in expectations between western migrants and native Dutch patients.

Conclusion: The main motives and expectations of migrants are similar to native Dutch patients, yet non-western migrants more often wanted action from the GP, e.g. examination or prescription, and less often passive forms of assistance such as giving information. At the same time they experience problems accessing their own GP. We recommend stimulation of self-care, education about the purpose of a GP cooperative, and examination and improvement of accessibility of daytime primary care.

Keywords: After hours care, Primary health care, Motivation, Expectations, Migrants

* Correspondence: ellen.keizer@radboudumc.nl
[1]Scientific Center for Quality of Healthcare (IQ healthcare), Radboud Institute for Health Sciences, Radboud University Medical Center, P.O. Box 9101, 6500, HB, Nijmegen, The Netherlands
Full list of author information is available at the end of the article

Background

There is a worldwide increase in migration flows between countries [1]. The Netherlands has also experienced an increase in the number of migrants. In 2015, 3.7 million inhabitants were migrants or children of migrants, which constituted 22% of the Dutch population [2]. Of these migrants, 56% have a non-western background and 44% a western background. By 2060, the proportion of these migrants is expected to have increased up to 31% [3].

Migrants' utilisation of healthcare services has often been investigated, showing a variety of results. Most studies found that migrants have a relatively high use of both primary care and some types of specialist care, while preventive care and other forms of healthcare are used less frequently [4–7]. Studies also showed differences in healthcare use between various migrant groups [8, 9], most notably between migrants with a non-western and a western origin. Non-western migrants also appear to have a higher use of primary healthcare services compared to western migrants. The demand of out-of-hours primary care turned out to be higher in deprived areas, where a relatively higher number of non-western migrants reside [10]. Moreover, general practices with a larger number of migrants in their patient population were found to have higher out-of-hours primary care use [11].

Previous studies at the Emergency Department (ED) and out-of-hours primary care showed that migrants more often use care for problems that are unnecessary from a medical perspective [12–14]. A possible explanation is that non-western migrants differ in help-seeking behaviour and have other expectations of healthcare than native citizens, because they are used to a different healthcare system in their country of origin, have a poorer health status [15–17] and have lower health literacy skills [18, 19]. Another reason could be linked to differences in the perception of urgency. Problems that may well be considered as nonurgent in the Netherlands, are often considered as urgent in other countries. This is likely to be caused by higher morbidity and mortality rates from infectious diseases in non-western countries compared to western countries [20].

In the Netherlands, each patient has to be registered in a general practice of his own choice, with general practitioners (GP) acting as gatekeepers for secondary care. Referrals are needed for visits to medical specialists in hospitals and are initiated and coordinated by the GP [21]. Migrants with residence permit have the same entitlements to GP care as all other Dutch people. Out-of-hours primary care is provided by 120 large-scale GP cooperatives [22]. The cooperatives serve 99% of the Dutch population of 17 million and are available every evening, night, weekend and during the holidays. Each GP cooperative has 50 to 250 GPs who provide care to 100,000 to 500,000 citizens. Every GP has to do a minimum number of shifts at the GP cooperative to maintain his/her registration as a GP. Patients are classified in urgency categories from high to low urgency. Key features of GP cooperatives in the Netherlands are listed in Table 1.

The GP cooperative is intended for urgent help requests that cannot wait until the regular consultation hours of the patient's own GP. However, in practice, a large part of the help requests proved to be nonurgent from a medical perspective (45%) [23]. As (non-western) migrants are more likely to use care for nonurgent problems, gaining insight into the motives and expectations of migrants for contacting GP cooperatives can be of value.We expect that their motives are often worry and a perceived need to see a doctor for a physical examination, because of the differences in contextual circumstances in their country of origin, such as morbidity and mortality from infections. Previous research has also shown that migrants more often perceive problems with their own GP's accessibility [24]. Therefore, low accessibility to daytime general practice could also be a motive for contacting out-of-hours primary care.

Since the migrant population is increasing, it is clearly relevant to understand the motives and expectations of this particular population. The objective of our study is to examine the motives and expectations of migrants for contacting out-of-hours primary care.

Methods

Design, setting and population

We used an existing dataset of survey studies on patient experiences, which we performed in stratified samples of patients who contacted a GP cooperative between 2009 and 2014. Data from 11,483 patients were available (response rate 45.6%). Stratification was based on the type of contact: equal numbers of questionnaires were distributed to patients who only had a telephone contact, patients who had a GP consultation at the GP cooperative, and patients who had a GP home visit. Data from a convenience sample of 42 GP cooperatives (from a total of approximately 120) spread across the Netherlands were used.

Questionnaire

For our study, we used the Consumer Quality Index (CQI) GP cooperatives [25]. This Dutch questionnaire was developed by the department of IQ healthcare of the Radboud University Medical Center Nijmegen and validated in the general population of the GP cooperative [26]. The questionnaire included questions about patient characteristics, expectations of healthcare, motives for seeking healthcare, and patient experiences in healthcare. In this study we used only a part of the questionnaire, namely the motives and expectations for contacting the GP cooperative as well as

Table 1 Features of general practitioner (GP) cooperatives in the Netherlands and charging system [22, 23, 44]

Theme	Feature
General	Out-of-hours primary care has been provided by large-scale general practitioner (GP) cooperatives since the year 2000
	Every GP has to do a minimum number of shifts at the GP cooperative to maintain his/her registration as a GP.
	Participation of 50–250 GPs per cooperative with a mean of 4 h on call per week with a compensation of about €65/h
	About 120 GP cooperatives in the Netherlands
	Population of 100,000 to 500,000 patients with an average care consumption of 250 contacts/1000 inhabitants per year
	Out-of-hours defined as daily from 5 p.m. to 8 a.m., all public holidays and the entire weekend
	Per shift GPs have different roles: supervising telephone triage, doing centre consultations or home visits
	The triage is supervised by telephone consultation doctors who can be consulted in case of doubt, while also checking and authorising all calls
Location	GP cooperative usually situated in or near a hospital
	Distance of patients to GP cooperative is 30 km at most
Accessibility	Access via a single regional telephone number, meaning the first contact is mostly with a triage nurse (only 5–10% walk in without a call in advance)
	Telephone triage by nurses supervised by GPs: contacts are divided into telephone advice (38%), centre consult (52%), or GP home visit (9%)
Facilities	Home visits are supported by trained drivers in identifiable fully equipped GP cars (e.g. oxygen, intra venous drip equipment, automated external defibrillator, medication for acute treatment)
	Information and communication technology (ICT) support including electronic patient files, online connection to the GP's car, and sometimes connection with the electronic medical record in the GP's daily practice
Charging system	Healthcare is largely covered by health insurance
	All residents over 18 years pay a monthly premium to their health insurance provider. There is no premium for children
	Employers pay a part of their employee's income to the tax administration for healthcare costs
	Patients do not have to pay an additional amount for GP care, both during and outside office hours
	Residents over 18 years must an annual deductible (385 euro in 2016) in case of use of healthcare (including emergency departments). This deductible is neither applicable to GP care, nor to children

the origin of the patient and his/her parents. Patients had to indicate for each motive and expectation whether it actually applied to them. These motives and expectations were the outcome measures in our study. Age, gender, education and health status of patients were used for case-mix adjustment in data analysis. Health status was measured with a 5-point Likert scale by asking patients to describe their own health (very good, good, fair, bad, very bad).

Procedure

At each GP cooperative, a representative sample of 600 patients received the questionnaire by post in a four-week period from 2009 to 2014. Patients received the questionnaire between four and ten days after their contact with the GP cooperative, while a reminder was sent after one week and after three weeks.

We asked the parents of patients aged under 12 to fill in the questionnaire. The following exclusion criteria were used: dying or deceased patients; patients who contacted the GP cooperative for administrative reasons or for confidential problems; patients residing abroad; exceptional telephone stalkers (calling several times without a help request) and patients who declared not to be willing to participate in research.

The three questions in the questionnaire about the origin of the patient, his/her father and his/her mother were used to determine whether a patient was a western migrant, a non-western migrant or a native Dutch patient. Migrants were defined in accordance with Statistics Netherlands, meaning that at least one parent was born abroad [27]. The patients were divided into three groups: non-western migrants (originating from Africa, Latin America, Asia -except Indonesia and Japan- or Turkey), western migrants (originating from European countries -except Turkey-, North America and Oceania, Indonesia or Japan) and native Dutch patients (both parents born in the Netherlands). If the parents were born in different countries outside the Netherlands, we used the mother's country of birth to determine the patient's origin. When the country of birth of the parents was unknown, we used the country of birth of the patient to define the origin. If the parents completed the questionnaire for their child we used their data to determine the origin.

Statistical analysis

Missing data occurred on the outcome variables motives ($N = 416$; 3.6%) and expectations ($N = 155$; 1.3%), as well as origin ($N = 629$; 5.5%), gender ($N = 1060$; 9.2%), age

(N = 1050; 9.1%), education (N = 1321; 9.1%) and self-reported health status (N = 1544; 13.4%). Results from a MNAR (missing not at random) test showed that the missing data appeared to be at random. We used multiple imputation (MI) to impute missing values (five imputation sets).

Descriptive statistics were used to describe patient characteristics, motives and expectations for contacting the GP cooperative. For each motive and expectation, differences between migrants and natives were tested with logistic regression analysis, while pooled odds ratios were calculated (pooling of all odds ratios of the single imputation sets into one overall odds ratio). To account for clustering of patients within GP cooperatives, the variable GP cooperative was added as a covariate in the analyses. In the analyses, we corrected for age, gender, education and self-reported health status, as these patient characteristics might influence the response tendencies of the respondents [28, 29]. Differences between migrants and natives were tested for motives and expectations with sufficient response heterogeneity (at least 5% /95%). This means that enough discrimination between the yes and no group was needed. Models were constructed for the following motives: urgent need for a GP, worry, need for medical information, own GP could not be contacted during office hours, and for all expectations. In order to account for multiple testing, we used $p < 0.01$ (99% CI) to determine the significance of the differences between the groups of origin.

Goodness of fit between the observed and predicted outcomes of the logistic models were assessed based on the Hosmer-Lemeshow test and its discrimination ability was assessed based on the area under the receiver operating curve (AUC). Since it is not possible in SPSS to pool the Hosmer-Lemeshow test and the AUC results, we presented the results of one single imputation set. Data were analysed using the Statistical Package for the Social Sciences (SPSS) 22.

Results

Multiple imputation

After multiple imputation of our data, we compared the descriptive statistics of the patient characteristics, motives and expectations of the original data with the pooled data. As the results were almost similar, we decided to present the results of the pooled data.

Patient characteristics

Table 2 shows a description of the study population for the different groups of origin. Of the respondents, 4.1% (N = 475) were non-western migrants, 6.1% (N = 700) western migrants and 89.8% (N = 10,308) native Dutch patients. We noticed a few minor differences between the origins of the groups regarding distribution in gender, education and self-reported health status. Compared to native Dutch patients, the non-western migrants in our sample seemed younger.

Motives for seeking healthcare

The most frequently mentioned motives for both non-western and western migrants to contact a GP cooperative were urgent need for a GP (54.9% - 52.4%), worry (49.3% - 43.0%) and need for medical information (21.3% - 26.2%) (Table 3). These motives were also most often mentioned by native Dutch patients. We found some minor differences between migrants and native Dutch patients (Table 4). Non-western migrants more often perceived an urgent need for contact with a GP as opposed to native Dutch patients (OR 1.65, 99% CI 1.27–2.16, corrected for gender, age, education and self-reported health status). They less often mentioned a need for medical information as a motive for contacting a GP cooperative (OR 0.59, 99% CI 0.43–0.81). They also reported more often that they could not contact their own GP during office hours (OR 1.71, 99% CI 1.21–2.43). Western migrants also mention more often that they could not contact their own GP during office hours (OR 1.38, 99% CI 1.04–1.84). We found no other differences in motives between western migrants and native Dutch patients. All four logistic models achieved sufficient calibration (Hosmer-Lemeshow test's P range of 0.129–0.171 in a single imputation set) and discrimination (AUC range of 0.606–0.651 in a single imputation set).

Expectations of healthcare

The expectations most often mentioned for both non-western and western migrants were seeing a doctor (46.2% - 46.6%) and getting advice (39.6% - 41.5%) (Table 3). Native Dutch patients also mentioned these expectations most often. A smaller group of non-western migrants expected to get a physical examination (27.4%), or expected prescription or medication (24.5%), or to be reassured (24.0%). A small group of non-western and western patients expected to be referred to a hospital (12.2% - 13.2%) or to receive treatment (e.g. a stitch) (both 7.4%). There were two significant differences between non-western migrants and native Dutch patients and no differences between western migrants and native Dutch patients (Table 4). Non-western migrants more often expected get a physical examination (OR 1.53, 99% CI 1.14–2.04) and to get a prescription or medication (OR 1.37, 99% CI 1.00–1.88) compared to native Dutch patients. All seven logistic models achieved both calibration (Hosmer-Lemeshow test's mean P range of 0.173–0.966 in a single imputation set) and discrimination (AUC range of 0.576–0.664 in a single imputation set).

Table 2 Description of study population (%)

Characteristic	Non-western (*N* = 475)	Western (*N* = 700)	Native dutch (*N* = 10,308)
Gender			
Male	39.9	40.1	42.9
Female	60.1	59.9	57.1
Age groups			
0–4	11.7	5.8	8.2
5–17	36.6	17.4	18.3
18–44	36.4	42.1	36.5
45–64	9.1	24.0	25.3
≥ 65	6.2	10.7	11.7
Education			
Low (≤ 10 years education)	38.2	35.8	42.7
Medium (11–14 years education)	38.2	33.4	32.4
High (≥ 15 years education)	23.6	30.8	24.9
Self-reported health status			
Excellent / very good	26.2	35.0	37.1
Good	46.7	37.2	38.8
Moderate / poor	27.1	27.8	29.4

Subgroup analyses

Due to a relatively small number of migrants, we showed the results for two main groups of migrants: non-western and western. These two groups being heterogeneous, we performed subgroup analyses for the largest countries of origin. We found no major differences in motives and expectations between the countries.

Discussion

Principal findings and interpretation

The most important motives for contacting a GP cooperative were similar for both migrants and native Dutch patients, namely worry, an urgent need for a GP and a need for medical information. We also found some differences, especially between non-western migrants

Table 3 Motives and expectations of patients for contacting a GP cooperative (%)

	Non-western (*N* = 475)	Western (*N* = 700)	Native dutch (*N* = 10,308)
Motive[1]			
I urgently needed a GP	54.9	52.4	48.2
I was worried	49.3	43.0	45.3
I needed medical information	21.3	26.2	27.2
My own GP could not be contacted during office hours	18.7	15.7	12.2
I had been referred to the GP cooperative by another caregiver	3.6	3.5	4.6
I did not have time to go to the GP during the day	3.3	1.9	1.3
The ED was not prepared to help me	3.0	2.1	0.8
I needed a second opinion	2.6	1.1	0.8
Expectation[1]			
Seeing a doctor	46.2	46.6	44.5
Advice	39.6	41.5	39.7
Physical examination	27.4	18.6	19.3
Prescription or medication	24.5	20.3	17.1
Reassurance	24.0	19.8	16.6
Referral to a hospital	12.2	13.2	12.0
Treatment (e.g. a stitch)	7.4	7.4	7.5

[1]Multiple answers were possible

Table 4 Logistic regression of motives and expectations of patients for contacting a GP cooperative ($N = 11,483$)

	OR Non-western[a, b] (99% CI)	OR Western[a, b] (99% CI)
Motive		
I urgently needed a GP	**1.65 (1.27–2.16)***	1.13 (0.91–1.41)
I was worried	0.96 (0.73–1.28)	0.92 (0.74–1.14)
I needed medical information	**0.59 (0.43–0.81)***	0.96 (0.74–1.25)
My own GP could not be contacted during office hours	**1.71 (1.21–2.43)***	**1.38 (1.04–1.84)***
Expectation		
Seeing a doctor	1.23 (0.96–1.59)	1.09 (0.87–1.35)
Advice	0.79 (0.59–1.07)	1.09 (0.87–1.35)
Physical examination	**1.53 (1.14–2.04)***	0.94 (0.71–1.23)
Prescription or medication	**1.37 (1.00–1.88)***	1.22 (0.94–1.59)
Reassurance	1.34 (0.96–1.85)	1.28 (0.99–1.67)
Referral to a hospital	1.28 (0.87–1.90)	1.10 (0.81–1.49)
Treatment (e.g. a stitch)	1.00 (0.60–1.67)	0.98 (0.64–1.50)

OR Odds Ratio, *CI* Confidence Interval
[a]Reference category: Native Dutch patients
[b]Corrected for gender, age, education and self-reported health status
*$p < 0.01$, in bold

and native Dutch patients. Compared to native Dutch patients, non-western migrants more often perceived an urgent need for contact with a GP. On the other hand, they less often mentioned a need for medical information. This could be explained by the fact that non-western migrants may have lower health literacy skills, resulting in poorer knowledge of healthcare services [18] and not knowing when to contact a GP cooperative [19, 30].

Migrants also reported more often that they could not contact their own GP during office hours. The accessibility of daytime general practice could be worse for migrants, because they are residing more often in urban areas where telephone accessibility in daytime general practices is generally poorer than in rural areas [31]. Moreover, longer telephone waiting times in daytime primary care are known to be associated with a higher use of out-of-hours primary care [11]. In addition, due to language barriers, migrants may have poorer negotiation skills, leading to barriers of accessing daytime general practice [32, 33].

Regardless of origin, most patients expected to see a doctor or to get advice. Non-western migrants more often expected to get a physical examination or to get a prescription or medication as opposed to native Dutch patients. Whenever migrants went to a physician in their country of origin, they were used to getting a physical examination or prescription and were reassured by these actions [34]. This could be possibly account for these differences.

Comparison with existing literature

To our knowledge, the motives or expectations of migrants for contacting a GP cooperative have not been studied previously. The most often mentioned motives for contacting a GP cooperative mentioned in our study are in accordance with a British study on motives of the general public for contacting a primary care out-of-hours service [35]. Moreover a Dutch study about non-urgent contacts found worry, the perceived need for urgent contact with a GP and the need for medical information as most important motives for contacting a GP cooperative [14]. The importance of a physical examination in medical encounters, especially with migrants, is known from national as well as international qualitative studies [34, 36, 37].

Our finding that migrants experience difficulties in the accessibility of their own GP is consistent with a British study, which found that patients in deprived areas perceived more difficulties in accessing their GP during consultation hours [32]. A Danish study found that migrants more often reported going to the ED because they could not contact a GP, or were not able to explain their problem on the telephone [33]. A Norwegian study reported that migrants were less likely to consider contacting a GP before attending the ED, because they thought it would take too long to make an appointment to consult a GP and they expected the ED to be better able to deal with their problem than a GP [38].

Strengths and limitations

A strength of our study is that we used a large dataset for this research, with a large group of patients from different GP cooperatives spread across the Netherlands. About one third of all Dutch GP cooperatives participated in this research. Our analyses were controlled for patient characteristics and cluster effects, while missing values had been imputated. The response rate was 45.9%, which is similar to response rates in other patient questionnaires in the setting of out-of-hours primary care services (39.7% to 45.7%) [39].

A limitation of our study is that we were not able to perform a non-response analysis; therefore it is difficult to determine whether our results are representative of all patients contacting a GP cooperative. The proportion of migrants was low compared to the proportion of migrants in the Dutch population, especially non-western migrants (4.1% versus 12.1%). Possibly, less integrated migrants were less likely to answer the questionnaire, due to language barriers [40]. Compared to the Dutch population, the distribution of the educational level of non-western migrants in our sample was the same. Even so, this is not representative of the whole non-western migrant community in the Netherlands (lower educational level) [41]. Moreover, it is unlikely that this is representative of the population who contacted a GP cooperative. This bias is due to the research method used: a written questionnaire in Dutch. Therefore, the migrants in our sample are not representative of all migrants in the Netherlands. Based on literature we can assume that lower educated non-western migrants face even more barriers in consulting their GP during daytime, due to limited health literacy [42]. In the analyses we corrected for self-reported health status, which is a subjective health measure reflecting a person's general perception of health. However, self-reported health status is widely used in several studies, also among migrants, being a good predictor of objective health status [43].

The number of migrants being small, we showed the results for two main groups of migrants: non-western and western. We are aware that these are two heterogeneous groups. Subgroup analyses for the largest countries of origin in the Netherlands showed that no major differences existed between those countries. In our study we did not have information about the urgencies of the contacts, neither about the medical history of the patients. Therefore it was not possible to relate the motives and expectations to the medical urgency (according medical professionals) of the contacts, which may (partly) explain the differences in motives and expectation between non-western migrants and native Dutch patients.

Implications for practice and future studies

Our results provide us with leads for practice and further research. It is important that migrants are informed about the healthcare system in the country in which they currently reside. Migrants are known not to be always very well-informed about the system [30]. Information on the purpose of the GP cooperative can be provided in general practices, during integration courses or in social meetings of migrants.

In addition, tailored communication by the patients' own GPs is essential, breaking down possible language barriers and taking into account low literacy. GPs could examine the expectations of their patients during consultations, give self-care advice if possible and inquire whether their patients accept and understand the advice given. This can be combined with an explanation about the Dutch healthcare system. The accessibility of daytime general practice could be a subject of further study. We recommend to examine whether the daytime GP practice is less accessible for migrants, and if so, how this can be improved. We also recommend to study the health literacy of migrants to manage their (minor) problems at home, possibly with support of primary health care organisations. Their experiences can help other migrants to gain access to daytime general practice or to use self-care. For the future our advice would be to offer this questionnaire also orally and in other languages, to reach a larger and more representative group of migrants. Finally, an in-depth qualitative study could provide further insight into the motives, expectations, and circumstances that increase the likelihood of migrants accessing out-of-hours primary health care. Combining this qualitative information with our quantitative results could lead to more concrete recommendations for practice.

Conclusion

Worry, the perceived need for a GP and for medical information are the most important reasons for contacting a GP cooperative, regardless of the patient's ethnic background. Patients expect to see a doctor and to get advice. Compared to native Dutch patients, non-western migrants more often want their GP to undertake some kind of action, e.g. an examination or prescription, and not just provide passive forms of assistance such as medical information. At the same time, they experience problems accessing their own GP during office hours. We recommend the stimulation of self-care, educating migrants about the purpose of a GP cooperative and examining and improving access to daytime primary care, especially for migrants.

Abbreviations

CI: Confidence interval; ED: Emergency department; GP: General practitioner

Acknowledgements

We would like to thank all participants in the study as well as Anita Oude Bos for collecting the data.

Funding

This work was financially supported by the participating GP cooperatives. The funding sources had no involvement in the study design, collection, analysis or interpretation of data, nor in writing the article.

Authors' contributions
EK designed the study, performed the statistical analyses, interpreted the data and drafted the manuscript. PB participated in designing the study, the statistical analyses and interpretation of the data. FA advised on the statistical analyses and critically revised the manuscript. PG and MM designed the study, participated in the interpretation of the data and critically revised the manuscript. MS and MW participated in the interpretation of the data and critically revised the manuscript for important intellectual content. All authors read and approved the final manuscript.

Consent for publication
Not applicable

Competing interests
The authors declare that they have no competing interests.

Author details
[1]Scientific Center for Quality of Healthcare (IQ healthcare), Radboud Institute for Health Sciences, Radboud University Medical Center, P.O. Box 9101, 6500, HB, Nijmegen, The Netherlands. [2]Department of Primary and Community Care, Radboud Institute for Health Sciences, Radboud University Medical Center, P.O. Box 9101, 6500, HB, Nijmegen, The Netherlands. [3]Pharos, Centre of Expertise of Health Disparities, P.O. Box 13318, 3507, LH, Utrecht, The Netherlands.

References
1. International Organization for Migration (IOM): World Migration Report 2015. In Geneva: IOM; 2015.
2. Centraal Bureau voor de Statistiek [Statistics Netherlands]: Bevolking. generatie, geslacht, leeftijd en herkomstgroepering, 15 september 2016 [Population; generation, gender, age and origin, 15 September 2016] [http://statline.cbs.nl/StatWeb/publication/?DM=SLNL&PA=37325&D1=0&D2=a&D3=0&D4=0&D5=a&D6=l&HDR=G2,G3&STB=G1,G5,T,G4&VW=T]. Accessed 11-11-2016.
3. van Duin C, Stoeldraijer L: Bevolkingsprognose 2014–2060: groei door migratie [Population prognosis 2014–2060: growth through migration]. In. Den Haag: Centraal Bureau voor de Statistiek [Statistics Netherlands]; 2014.
4. Norredam M, Nielsen SS, Krasnik A. Migrants' utilization of somatic healthcare services in Europe–a systematic review. Eur J Pub Health. 2010;20(5):555–63.
5. Uiters E, Deville W, Foets M, Spreeuwenberg P, Groenewegen PP. Differences between immigrant and non-immigrant groups in the use of primary medical care; a systematic review. BMC Health Serv Res. 2009;9:76.
6. Sole-Auro A, Guillen M, Crimmins EM. Health care usage among immigrants and native-born elderly populations in eleven European countries: results from SHARE. Eur J Health Econ. 2012;13(6):741–54.
7. Uiters E, Deville WL, Foets M, Groenewegen PP. Use of health care services by ethnic minorities in The Netherlands: do patterns differ? Eur J Pub Health. 2006;16(4):388–93.
8. Sandvik H, Hunskaar S, Diaz E. Immigrants' use of emergency primary health care in Norway: a registry-based observational study. BMC Health Serv Res. 2012;12:308.
9. Norredam M, Krasnik A, Moller Sorensen T, Keiding N, Joost Michaelsen J, Sonne Nielsen A. Emergency room utilization in Copenhagen: a comparison of immigrant groups and Danish-born residents. Scand J Public Health. 2004;32(1):53–9.
10. Jansen T, Zwaanswijk M, Hek K, de Bakker D. To what extent does sociodemographic composition of the neighbourhood explain regional differences in demand of primary out-of-hours care: a multilevel study. BMC Fam Pract. 2015;16:54.
11. Smits M, Peters Y, Broers S, Keizer E, Wensing M, Giesen P. Association between general practice characteristics and use of out-of-hours GP cooperatives. BMC Fam Pract. 2015;16(52)
12. Philips H, Remmen R, De Paepe P, Buylaert W, Van Royen P. Out of hours care: a profile analysis of patients attending the emergency department and the general practitioner on call. BMC Fam Pract. 2010;11:88.
13. Padela AI, Punekar IR. Emergency medical practice: advancing cultural competence and reducing health care disparities. Acad Emerg Med. 2009;16(1):69–75.
14. Keizer E, Smits M, Peters Y, Huibers L, Giesen P, Wensing M. Contacts with out-of-hours primary care for nonurgent problems: patients' beliefs or deficiencies in healthcare? BMC Fam Pract. 2015;16(1):157.
15. Stirbu I, Kunst AE, Bos V, Mackenbach JP. Differences in avoidable mortality between migrants and the native Dutch in The Netherlands. BMC Public Health. 2006;6:78.
16. Devillé W, Uiters E, Westert GP, Groenewegen P: Perceived health and consultation of GPs among ethnic minorities compared to the general population in the Netherlands. In: In: Westert GP, Jabaaij L, François G, editors Morbidity, performance and quality in primary care. edn. Oxford: Radcliffe Publishing Ltd; 2006: 85–96.
17. Rechel B, Mladovsky P, Ingleby D, Mackenbach JP, McKee M. Migration and health in an increasingly diverse Europe. Lancet. 2013;381(9873):1235–45.
18. Berkman ND, Sheridan SL, Donahue KE, Halpern DJ, Viera A, Crotty K, Holland A, Brasure M, Lohr KN, Harden E, et al. Health literacy interventions and outcomes: an updated systematic review. Evid Rep Technol Assess (Full Rep). 2011;199:1–941.
19. Willems S, Peersman W, De Maeyer P, Buylaert W, De Maeseneer J, De Paepe P. The impact of neighborhood deprivation on patients' unscheduled out-of-hours healthcare seeking behavior: a cross-sectional study. BMC Fam Pract. 2013;14(1):136.
20. Dye C, O'Garra A. Preface. The science of infectious diseases. Philos Trans R Soc Lond Ser B Biol Sci. 2014;369(1645):20140055.
21. Faber MJ, Burgers JS, Westert GP. A sustainable primary care system: lessons from the Netherlands. J Ambul Care Manage. 2012;35(3):174–81.
22. Smits M, Rutten M, Keizer E, Wensing M, Westert G, Giesen P. The development and performance of after-hours primary Care in the Netherlands: a narrative review. Ann Intern Med. 2017;166(10):737–42.
23. Ineen: Benchmarkbulletin huisartsenposten 2015 [Benchmark report GP cooperatives 2015]. In.; 2016.
24. Hanssens LG, Detollenaere J, Hardyns W, Willems SJ. Access, treatment and outcomes of care: a study of ethnic minorities in Europe. Int J Public Health. 2016;61(4):443–54.
25. Delnoij DM, Rademakers JJ, Groenewegen PP. The Dutch consumer quality index: an example of stakeholder involvement in indicator development. BMC Health Serv Res. 2010;10:88.
26. Hammink A, Giesen P: CQ-index huisartsenposten. Meetinstrumentontwikeling en onderzoek naar discriminerend vermogen [CQ-index GP cooperatives. Development and discriminative power]. In. Nijmegen: Scientific Institute for Quality of Healthcare (IQ healthcare), Radboudumc; 2010.
27. Centraal Bureau voor de Statistiek [Statistics Netherlands]: Standaarddefinitie allochtonen [Standard definition migrants]. In. Voorburg: Centraal Bureau voor de Statistiek [Statistics Netherlands]; 2000.
28. Smits M, Huibers L, Oude Bos A, Giesen P. Patient satisfaction with out-of-hours GP cooperatives: a longitudinal study. Scand J Prim Health Care. 2012; 30(4):206–13.
29. Paddison C, Elliott M, Parker R, Staetsky L, Lyratzopoulos G, Campbell JL, Roland M. Should measures of patient experience in primary care be adjusted for case mix? Evidence from the English general practice patient survey. BMJ Qual Saf. 2012;21(8):634–40.
30. Rechel B, Mladovsky P, Deville W, Rijks B, Petrova-Benedict R, McKee M. Migration and health in the European Union. In. McGras-Hill Education. European Observatory on Health Systems and Policies Series: Maidenhead; 2011.
31. Inspectie voor de Gezondheidszorg (IGZ) [Dutch Health Care Inspectorate]: Telefonische bereikbaarheid huisartsen nog steeds onder de maat [Telephone accessibility of GPs still below standard]. In. Den Haag: Ministerie van Volksgezondheid en Sport; 2011.
32. Drummond N, McConnachie A, O'Donnell CA, Moffat KJ, Wilson P, Ross S. Social variation in reasons for contacting general practice out-of-hours: implications for daytime service provision? Br J Gen Pract. 2000;50(455):460–4.
33. Norredam M, Mygind A, Nielsen AS, Bagger J, Krasnik A. Motivation and relevance of emergency room visits among immigrants and patients of Danish origin. Eur J Pub Health. 2007;17(5):497–502.
34. O'Donnell CA, Higgins M, Chauhan R, Mullen K. Asylum seekers' expectations of and trust in general practice: a qualitative study. Br J Gen Pract. 2008;58(557):e1–11.

35. Shipman C, Dale J. Using and providing out-of-hours services: can patients and GPs agree? Health Soc Care Community. 1999;7(4):266–75.
36. Hemke F. Onbekend maakt onbemind. Huisartsenzorg voor migranten. Knelpunten & mogelijke oplossingen [Unknown, unloved. GP care for migrants. Problems and possible solutions]. In. Pharos, Julius Centrum - afdeling huisartsengeneeskunde: Utrecht; 2010.
37. Teunissen E, Sherally J, van den Muijsenbergh M, Dowrick C, Van Weel-Baumgarten E, van Weel C. mental health problems of undocumented migrants (UMs) in The Netherlands: a qualitative exploration of help-seeking behaviour and experiences with primary care. BMJ Open. 2014;4(11):e005738.
38. Mahmoud I, Eley R, Hou XY. Subjective reasons why immigrant patients attend the emergency department. BMC Emerg Med. 2015;15:4.
39. Garratt AM, Danielsen K, Hunskaar S. Patient satisfaction questionnaires for primary care out-of-hours services: a systematic review. Br J Gen Pract. 2007; 57(542):741–7.
40. Centraal Bureau voor de Statistiek [Statistics Netherlands]: Enqueteonderzoek onder allochtonen. Problemen en oplossingen [Survey research among migrants. Problems and solutions]. In. Voorburg/Heerlen: CBS; 2005.
41. Centraal Bureau voor de Statistiek [Statistics Netherlands]: Bevolking; hoogst behaald onderwijsniveau; geslacht, leeftijd en herkomst, 17 mei 2016 [Population; highest education level; gender, age and origin, 17 May 2016] [http://statline.cbs.nl/Statweb/publication/?DM=SLNL&PA=82275NED&D1=0&D2=0&D3=0&D4=a&D5=1-3,l&D6=39,44,49,54,59&VW=T]. Accessed 11-11-2016.
42. Heijmans M, Zwikker H, van der Heide I, Rademakers J. Hoe kunnen we de zorg beter laten aansluiten bij mensen met lage gezondheidsvaardigheden? [How can we make healthcare better attuned to people with low health literacy?]. In. NIVEL: Utrecht; 2016.
43. Wu S, Wang R, Zhao Y, Ma X, Wu M, Yan X, He J. The relationship between self-rated health and objective health status: a population-based study. BMC Public Health. 2013;13:320.
44. Mossialos E, Wenzl M, Osborn R, Anderson C: International profiles of health care systems, 2014. In: The Commonwealth Fund; 2015.

12

Prevalence, aetiologies and prognosis of the symptom dizziness in primary care

Stefan Bösner*, Sonja Schwarm, Paula Grevenrath, Laura Schmidt, Kaja Hörner, Dominik Beidatsch, Milena Bergmann, Annika Viniol, Annette Becker and Jörg Haasenritter

Abstract

Background: Dizziness is a common reason for consulting a general practitioner and there is a broad range of possible underlying aetiologies. There are few evidence-based data about prevalence, aetiology and prognosis in primary care. We aimed to conduct a systematic review of symptom-evaluating studies on prevalence, aetiology or prognosis of dizziness in primary care.

Methods: We systematically searched MEDLINE and EMBASE. Two independent researchers screened titles and abstracts according to predefined criteria. We included all studies evaluating the symptoms 'dizziness' or 'vertigo' as a reason for consultation in primary care. We extracted data about study population and methodology and prevalence, aetiology and prognosis. Two raters independently judged study quality and risk of bias. We investigated the variation across studies using forest plots, I^2 and prediction intervals. Since we anticipated a great amount of clinical and unexplained statistical heterogeneity, we provided qualitative syntheses instead of pooled estimates.

Results: We identified 31 studies (22 on prevalence, 14 on aetiology and 8 on prognosis). Consultation prevalence differs between 1,0 and 15,5%. The most common aetiologies are vestibular/peripheral (5,4-42,1%), benign peripheral positional vertigo (4,3-39,5%), vestibular neuritis (0,6-24,0%), Menière's disease (1,4-2,7%), cardiovascular disease (3,8-56,8%), neurological disease (1,4-11,4%), psychogenic (1,8-21,6%), no clear diagnosis (0,0-80,2%). While studies based on subjective patient assessment reported improvement rates from 37 to 77%, these findings could not be confirmed when applying instruments that measure symptom severity or quality of life.

Conclusion: There is a broad variety of possible underlying diseases for the symptom dizziness. There exist only few methodologically sound studies concerning aetiology and prognosis of dizziness.

Keywords: Family practice, Dizziness, Vertigo, Diagnosis, Systematic review

Background

Dizziness is a common complaint and frequent reason for consultation in primary care virtually affecting every person once in his or her lifetime [1]. While dizziness is a more subjective and vague symptom referring to a sense of spatial disorientation, motion of the environment, or light headedness, vertigo (as a subcategory of dizziness) is described as an illusion of movement, either of the external world revolving around the individual or of the individual revolving in space. Both symptoms can be caused by a broad spectrum of diseases ranging from benign and self-limiting (e.g. neuritis vestibularis) to severe and potentially life-threatening causes (e.g. cardiac arrhythmias or acute cerebral-vascular events) [2].

Dizziness affects patients in many ways. It is one of the most important single symptoms with a negative influence on well-being in old age [3]. While life-threatening illness is rare, many patients with dizziness do have serious functional impairment, such as increased risks for falls, significant disability, handicap and

* Correspondence: boesner@staff.uni-marburg.de
Department of General Practice / Family Medicine, University of Marburg, Karl-von-Frisch-Str, 435043 Marburg, Germany

increased incidence of symptom-related fears, anxiety or depression [4, 5].

For most patients with dizziness the general practitioner (GP) is the first contact person within the official healthcare system. In comparison to different specialists like neurologists, ENT doctors or cardiologists who would only provide a workup for selected underlying diseases, GPs are trained to identify the whole range of possible aetiologies for the symptom dizziness. Hereby it is not always necessary to make an exact diagnosis as GPs in their role as gatekeepers first of all need to identify patients with uncomplicated diseases (which are often self-limiting, needing only symptomatic relief) while not overseeing potential serious diseases, which need further investigation and at times immediate therapy. In this process, GPs base their decisions predominantly on history and clinical examination. In order to do so effectively, they need setting specific knowledge about the prevalence, possible underlying aetiologies and their respective frequencies (pre-test probabilities) and the prognosis of the respective symptom to reach an acceptable diagnostic decision. Because of already selected patients and consequently resulting differing pre-test probabilities, data generated in secondary care are not applicable for the primary care context.

There has been a recently published systematic review about health care utilization, prognosis and outcomes of vestibular disease in primary care [6]. As far as we know there are no systematic reviews summarizing current evidence concerning prevalence, aetiology and prognosis of dizziness in primary care.

We aimed to answer three questions: 1) How often do patients present with dizziness in primary care, i.e. what is the prevalence/ incidence of the symptom in this setting? 2) What are the underlying aetiologies and their respective frequencies? 3) What is the prognosis of these patients?

Methods

Types of studies

We performed a systematic review including symptom evaluating studies about dizziness in a primary care setting. Symptom evaluating studies are defined as studies that examine patients presenting with a defined symptom in a given health care setting. These studies seek to investigate prevalence/incidence, underlying aetiologies and prognosis for patients presenting with this symptom [7].

Inclusion- and exclusion criteria

We included all original research articles evaluating the symptoms "dizziness" and "vertigo" as a primary or a secondary consulting reason at a primary care setting. We did not limit our search to the date of publications, patient age or study quality. All types of studies except qualitative studies, case reports and narrative reviews could be included.

The findings of the studies had to include at least one of the following estimates: prevalence or incidence of dizziness and/or vertigo, information about underlying diagnoses and/or prognoses. There was no restriction regarding to the kinds of data assessment, outcome measurement or the study quality. We excluded studies that evaluated other settings than primary care (e.g. hospital care, emergency centres, secondary care) and studies, in which patients were selected before recruitment, for example because of an increased probability for a specific underlying diagnosis.

Search strategy

In January 2015, we did a computer-based search of the PUBMED and EMBASE databases. The authors also screened the reference list of all relevant studies (snow ball search). Studies published in English, German, Dutch, Italian, Russian, Swedish, French and Spanish were included.

We used the following search syntax for electronic searches:

We defined two main search concepts ("dizziness" and "primary care") and combined them by "AND". To operationalize "dizziness", we used the terms "dizziness", "vertigo", "giddiness" and "light headedness" in different ways of notations (in title or abstract) OR the MESH terms "dizziness" and "vertigo". To operationalize "primary care", we used four different strategies and combined them by OR: (1) the terms "primary care", "general practice" or "general practitioner" in different ways of notations in title or abstract, (2) the MESH terms "family practice", "physicians, family", "primary Health care" and "rural health", (3) paper was published in a journal, which typically covers primary care research OR (4) the term "primary care" in different ways of notations appeared in the affiliation of at least the main author. The whole syntax can be found in Additional file 1.

Selection of publications

All identified studies went through a two-step selection process. First, we screened titles and abstracts. Studies meeting all three selection criteria "original research article", "inclusion of patients because of dizziness and/ or vertigo" and "primary care setting" were applied as potential appropriate. In the next step, we analysed the full texts of the selected articles regarding to inclusion- and exclusion criteria. Reasons for exclusion were documented.

Two independent review authors (SS/PG or SS/LS for title/abstracts; SS/DB or SS/MB for full texts) did the whole selection process. Disagreements were resolved by discussion between the respective two review authors (SS, PG, LS, DB, and MB). A third review author (either JH or SB) was consulted if disagreement persisted.

Data extraction

We extracted bibliographic data (author, publication year, title and journal), country, setting, study design, inclusion- and exclusion criteria, kind of recruitment, study population (age, gender distribution), study duration. To answer the first research question (prevalence/incidence), we registered the number of dizziness cases and the number and type of the population from which the cases descended from (e.g. number of all practice consultations or all registered patients of a practice). Furthermore, we extracted all diagnostic categories and their absolute and relative frequencies (second research question "aetiology"). Finally, we documented every kind of prognostic outcome (third research question). In addition, we differentiated in our sub-analysis, where data allowed doing so, patients with dizziness from patients suffering from vertigo.

Quality assessment

To our knowledge, no tools exist yet to assess the risk of bias in symptom evaluating studies. Therefore, we developed a standardized tool, based on the sparse methodological literature [7, 8] and own previous experience in the area [9, 10]. Two reviewers (SS and KH) independently answered signal questions and assessed the risk of bias separately for four key domains: selection of patients and GPs, data collection and patient flow, determination of the underlying aetiology, and determination of the prognosis. The characteristic values were documented with "yes", "no" or "unclear". In addition, reviewers rated their concern that the selection of patients and GPs might had introduced clinical heterogeneity. A detailed description of the tool can be found in Additional file 2.

Data analysis

Studies can use different measures to report the prevalence or incidence of the symptom in a particular setting, e.g. patients presenting with the symptom in relation to all patients presenting in a specified time period; number of consultations due to the particular symptom in relation to all consultations in a specified time period etc. Since the definition of the nominator and denominator of the frequency measure has a major influence on the results, we grouped studies according to the frequency measure and plotted the results using forest plots. To answer question 2 (aetiologies and respective frequencies), we aimed to estimate how often dizziness and/or vertigo were caused by a particular aetiology. For each study presenting data for a particular condition, we calculated the respective proportion and the 95% confidence interval using the Wilson procedure with a correction for continuity. [11] We grouped all eligible studies by underlying aetiologies and plotted the results using forest plots.

We used different measures to quantify the variability across studies: I^2 quantifies the percentage of variation that is not due to chance [12]. Tau^2 is an estimate of the between-study variance in a random-effects meta-analysis [12]. Note that in our case the term 'effect' refers to a proportion, e.g. proportion of patients with a particular condition. The interpretation of tau^2 is not intuitive. However, it allows the calculation of prediction interval. Prediction intervals can be interpreted as a range within the "true" proportion of a future study that is similar to those included in the analysis will lie with a probability of 95% [13]. Besides the number of studies, the heterogeneity across studies determines the width of the interval.

Since we expected substantial variation across studies due to different sources (methodological heterogeneity as well as clinical heterogeneity caused by different definitions of the symptom, of underlying conditions, differences in the diagnostic and prognostic work-up, case-mix, health care system and time period), we aimed to provide only qualitative summaries instead of pooled estimates.As there was only a limited number of studies that contributed data to our third research question (prognosis), we analysed these data only descriptively.

Data analysis was done by the statistical program R 3.1.2 (R Foundation for statistical analysis, Vienna, Austria).

Results

Search result and study selection

Our initial search identified 1598 references in EMBASE and 903 in PUBMED. The snowball search identified eleven references. After extraction of 332 duplicates, 2501 unique references remained. The title and abstract screening of these references detected 120 studies as potential appropriate. Finally, the full text analysis of these trials produced 31 studies, which met the inclusion criteria. Further details are given in a flow chart (Fig. 1).

Included studies

Data accrue mainly from Europe (21 studies) and USA (five studies). Time of publications varied between 1972 and 2014. Twenty three studies took place in general practice, five in primary health care centres and the remaining three in hospital based

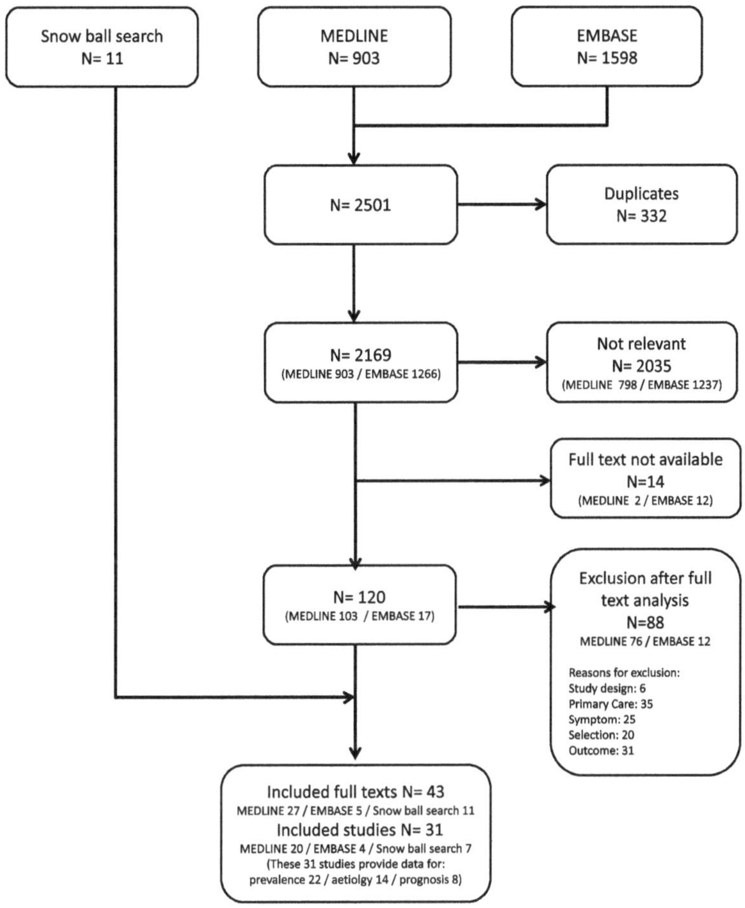

Fig. 1 Flow chart

primary care centres. Studies varied widely concerning the number on included patients with dizziness ranging from 30 to 10,871. The percentage of women included was mentioned in 16 studies ranging from 58 to 80%. Nineteen of the included studies recruited patients prospectively during the consultations; the other studies were based on chart review and routine data. Further details of the included studies are shown in Table 1.

Quality of included studies

Quality assessment happened for four distinctive domains. For domain A (selection of patients and GPs), 14 studies had a low, three an unclear and 12 a high risk of bias. For domain B (data collection and patient flow), 19 studies had a low, one an unclear and ten a high risk of bias. For domain C (assessment of aetiology), two studies had a low, two an unclear and ten a high risk of bias. For domain D (assessment of prognosis), five studies had a low, two an unclear and one a high risk of bias. Table 2 summarizes the quality assessment of all included studies.

Prevalence of the symptoms "dizziness" and "vertigo" in primary care

Twentry two studies commented on prevalence data, nine of them had a low risk of bias. Depending on numerator and denominator, results for prevalence can be grouped in four categories. Four studies describe the number of patients who have contacted a physician at least once because of dizziness/vertigo in relation to all listed patients. Prevalence ranges from 0,8% [14] to 7,9% (DNSGP-2) [15]. Seven studies describe the number of patients with dizziness in relation to all patients seen in consultation. Prevalence ranges from 1,2% [16] to 8,1% [17]. Five studies describe the number of consultations due to the symptom dizziness in relation to all consultations (e.g. if the same patient has more than one consultation he is here counted more than one time). Prevalence ranges from 1,0% (BEACH) [18] to 15,5% [19]. In four of the five studies results are below 2%, only the study done by Wun et al. represents with 15,5% an outlier. 50% of the patients seen in this study suffered from hypertension. The authors assume that patients utilized the symptom "dizziness" as a kind of entrance

Table 1 Brief description of the included studies

Studies	Time of recruitment	Country	Setting	Number of dizzy patients	Mean Age of study sample (range)	Female (%)	Data collection	Inclusion criteria	Exclusion criteria	Answered research questions[b]
BEACH 2014 [18]	04/2013 - 03/2014	Australia	959 general practitioners	993	n.r.	n.r.	prospective	all patients contacts ICPC: Reason for encounter vertigo/ dizziness		1
Bird 1998 [39]	08/1993 - 071995	Great Britain	3 general practices	503	median 58 (3-99)	n.r.	retrospective	complaining of symptoms allied to dizziness ➔ stratified sample was studied in more detail	patients had seen their GP about the same problem within the past 12 months	1,2
CONTENT 2007 [1]	04/2005 - 12/2006	Germany	17 general practices	607	n.r.	70.8[a]	prospective	all patients contacts ICPC: Reason for encounter N17 – vertigo/ dizziness		1
DNSGP-2 2010 [15]	01/2001 - 12/2001	Netherlands	96 family practices	3990	76.1 (SEM 0.11) (65+)	65.9	prospective	database with presented symptoms recorded as freetext: Dutch synonyms for dizziness		1,2
Ekvall 2004 [16]	1998 and 2000	Sweden	2 health care centres (14 GPs)	311	range 12-94	74.9[a]	retrospective	ICD9/10: 780.4 / R 42 and 386 / H81		1
Ekvall 2005 [3]	01/2003 - 12/2003	Sweden	6 primary health care centres	prev: 197 aet: 38	prev: range 65-99 aet: Median 83 (65-94)	prev: 70.1[a] aet: 65.8[a]	prev: retrospective aet: prospective	prev: 65 years or older diagnosis R42 (ICD 10) aet: study participants; ICD 10 Code R 42		1,2
Fink 2007 [40]	10/1989 - 09/1999	Austria	1 general practitioner	408[a]	n.r.	n.r.	prospective	all Episodes of Cares: dizziness as reason for encounter		1
Garrigues 2008 [41]	11/2003 - 11/2004	Spain	6 primary care centres	191	55.8 (SD 17.6) (range 10+)	68.6	prospective	vertigo crisis (illusion of unequivocal rotary movement)	under 10 years	1
Gerber 1992 [42]	15 months	USA	general internal medicine group practice (4 general internists)	46	range 18+	n.r.	prospective	all physical complaints reported complaint of dizziness		1
Hanley 2002 [43]	10/1999 - 03/2000	Ireland	13 general practitioners	70	n.r.	n.r.	prospective	vertigo (do you see the world spin around you as if you had got off a playground roundabout)		2
Harding 1980 [44]	n.r.	Colombia, India, Sudan, Philippines	primary health facilities	90	range 16+	n.r.	prospective	reason for encounter of all patients aged 16 or older: dizziness	so seriously ill or required such urgent medical care that it would be unreasonable to administer the research questionnaires pat. Who refused to take part pat. Who had already attended once	1
Hopkins 1989 [45]	1981 - 1982	Great Britain	48 general practices (143 doctors)	n.r.	n.r.	n.r.	unclear	patients consulting for ICD 9: 780.4 and 386		1
Jayarajan 2003 [14]	08/2000 - 07/2001	Great Britain	53 general practitioners	62,6 average (3318)	range 5+ 5-20: 1.3% 20-40: 13.5% 40-60: 24.7% 60-80: 40.5% > 80: 20%	n.r.	retrospective	dizziness		1

Table 1 Brief description of the included studies *(Continued)*

Studies	Time of recruitment	Country	Setting	Number of dizzy patients	Mean Age of study sample (range)	Female (%)	Data collection	Inclusion criteria	Exclusion criteria	Answered research questions[b]
Kroenke 1989 [25]	08/1984 – 07/1987	USA	Internal Medicine clinic at Brooke Army Medical Center (primary care)	55	n.r.	n.r.	retrospective	dizziness (new complaint or recurrent complaint that prompted a new diagnostic workup)	chronic dizziness	1,2,3
Kroenke 1998 [26]	n.r.	USA	Walter Reed Army Medical Center general medicine walk-in clinic	30	adults	n.r.	prospective	adult outpatients presenting with physical complaints (excl. Upper respiratory infection) dizziness		3
Kwong 2005 [4]	02/2001 – 01/2003	Canada	1 family practice center	50	range 65-91 < 80: 38% > = 80 62%	58	retrospective	ICD 9 code of "780" (dizziness) 65 years of age or older random sample of eligible charts	Patients who are discharged from service or died	2
Lawson 1999 [35]	a 3 month period	Great Britain	general practitioners from 4 practices	50	74 (61-78)	74[a]	prospective	patients presenting with dizziness more than 60 years of age		1,2
Maarsingh 2010 [23, 36]	06/2006 - 01/2008	Netherlands	45 family physicians in 24 family practices	417	78.5 (65-95)	74	prospective	dizziness being present for at least 2 weeks main reason for consultation 65 years or older	inability to speak Dutch or English, severe cognitive impairment, severe visual impairment (i.e. corrected visual acuity of less than 3/60 for the best eye), severe hearing impairment (i.e. verbal communication impossible), wheelchair dependency	2,3
Mash 2012 [46]	n.r.	South Africa	240 health workers (nurses saw 86,1% of the patients) in mobile clinics, fixed clinics and community health centres	299	n.r.	n.r.	prospective	all patients contacts ICPC: Reason for encounter N17 – vertigo/ dizziness		1
MedViP 2008 [47]	04/2001 - 12/2002	Germany	138 primary care practices	10,871	59	67.2	retrospective	ICD 10 Codes (H81, H82, A88, R42) dizziness medication synonyms for dizziness diagnoses		1,2
Morrell 1972 [48, 49]	1 year	Great Britain	1 general practice (3 doctors)	74	0-4: 1.4[a] % 5-14: 10.8[a] % 15-24: 17.6[a] % 25-44: 21.6[a] % 45-64: 25.7[a] % > 65: 23.0[a] %	70.3[a]	prospective	patients with a new symptom (which had not been presented to any doctor in the previous 12 months) disturbance of balance		1,2
NAMCS 1989 [50]	1981 and 1985	USA	family physicians, general practitioners and general internists	531	61.3 (25+)	66.7	prospective	all patients contacts Reason for encounter: S225.0 vertigo – dizziness		1
PCD 1994 [27, 51]	01-06 and 08-10 1991	USA	4 family group practices, 1 internal medicine group practice, 1 university family practice center, 1 solo general internist, 1 solo family physician, 1 county hospital emergency department	142	58.6 (17-90) > 60: 59.2% < 60: 40.8%	71.8	prospective	dizziness as chief complaint or part of a symptom complex that represented the principal reason for visit at least 18 years		2,3

Table 1 Brief description of the included studies *(Continued)*

Studies	Time of recruitment	Country	Setting	Number of dizzy patients	Mean Age of study sample (range)	Female (%)	Data collection	Inclusion criteria	Exclusion criteria	Answered research questions[b]
Rieger 2014 [52]	01/2008 - 12/2008	Germany	general practitioners	489598[a]	range 18-74	n.r.	retrospective	ICD H81, H82, R42, A88.1, E53.8, F45.8, G11.8, G43.1, G45.0-, G62, G63, G90.3, H55, H83.0– 2, I95.1, N95.1 and R26 without R26.1		1
Sicras 2007 [17]	2006	Spain	5 primary health care centers	6504	n.r.	n.r.	retrospective	ICPC diagnosis N17 vertigo/ dizziness		1
Sczepanek 2011 [24]	n.r.	Germany	21 primary care practices	69	76.19 (SD 6.64) (range 65-95)	69.6	prospective	incident dizziness (less than six months) as main reason for encounter age at least 65 years	insufficient command of the German language, dementia, terminal diseases	2,3
Transition Project 2012 [53]	1995 - 2005	Netherlands, Malta, Serbia	59 general practices (69 doctors)	n.r.	n.r.	n.r.	prospective	all patients contacts ICPC: Reason for encounter N17 – vertigo/ dizziness		1
Wun 2000 [19]	12/1997 - 03/1998	China	28 commune clinics = general practice clinics (42 primary care doctors)	1331	60.8 (SD 13.5)	n.r.	prospective	all patients contacts ICPC: Reason for encounter N17 – vertigo/ dizziness		1
Yardley 1998 [22]	n.r.	Great Britain	10 general practices	aet: 143 prog: 76	aet: 59.8[a] (18+) prog: 59.6[a]	aet: 80.4[a] prog: 82.9[a]	aet: retrospective prog: prospective	study participants 18 years and older with a complaint of dizziness patient still symptomatic	non-vestibular cause for dizziness performance of vigorous head or body movements during exercise therapy was contraindicated multiple, life-threatening or progessive central disorders	2,3
Yardley 2004 [21]	2001 - 2002	Great Britain	20 general practices	aet: 170 prog: 87	aet: 61.9[a] (18+) prog: 61.0 SD 14.42	aet: 71 prog: 71	aet: retrospective prog: prospective	study participants 18 years and older with a complaint of dizziness	Patients no longer found to be dizzy duration of dizziness less than 2 months during the past 2 years nonlabyrinthine cause of dizziness in patient records, none of the rehabilitation exercises provoked dizziness, medical contraindications for making required head movements serious comorbid conditions	2,3
Yardley 2012 [20]	10/2008 - 07/2009	Great Britain	35 general practices	112	58.2 (18 +)	75	prospective	study participants 18 years and older with a complaint of dizziness during the past two years	patients who were no longer dizzy, non vestibular causes of dizziness, dizziness was not aggravated by rapid head movements, contraindications to treatment by vestiublar rehabilitation inability to speak English	3

[a]Data not directly available in publication, but could be calculated
[b]First research question: Prevalence of the consulting reason dizziness at general practice
Second research question: Aetiology of the consulting reason dizziness at general practice
Third research question: Prognosis of the consulting reason dizziness at general practice
n.r Not reported, *prev* Prevalence, *aet* Aetiology, *prog* Prognosis, *BEACH* Bettering the Evaluation and Care of Health, *CONTENT* **CONT**inuous morbidity registration **E**pidemiologic **NeT**work, *DNSGP-2* Second Dutch National Survey of General Practice, *MedViP* Medizinische Versorgung in der Praxis, *NAMCS* National Ambulatory Medical Care Survey, *PCD* Primary Care Dizziness Study

card to get their blood pressure monitored. Finally, four studies describe the number of consultations due to the symptom dizziness in relation to all reasons for encounter. Prevalence ranges from 0,7% (BEACH) [18] to 9,9% [19]. Forest plots and measures of heterogeneity are presented in Additional file 3.

Aetiologies of the symptoms "dizziness" and "vertigo" in primary care

We identified 14 studies assessing data on the aetiology of dizziness and/or vertigo. The most common categories for dizziness were cardiovascular (3,8-56,8%) and otologic peripheral (5,4-42,1%) problems

Table 2 Risk of bias

Study	Domain A: selection of patients and GPs	Domain B: Data collection and patient flow	Domain C. diagnostic work-up	Domain D: prognostic work-up
BEACH	low	low	n.r.	n.r.
Bird 1998	?	?	high	n.r.
CONTENT	low	low	n.r.	n.r.
DNSGP-2	low	low	high	n.r.
Ekvall 2004	high	high	n.r.	n.r.
Ekvall 2005	high	high	high	n.r.
Fink 2007	high	low	n.r.	n.r.
Garrigues 2008	low	low	n.r.	n.r.
Gerber 1992	high	low	n.r.	n.r.
Hanley 2002	low	low	?	n.r.
Harding 1980	low	low	n.r.	n.r.
Hopkins 1989	high	high	n.r.	n.r.
Jayarajan 2003	high	high	n.r.	n.r.
Kroenke 1989	high	high	high	high
Kroenke 1998	low	low	n.r.	?
Kwong 2005	?	high	high	n.r.
Lawson 1999 – prev.	?	low	n.r.	n.r.
Lawson 1999 – aet.	low	low	low	n.r.
Maarsingh 2010	low	low	low	low
Mash 2012	low	low	n.r.	n.r.
MedViP –prev.	low	high	n.r.	n.r.
MedViP –aet.	high	high	high	n.r.
Morrell 1972	?	low	high	n.r.
NAMCS	low	low	n.r.	n.r.
PCD	low	low	?	?
Rieger 2014	high	high	n.r.	n.r.
Sczepanek 2011	low	low	high	low
Sicras 2007	high	high	n.r.	n.r.
Transition Project	low	low	n.r.	n.r.
Wun 2000	low	low	n.r.	n.r.
Yardley 1998	high	high	high	low
Yardley 2004 – aet.	high	high	high	n.r.
Yardley 2004 – prog.	high	low	n.r.	low
Yardley 2012	high	low	n.r.	low

Risk of bias was rated as low, high or unclear (?)
n.r Not relevant, because the respective study provided no data in regard to aetiologies and/ or prognosis
prevalence, *aet* Aetiology, *prog* Prognosis

including Benign Positional Paroxysmal Vertigo (BPPV) and vestibular neuritis. Frequent reasons for vertigo were as well otologic peripheral causes, BPPV and vestibular neuritis, whereas cardiovascular disease did not play any role. It is noteworthy that 13 out of 14 studies used a category like "no specific diagnosis possible" and that up to 80% of cases were assigned to that category. Table 3 summarizes the results for several differential diagnoses separated for the symptoms dizziness and vertigo. Forest plots and measures of heterogeneity are presented in Additional file 4.

We could identify only two studies with a low risk of bias. Both looked at older patients with the symptom dizziness and identified cardiovascular disease as main aetiology followed by peripheral vestibular disease (see Table 4).

Prognosis of the symptoms "dizziness" and "vertigo" in primary care

Prognostic parameters were assessed in eight studies (two of them with a low risk of bias) using different end-points. Three studies all conducted by Yardley et al. [20–22] used the short form of the vertigo symptom scale (ranging from 0 to 60 points). All studies were intervention studies in the field of vestibular rehabilitation. In none of the studies, the respective control groups showed a significant change of 3 points (5%) at the end of the one-year follow up period.

Five studies [20–24] looked with the help of different instruments like the dizziness handicap inventory, the vertigo handicap questionnaire or the SF 36 (short version) at changes in quality of life. All studies only showed slight improvement, which was in most instances regarded as clinically non-significant.

Five studies [20, 22, 25–27] measured subjective patient assessment. Patients reported subjective improvement in al studies ranging from 37% [5] to 77% [26].

Discussion

Summary of principal findings

This systematic review identified 31 studies of the symptoms dizziness and/or vertigo at the primary care setting. In regard to all research questions results were very heterogeneous. The most common reasons for dizziness were cardiovascular (3,8-56,8%) and otologic peripheral problems (5,4-42,1%). Frequent reasons for vertigo were as well otologic peripheral causes, BPPV and vestibular neuritis, whereas cardiovascular disease did not play any role. In up to 80% of cases no specific diagnosis could be made. Regarding prognosis, most studies only showed slight, often non-significant improvement.

Table 3 Aetiologies of dizziness and vertigo (all studies)

Dizziness				
Aetiology	Number of studies	Number of patients	Results (range)	Heterogeneity I^2 (95% CI)/prediction interval
Otologic peripher	10	10,658	5,4-42,1%	95.5% (93.4-96.9%) 7.7-51.6%
BPPV *(subcategory)*	6	7956	4,3-39,5%	93.2% (88.0-96.2%) 0.5-73.8%
Vestibular neuritis *(subcategory)*	6	7956	0,6-24,0%	98.4% (97.6-98.9%) 0.0-98.6%
Ménière's disease *(subcategory)*	4	7802	1,4-2,7%	0.0% (0.0-0.0%) 1.4-2.8%
Cardiovascular	8	3011	3,8-56,8%	98.5% (98.0-98.9%) 0.4-89.1%
Neurological central	9	10,620	1,4-11,4%	78.7% (60.0-88.7%) 2.1-12.7%
Psychogenic	8	3016	1,8-21,6%	88.5% (79.7-93.5%) 1.1-31.2%
No specific diagnosis	11	10,713	0,0-80,2%	99.4% (99.3-99.5%) 1.6-90.5%
Vertigo				
Aetiology	Number of studies	Number of patients	Results (range)	Heterogeneity I^2 /prediction interval
Otologic peripher	3	383	27.3-92.9%	96.2% (91.8-98.2%) 0.0-100.0%
BPPV *(subcategory)*	3	383	4.9-42.9%	96.4% (92.5-98.3%) 0.0-100.0%
Vestibular neuritis *(subcategory)*	3	383	8.4-40.0%	94.3% (86.8-97.6%) 0.0-100.0%
Ménière's disease*(subcategory)*	3	383	4.2-10.0%	43.5% (0.0-83.1%) 0.0-94.1%
Cardiovascular	0			
Neurological central	1	70	4.3%	n/a
Psychogenic	1	70	1.4%	n/a
No specific diagnosis	3	383	1.4-72.7%	92.3% (80.7-96.9%) 0.0-100.0%

Prevalence

Prevalence of dizziness varied markedly between studies. One reason might be that dizziness as a symptom depends on capturing and judging various sensations [2] and therefore epidemiological research faces difficulties describing and standardizing this symptom [28]. Furthermore, for identification of patients presenting with dizziness some studies counted every dizzy patient prospectively or used databases that provide data on reasons for encounter for every consultation. In contrast, other studies used routine data, with a high risk of overlooking dizzy patients with diagnoses that are not necessarily accompanied by dizziness. Both might explain heterogeneity of prevalence data.

Compared to data from emergency departments, where dizziness accounts for 2,5% [29] and 3,3% [30] of consultations, our findings provide similar figures.

Aetiology

At primary care level GPs do not necessarily need to know the exact diagnoses. This is in accordance with studies based on routine data, where in 46,0 to 80,2% of the cases an explicit diagnosis is missing. For a symptom, that according to Sloane et al. [2] resolves for most patients spontaneously, this seems to be a reasonable approach as long as avoidable life-threading conditions can be reliably identified. On the other hand, GPs describe dizziness as a confusing and difficult problem to deal with [4]. Geser et al. [31]

Table 4 Aetiology of dizziness (only studies with low risk of bias)

	Maarsingh 2010	Lawson 1999
Peripheral vestibular	14.4% [11.2; 18.2]	34.0% [21.6; 48.9]
BPPV		8.0% [2.6; 20.1]
Vestibular neuritis		24.0% [13.5; 38.5]
Morbus Meniere	–	2.0% [0.1-12.0]
Cardiovascular	56.8% [51.9; 61.6][a]	48.0% [33.9; 62.4]
Neurological central	2.9% [1.6; 5.1][b]	10.0% [3.7; 22.6]
Cerebrovascular	–	4.0% [0.7; 14.9]
Psychogenic	9.8% [7.2; 13.2]	–
Musculosceletal	3.6% [2.1; 6.0]	4.0% [0.7; 14.9]
Other internistic diseases	0.7% [0.2; 2.3]	–
Drug effects	2.4% [1.2; 4.5]	–
Other	1.2% [0.4; 2.9]	–
No specific diagnosis	8.2% [5.8; 11.3]	22.0% [12.0; 36.3]

[a]incl. Cerebrovascular; [b]excl. cerebrovascular

report that in most of the patients referred to a specialized dizziness clinic neuro-otological disorders were underdiagnosed. However, with a diagnostic approach, substantially based on medical history and clinical examination, GPs could be successfully trained to provide a better work up. Our findings support this suggestion: The proportion of unclear diagnoses decreases to 0,0-22,0%, if only prospective studies exclusively on the symptom dizziness were considered, where participating GPs presumably had to deal in one way or another with diagnostic strategies to provide a work up of their patients.

Two reviews, including studies from primary care and other settings find 4 to 48% peripheral vestibular diseases [2] and a quality-adjusted mean for peripheral vestibular diseases of 44% [32]. Studies from specialized dizziness clinics show 40,9% [33] and 46,8% [34] peripheral vestibular disease. These findings are higher than ours (5,4-42,1% peripheral vestibular diseases).

Regarding cardiovascular diseases, we found a higher proportion in older patients, especially in studies with a low risk of bias. For patients of 60 or 65 years and older the two studies with a low risk of bias showed 48,0% [35] and 56,8% ([36] cardiovascular problems. In comparison, the results of studies with a high risk of bias that included only older patients range from 10,0% [4] to 13,0% [24].

It is interesting to note that in one study conducted in the emergency department, 21,1% of dizzy patients suffered from a cardiovascular disease [30, 37], whereas in dizziness clinics cardiovascular diseases do not rank among the mentioned frequent aetiologies [31, 33, 34]. Dizziness due to cardiovascular problems might go along with other symptoms like angina pectoris that rather warrant a visit to the emergency department.

Prognosis

Knowledge of prognosis is helpful in the context of further decision making in primary care. If dizziness in this setting has a good prognosis and will disappear in most patients from alone then it would not be necessary to always make an exact diagnosis provided red flags are taken into account. Symptomatic therapy would suffice.

While in the included studies there could be shown improvement based on subjective patient assessment, this could not be confirmed when applying instruments that measure quality of life.

In comparison, at a specialized dizziness clinic the mean score of the Dizziness Handicap Inventory (DHI) improved significantly after two year follow-up [38]. Possible explanations for this difference could be that treatment interventions in specialized clinics are more effective. Another explanation would be the shorter follow up in the primary care studies.

Overall, there is a scarcity of studies, which investigate prognosis of dizziness in primary care: Two of the four studies using the DHI include only patients of a minimum age of 65 years. The other two are intervention studies. Yardley et al. reported that about 90% of the invited patients did not participate in the study assuming that the majority of these patients were no longer dizzy [20]. This selection effect could be one explanation for the rather bad prognosis in primary care.

Quality of included studies

The quality of the results of a systematic review depends on the quality of the included studies. Although we found 9 studies of high quality (low risk of bias for the domains A and B), which provide data on prevalence, we decided, that a meta-analysis was not reasonable because of the high clinical and methodical heterogeneity between these studies. For example, studies differ in outcomes (numerator and denominator), duration of dizziness, patient ages, proportion of women, number and type of health care institutions (practices, health care centre). Furthermore, study results depend on cultural variances, regarding, inter alia, health care systems and definition of dizziness in different countries.

Regarding aetiology we found only two studies with a low overall risk of bias (low risk of bias for the domains A, B and C). The majority of studies considers just the GPs diagnosis without follow up or standardised diagnostic approach. Moreover they do not define aetiological categories and therefore the forming of categories was difficult and at risk of overlapping. For example, some studies provided no information, under which category cerebrovascular diseases were grouped (neurological or cardiogenic).

Dizziness may have a multifactorial origin and therefore some studies allow more than one diagnosis per patient, resulting in a sum of all diagnoses over 100% and accordingly higher percentages in all aetiological categories. Other studies have a high proportion of unclear diagnosis, leading to lower percentages in other categories.

Due to the small number of trustworthy studies we could not assess, how duration of dizziness, patients age or gender influenced the proportion of underlying etiologies.

Limitations

There are limitations to our study, influenced by three factors, which could lead to a bias in interpretation:

First, factors which influence the internal validity of the included studies like incomplete recruitment or imprecise inclusion criteria. We controlled this type of bias with rigorous quality assessment and defined clear inclusion criteria for all included studies.

Second, factors which might influence the external validity of the included studies like setting or recruitment characteristics that influence transferability to the local health care system.

Third, factors which influence the internal validity of this systematic review like mistakes in the screening process or full text analysis. Both processes were performed by two independent reviewers, which minimized this risk.

The majority of the included studies have been conducted in health care systems with a gatekeeper, some studies are from countries with direct access to specialists care. This lack of a filter might have an impact on the aetiology of the symptoms and adds an additional source of heterogeneity. These differences cannot only be seen between countries but also within one country. Germany, for example, has not an official gate keeping system but some counties have implemented a voluntary gate keeping system. Additionally, in rural areas patients tend always to contact their GP first while in urban areas specialist are contacted directly in comparatively higher frequency.

In regard to our third research question (prognosis) we could only include data looking at 'usual care' and did not perform an evaluation of the effectiveness of available treatments which limits the *practical application of our findings.*

Due to the missing quality standard for symptom evaluating studies we developed a more comprehensive catalogue of criteria that, when applied to the included studies, showed a broad spectrum from low to high risk of bias. As this also may introduce variance across studies, we did not pool data.

Although we have decided on structured steps concerning our search strategy, data extraction and analysis, we have not published a review protocol.

Conclusions

In conclusion, we have shown that vertigo and dizziness are common reasons for consultation in general practice. The review identified only few studies that were pointing with a low risk of bias to the aetiology of dizziness. It would be desirable to develop better methodological procedures that allow conducting studies with a lower risk of bias. As there are already enough reliable data on prevalence, future studies should concentrate on assessing aetiology of dizziness. Many studies included in this review grouped a considerable number of patients in the category 'diagnosis not possible'. While this surely reflects the reality in a certain percentage of patients, future research should concentrate on developing an internationally unified and accepted reference standard for the main underlying aetiologies of dizziness.

As prognosis often is not very good, rehabilitative aspects in patients with dizziness seem to be important for both research and practical implementation.

Furthermore, in many cases the underlying cause of the complaints remains unexplained. Here we can see the need of developing practical guidelines for the work up of dizziness and vertigo in primary care.

Additional files

Additional file 1: Search strategy: contains detailed information regarding the search strategy used for this systematic review.

Additional file 2: Study quality: contains detailed information on the assessment of risk of bias and sources of clinical heterogeneity.

Additional file 3: Details prevalence: contains detailed information on the prevalence of dizziness.

Additional file 4: Details aetiology: contains detailed information on the aetiology of dizziness.

Abbreviations

BPPV : Benign Positional Paroxysmal Vertigo; DHI: Dizziness Handicap Inventory; ENT: Ear Nose and Throat; GP: General practitioner

Acknowledgements

Not applicable

Funding

The study was funded by our own department.

Authors' contributions

SB, JH, SS, PG, LS, KH, DB, MB, AV and AB participated in the study design and analyses. SS and JH performed the search. SB wrote a first draft of the manuscript. JH, SS, PG, LS, KH, DB, MB, AV and AB commented on this draft and performed critical revisions. All authors have read and approved the manuscript.

Consent for publication
Not applicable.

Competing interests
The authors declare that they have no competing interests.

References

1. Laux G, Rosemann T, Korner T, Heiderhoff M, Schneider A, Kuhlein T, Szecsenyi J. Detailed data collection regarding the utilization of medical services, morbidity, course of illness and outcomes by episode-based documentation in general practices within the CONTENT project. Gesundheitswesen. 2007;69:284–91. https://doi.org/10.1055/s-2007-976517.
2. Sloane PD, Coeytaux RR, Beck RS, Dallara J. Dizziness: state of the science. Ann Intern Med. 2001;134:823–32.
3. Ekvall Hansson E, Mansson N-O, Hakansson A. Benign paroxysmal positional vertigo among elderly patients in primary health care. Gerontology. 2005;51:386–9. https://doi.org/10.1159/000088702.
4. Kwong ECK, Pimlott NJG. Assessment of dizziness among older patients at a family practice clinic: a chart audit study. BMC Fam Pract. 2005;6:2. https://doi.org/10.1186/1471-2296-6-2.
5. Yardley L, Owen N, Nazareth I, Luxon L. Prevalence and presentation of dizziness in a general practice community sample of working age people. Br J Gen Pract. 1998;48:1131–5.
6. Grill E, Penger M, Kentala E. Health care utilization, prognosis and outcomes of vestibular disease in primary care settings: systematic review. J Neurol. 2016;263(Suppl 1):36–44. https://doi.org/10.1007/s00415-015-7913-2.
7. Donner-Banzhoff N, Kunz R, Rosser W. Studies of symptoms in primary care. Fam Pract. 2001;18:33–8.
8. Richardson WS, Wilson MC, Guyatt GH, Cook DJ, Nishikawa J. Users' guides to the medical literature: XV. How to use an article about disease probability for differential diagnosis. Evidence-Based Medicine Working Group. JAMA. 1999;281:1214–9.
9. Viniol A, Beidatsch D, Frese T, Bergmann M, Grevenrath P, Schmidt L, et al. Studies of the symptom dyspnoea: a systematic review. BMC Fam Pract. 2015;16:152. https://doi.org/10.1186/s12875-015-0373-z.
10. Haasenritter J, Biroga T, Keunecke C, Becker A, Donner-Banzhoff N, Dornieden K, et al. Causes of chest pain in primary care–a systematic review and meta-analysis. Croat Med J. 2015;56:422–30.
11. Newcombe RG. Two-sided confidence intervals for the single proportion: comparison of seven methods. Stat Med. 1998;17:857–72.
12. Higgins JPT, Green S. Cochrane Handbook for Systematic Reviews of Interventions: Version 5.1.0 [updated March 2011]. 5th ed: The Cochrane Collaboration; 2011.
13. Higgins JPT, Thompson SG, Spiegelhalter DJ. A re-evaluation of random-effects meta-analysis. J R Stat Soc Ser A Stat Soc. 2009;172:137–59. https://doi.org/10.1111/j.1467-985X.2008.00552.x.
14. Jayarajan V, Rajenderkumar D. A survey of dizziness management in General Practice. J Laryngol Otol. 2003;117:599–604. https://doi.org/10.1258/002221503768199915.
15. Maarsingh OR, Dros J, Schellevis FG, van Weert HC, Bindels PJ, van der Horst HE. Dizziness reported by elderly patients in family practice: prevalence, incidence, and clinical characteristics. BMC Fam Pract. 2010;11:2. https://doi.org/10.1186/1471-2296-11-2.
16. Ekvall, Hansson E, Mansson N-O, Hakansson A. What happens with the dizzy patient in primary health care? Does education influence treatment? Adv Physiother. 2004;6:93–6. https://doi.org/10.1080/14038190310016625.
17. Sicras-Mainar A, Velasco-Velasco S. Patterns of health resources use and costs in patients with neurological disorders in primary care. [Spanish]. Rev Neurol. 2007;45:641–6.
18. Britt H. General practice activity in Australia 2013–14: BEACH : bettering the evaluation and care of health.
19. Wun Y, Lu X, Liang W, Dickinson J. The work by the developing primary care team in China: a survey in two cities. Fam Pract. 2000;17:10–5.
20. Yardley L, Barker F, Muller I, Turner D, Kirby S, Mullee M, et al. Clinical and cost effectiveness of booklet based vestibular rehabilitation for chronic dizziness in primary care: single blind, parallel group, pragmatic, randomised controlled trial. BMJ. 2012;344:e2237. https://doi.org/10.1136/bmj.e2237.
21. Yardley L, Donovan-Hall M, Smith HE, Walsh BM, Mullee M, Bronstein AM. Effectiveness of primary care-based vestibular rehabilitation for chronic dizziness. Ann Intern Med. 2004;141:598–605.
22. Yardley L, Beech S, Zander L, Evans T, Weinman J. A randomized controlled trial of exercise therapy for dizziness and vertigo in primary care. Br J Gen Pract. 1998;48:1136–40.
23. Dros J, Maarsingh OR, Beem L, van der Horst, Henriette E, ter Riet G, Schellevis FG, van Weert, Henk CPM. Functional prognosis of dizziness in older adults in primary care: a prospective cohort study. J Am Geriatr Soc. 2012;60:2263–9. https://doi.org/10.1111/jgs.12031.
24. Sczepanek J, Wiese B, Hummers-Pradier E, Kruschinski C. Newly diagnosed incident dizziness of older patients: a follow-up study in primary care. BMC Fam Pract. 2011;12:58. https://doi.org/10.1186/1471-2296-12-58.
25. Kroenke K, Mangelsdorff AD. Common symptoms in ambulatory care: incidence, evaluation, therapy, and outcome. Am J Med. 1989;86:262–6.
26. Kroenke K, Jackson JL. Outcome in general medical patients presenting with common symptoms: a prospective study with a 2-week and a 3-month follow-up. Fam Pract. 1998;15:398–403.
27. Bailey KE, Sloane PD, Mitchell M, Preisser J. Which primary care patients with dizziness will develop persistent impairment? Arch Fam Med. 1993;2:847–52.
28. Grill E, Müller M, Brandt T, Jahn K. Vertigo and dizziness: challenges for epidemiological research. OA Epidemiology. 2013;1(2):12.
29. Kerber KA, Meurer WJ, West BT, Fendrick AM. Dizziness presentations in U.S. emergency departments, 1995-2004. Acad Emerg Med. 2008;15:744–50. https://doi.org/10.1111/j.1553-2712.2008.00189.x.
30. Newman-Toker DE, Hsieh Y-H, Camargo, Jr CA, Pelletier AJ, Butchy GT, Edlow JA. Spectrum of dizziness visits to US emergency departments: cross-sectional analysis from a nationally representative sample. Mayo Clin Proc. 2008;83:765–75. https://doi.org/10.4065/83.7.765.
31. Geser R, Straumann D. Referral and final diagnoses of patients assessed in an academic vertigo center. Front Neurol. 2012;3:169. https://doi.org/10.3389/fneur.2012.00169.
32. Kroenke K, Hoffman RM, Einstadter D. How common are various causes of dizziness? A critical review. South Med J. 2000;93:160–7. quiz 168
33. Obermann M. Chronischer Schwindel aus neurologischer Sicht. Dtsch Med Wochenschr. 2013;138:269–74. https://doi.org/10.1055/s-0032-1332838.
34. Strupp M, Dieterich M, Brandt T. The treatment and natural course of peripheral and central vertigo. Dtsch Arztebl Int. 2013;110:505–15; quiz 515-6. https://doi.org/10.3238/arztebl.2013.0505.
35. Lawson J, Fitzgerald J, Birchall J, Aldren CP, Kenny RA. Diagnosis of geriatric patients with severe dizziness. J Am Geriatr Soc. 1999;47:12–7.
36. Maarsingh OR, Dros J, Schellevis FG, van Weert HC, van der Windt DA, ter Riet G, van der Horst HE. Causes of persistent dizziness in elderly patients in primary care. Ann Fam Med. 2010;8:196–205. https://doi.org/10.1370/afm.1116.
37. Moller H-J, Langer S, Schmauss M. Escitalopram in clinical practice: results of an open-label trial in outpatients with depression in a naturalistic setting in Germany. Pharmacopsychiatry. 2007;40:53–7. https://doi.org/10.1055/s-2007-970142.
38. Obermann M, Bock E, Sabev N, Lehmann N, Weber R, Gerwig M, et al. Long-term outcome of vertigo and dizziness associated disorders following treatment in specialized tertiary care: the Dizziness and Vertigo Registry (DiVeR) Study. J Neurol. 2015;262:2083–91. https://doi.org/10.1007/s00415-015-7803-7.
39. Bird JC, Beynon GJ, Prevost AT, Baguley DM. An analysis of referral patterns for dizziness in the primary care setting. Br J Gen Pract. 1998;48:1828–32.
40. Fink W, Haidinger G. Die Häufigkeit von Gesundheitsstörungen in 10 Jahren Allgemeinpraxis. Z Allg Med. 2007;83:102–8. https://doi.org/10.1055/s-2007-968157.
41. Garrigues HP, Andres C, Arbaizar A, Cerdan C, Meneu V, Oltra JA, et al. Epidemiological aspects of vertigo in the general population of the Autonomic Region of Valencia, Spain. Acta Otolaryngol. 2008;128:43–7. https://doi.org/10.1080/00016480701387090.
42. Gerber PD, Barrett JE, Barrett JA, Oxman TE, Manheimer E, Smith R, Whiting RD. The relationship of presenting physical complaints to depressive symptoms in primary care patients. J Gen Intern Med. 1992;7:170–3.
43. Hanley K, O' Dowd T. Symptoms of vertigo in general practice: a prospective study of diagnosis. Br J Gen Pract 2002;52:809–812.
44. Harding TW, de Arango, M V, Baltazar J, Climent CE, Ibrahim HH, Ladrido-Ignacio L, et al. Mental disorders in primary health care: a study of their frequency and diagnosis in four developing countries. Psychol Med 1980;10:231–241.

45. Hopkins A. Lessons for neurologists from the United Kingdom Third National Morbidity Survey. J Neurol Neurosurg Psychiatry. 1989;52:430–3.
46. Mash B, Fairall L, Adejayan O, Ikpefan O, Kumari J, Matheel S, et al. A morbidity survey of South African primary care. PLoS One. 2012; https://doi.org/10.1371/journal.pone.0032358.
47. Kruschinski C, Kersting M, Breull A, Kochen MM, Koschack J, Hummers-Pradier E. Frequency of dizziness-related diagnoses and prescriptions in a general practice database. Z Evid Fortbild Qual Gesundhwes. 2008;102:313–9.
48. Morrell DC. Symptom interpretation in general practice. J R Coll Gen Pract. 1972;22:297–309.
49. Morrell DC, Gage HG, Robinson NA. Symptoms in general practice. J R Coll Gen Pract. 1971;21:32–43.
50. Sloane PD. Dizziness in primary care. Results from the National Ambulatory Medical Care Survey. J Fam Pract. 1989;29:33–8.
51. Sloane PD, Dallara J, Roach C, Bailey KE, Mitchell M, McNutt R. Management of dizziness in primary care. J Am Board Fam Pract. 1994;7:1–8.
52. Rieger A, Mansmann U, Maier W, Seitz L, Brandt T, Strupp M, Bayer O. Management of patients with the cardinal symptom dizziness or vertigo. Gesundheitswesen. 2014;76:e32–8. https://doi.org/10.1055/s-0033-1357145.
53. Soler JK, Okkes I, Oskam S, van Boven K, Zivotic P, Jevtic M, et al. An international comparative family medicine study of the Transition Project data from the Netherlands, Malta and Serbia. Is family medicine an international discipline? Comparing incidence and prevalence rates of reasons for encounter and diagnostic titles of episodes of care across populations. Fam Pract. 2012;29:283–98. https://doi.org/10.1093/fampra/cmr098.

13

Nutrition care practices of primary care providers for weight management in multidisciplinary primary care settings in Ontario, Canada

Stephanie Aboueid[1*], Ivy Bourgeault[2] and Isabelle Giroux[3]

Abstract

Background: Despite the recommended guidelines on addressing diet for the management and prevention of obesity in primary care, the literature highlights that their implementation has been suboptimal. In this paper, we provide an in-depth understanding of current nutrition-related weight management practices of primary care providers (PCPs) working in relatively new multidisciplinary health care settings in Ontario.

Methods: Three types of multidisciplinary primary care settings were included (2 Family Health Teams, 3 Community Health Centres and 1 Nurse Practitioner-Led Clinic). Participants ($n = 20$) included in this study were nurse practitioners ($n = 13$) and family physicians ($n = 7$) supporting care for adult patients (18 years or older). In-depth interviews were transcribed, coded and the content was analyzed using an integrated approach.

Results: Our analysis showed that most PCPs used anthropometric measures such as weight for screening patients who would benefit from nutrition counselling with a dietitian. The topic of nutrition was generally brought up either during physical examinations, when patients were diagnosed with a chronic disease, or when blood markers were out of normal range. Participants also mentioned that physical examinations are no longer occurring annually, with most PCPs offering episodic care. All participants reported utilizing dietetic referrals, noting the enablers for providing the referral, which included access to an on-site dietitian. Nonetheless, dietetic referrals were mostly used when patients had an obesity-related co-morbidity. Participants mentioned that healthy eating advice was reinforced during follow-up visits with patients only when there was enough time to do so. Electronic Health Records (EHRs) were utilized to facilitate message reinforcement by PCPs, who perceived EHRs to be helpful for viewing what was discussed in the session with the dietitian.

Conclusions: PCPs mostly used objective measures to screen for patients who would benefit from nutrition counselling rather than diet assessment, which undermines the importance of dietary intake and overemphasizes weight. With physical examinations occurring less frequently, there will be additional missed opportunities for addressing nutrition-related concerns. The presence of a dietitian on site allowed for PCPs to refer patients to nutrition counselling. Having sufficient time during medical visits and EHRs seemed to facilitate message reinforcement by PCPs in follow-up visits with patients.

Keywords: Obesity, Primary health care, Qualitative research, Family medicine, Family physicians, Nurse practitioners, Weight management, Nutrition

* Correspondence: sabou095@uottawa.ca
[1]School of Public Health and Health Systems, Faculty of Applied Health Sciences, University of Waterloo, 200 University Avenue West, Waterloo, ON N2L 3G1, Canada
Full list of author information is available at the end of the article

Background

Obesity is multifactorial and is strongly associated with many chronic diseases [1, 2]. In 2014, roughly 5.3 million Canadian adults were living with obesity [3]. Obesity has been classified as a complex, chronic, relapsing condition, which highlights the importance of its prevention and management [4, 5]. Primary care is the first point of contact for all patients and thus is viewed as the ideal place to address obesity [6]. Given the complexity of obesity, multicomponent interventions (i.e., those addressing diet, exercise, and behavioural therapy) are required in primary care [7–9]. In terms of diet, it has been shown that an individualized medical nutrition therapy program is essential for adherence to nutrition counselling for weight management [10]. Registered dietitians (RDs) are health professionals whose services have been shown to be effective in managing excess body weight [11–13]. However, many patients who would benefit from nutrition counselling are not aware of this service or do not receive it [14–18]. Moreover, only 37% of Canadian patients report that they have received nutrition counselling in primary care [19].

There are, however, many barriers to accessing RD services due to lack of accessibility and in the Canadian context, cost of care [14–16]. In response to the sub-optimal care in health promotion practices - including nutrition care - there has been a shift towards multidisciplinary clinics as part of the primary health care reform in Canada [20]. This transition began in the year 2000 and included an objective to focus on the prevention and management of chronic diseases, including obesity [20]. This shift is seen as an enabler for better utilization of specialized health care professionals, including dietitians [20]. Some of the key multidisciplinary initiatives include Community Health Centres (CHCs), Family Health Teams (FHTs), and Nurse Practitioner-Led Clinics (NPLCs).

While CHCs, FHTs, and NPLCs were established at different times, for different reasons, and follow their own models, they share an important characteristic: the variety of health care professionals who work in the same location. Given the importance of preventing and managing obesity in primary care [6], it is critical to understand how primary care providers working in different types of multidisciplinary clinics deliver nutrition care to adult patients (18 years or older) with obesity. In light of this, our study was designed to understand nutrition-related weight management practices of family physicians (FPs) and nurse practitioners (NPs) working in multidisciplinary clinics. Although there are many approaches to weight management, this study focused on nutrition care in order to provide an in-depth understanding of this practice area while accounting for respondent burden. By capturing the underlying reasons for their practice and contexts in which they work, we can further our knowledge with the aim of improving weight management in primary health care facilities.

Methods

Settings and participants

Using a purposive sampling technique, we began by approaching the director of each clinical setting in proximity to the research institution. Once permission was obtained from the clinical director, all primary care providers (PCPs) at each site were contacted via email. If interested, a consent form outlining the details of the study was provided to the PCP. Out of 15 NPs and 10 FPs who were approached, 13 and 7 accepted, respectively. Our sample included NPs and FPs working in 2 FHTs, 3 CHCs, and 1 NPLC. The higher number of NPs involved in this study was due to the inclusion of the NPLC setting, which is primarily comprised of NPs. The ratio of NPs to FPs is the same for the two other settings (3 NPs and 3 FPs). The recruitment and data collection occurred in Fall 2016 and Winter 2017. Each participant was given a 50-dollar Canadian coffee card as a token of appreciation for taking the time to participate in the study.

To test the interview protocol, a pilot test that included 4 PCPs was conducted. Data from the pilot test were not included in this study because the interview protocol was refined based on participants' feedback to include more follow-up probes. The first inclusion criterion was: NPs and FPs who provide health care to adult patients. This is important as questions that were asked during the interview pertain to excess weight in adult patients. The second inclusion criterion was: NPs and FPs who had been working at the site for at least 6 months. This ensured that the health care professional had been working at the site for a considerable number of hours in order to accurately convey their practices at the clinical setting.

Data collection

This qualitative study was based on in-depth individual semi-structured interviews. In order to allow for comparability between participants while allowing the interviewer to explore subjects of interest, the combination approach recommended by Patton was used [21]. As such, the interview began by using a standardized open-ended approach and ended with the interviewer being free to explore any subjects of interest during the latter parts of the interview [21]. The main topic areas covered in the interview guide were: 1) the screening tools used for determining which patients would benefit from nutrition counselling, 2) approaching the topic of nutrition and providing initial advice, 3) providing dietetic referrals, and 4) understanding message reinforcement practices (i.e., reinforcing healthy eating advice over time).

Questions on barriers and enablers for approaching the topic of nutrition counselling for weight management and providing a dietetic referral were also asked. The interview guide was included as an additional file (Additional file 1).

The interviewer who conducted all the interviews (SA) was a dietitian and graduate student trained in qualitative research methods. A research assistant (RA) was also present during the interview and took detailed notes of the conversation as well as other context-information. The research assistant was an undergraduate student who wanted to gain experience in research. Her presence did not affect data collection as the research study mostly included notes taken by the interviewer (SA). Both notes were compared after the interviews for training purposes but RA notes were not used for the analysis. Interviews were recorded with each participant's written informed consent. Interview length ranged from 30 to 50 min. In the consent form, each participant had the option of providing a member check once data analysis was complete. Seven out of 20 participants were initially interested in member checking.

Data analysis

The interviews were transcribed verbatim and managed using NVivo software (QSR International Pty Ltd. Version 11). Investigator triangulation was used where researchers used various angles to interpret the data [22]. Two researchers (SA and IG) analyzed the data independently and discrepancies were resolved by including the perspective of a third researcher (IB). Emerging themes were discussed with the research team to minimize bias and maintain reflexivity [23]. An integrated approach was used where the literature review informed both the interview questions and deductive codes, while inductive codes emerged from the data collected. Examples of deductive codes under the theme "barriers for approaching the topic of nutrition" included "lack of time; lack of knowledge". Nevertheless, to avoid forcing data under predetermined codes, inductive codes were also generated based on the interviewees' responses.

Interviews from all clinical sites were coded together to achieve the main goal of understanding nutrition care practices in multidisciplinary settings, while maximizing diversity. The inductive analysis process consisted of starting with a line-by-line coding approach. Examples of line-by-line codes included "Body Mass Index and body weight". Once all descriptive codes were identified, similar codes were grouped under 4 main categories (i.e., screening, approaching the topic of nutrition, dietetic referrals, and reinforcing the healthy eating advice). For instance, the codes "Body Mass Index and body weight" were grouped under the category "screening". Codes changed and developed as more interviews were conducted and as field experience was gained. Constant comparative analysis was used to group major themes, which were then refined in an iterative process. Major themes and interpretations are provided with interview quotes along with the participant's profession and place of work. Out of the seven participants who were initially interested in a member check (i.e., verifying the way in which the data were analyzed), four participants completed the member check. There were no revisions that needed to be made.

Results

A total of 20 individual interviews were conducted with primary care providers working in different types of multidisciplinary primary care settings. Table 1 describes the sample in terms of characteristics and demographics.

Screening

Participants were asked about how they screened for patients who would benefit from nutrition counselling. Although a particular screening tool was not used, the following measures, markers, or questions were used to screen patients: body mass index (BMI) or body weight, general questions on food intake, blood work tests results, the presence of chronic disease, and waist circumference.

> "Dietary intake is always done in the context of weight. If the patient is skinny and has a poor diet we won't talk about it. If the person is normal weight, we will not bring it up." FHT, FP – participant 10

Most PCPs did not use an evidence-based screening tool to screen for patients who would benefit from nutrition

Table 1 Participant characteristics and demographics

Profession	n
Family physicians	7
Nurse Practitioners	13
Experience in profession (years)	n
≤5	6
6–15	9
15–25	2
≥25	3
Self-identified gender	n
Female	16
Male	4
Experience in organization (years)	n
≤1	2
2–5	8
6–10	7
≥11	3

counselling. Rather, participants mentioned asking general questions to assess diet. As one participant stated:

> "I don't use any tools because I am always dealing with multiple issues so it's more of a time thing. In the general assessment I ask: 'do you eat healthy?' and then they say yes so then I challenge them and ask 'what is healthy?' and then they would say 'I eat Wendy's instead of McDonald's and often it's not really what I am looking for." FHT, FP – participant 15

Approaching the topic of nutrition

Participants enumerated many instances in which the topic of nutrition would be brought up as well as how they provided initial advice. The topic of nutrition in terms of weight management was discussed during: physical examinations, when the patient was diagnosed with a chronic disease such as diabetes or hypertension, when blood work indicated hypercholesterolemia or hyperglycemia, if BMI was over 30. 0 kg/m^2, when patients brought it up, during menopause, every medical encounter, and during pregnancy.

As mentioned by most participants, the topic of nutrition was mostly brought up during physical examinations. Participants, however, also reported that these examinations were no longer conducted annually. Episodic care is now favoured where patients receive physicals every two to three years.

> "The topic is usually brought up either if they're in for an annual physical or a problem affected by obesity like diabetes, hypertension, or sleep apnea. Physicals are now every 2 or 3 years and I am going to stop them. Most family doctors are not doing them anymore and are moving towards episodic care." FHT, FP – participant 14

Most participants felt that nutrition was discussed more in terms of management of chronic diseases rather than prevention. Many reasons for this occurrence were identified including fear of offending patients. However, they believed that a patient's chronic disease diagnosis justified a discussion regarding nutrition.

> "Quite commonly if we're doing chronic disease management – diabetes, hypertension, lipid control – those types of things come up very early in the conversation. Some people associate weight discussion as a negative thing, instead of something that carries them forward into a positive role for their health management." NPLC, NP – participant 5

Blood work test results indicating elevated blood cholesterol and/or glucose concentrations, high blood pressure, and an elevated BMI were also indicators that prompted PCPs to bring up the topic of nutrition.

> "It's usually during physicals if I see that their BMI is above 30 or if their A1C is in the diabetic or pre-diabetic range or if they have dyslipidemia." CHC, FP – participant 21

The patients also seemed to play an important role in the discussion of nutrition as some were reported to be interested in learning more about healthy diets. This was especially the case when they were diagnosed with a chronic disease.

> "Obviously sometimes patients will bring it up and say that weight is an issue and will say that they have problems with good diets or what they should eat. It happens quite frequently when people have early pre-diabetes or diabetes. When they get diagnosed more often they are overweight and the first question they ask is what should I be eating." FHT, FP – participant 10

A patient being diagnosed with a chronic disease was the most mentioned enabler for approaching the topic of nutrition, whereas lack of time was the most important barrier. The enablers and barriers for approaching the topic of nutrition and supporting quotes are provided in Table 2.

Dietetic referrals

Approaching the dietetic referral

PCPs used many different approaches as well as a combination of approaches when suggesting a dietetic referral. These approaches included: assessing patients' level of readiness to change, proposing the referral while explaining the importance, explaining what a RD does, and providing general information on how their weight is affecting their health.

> "Explaining in more detail why the referral is being made and how important it is in disease management and prevention and explain that lifestyle changes can really affect a lot of organs and multiple diseases." FHT, FP – participant 15

> "If I think that their diabetes is out of control because of their weight I will explain that this is getting out of control because no matter what we give you {medication}, you're intake is going to super exceed that. ... We talk about the complications. ... So I think it's general counselling on what the weight is doing to their health." FHT, FP – participant 10

In particular, one participant elaborated on a new approach of not giving an option to the patient as it increased the likelihood of initiating nutrition counselling with a dietitian.

Table 2 Key enablers and barriers for approaching the topic of nutrition

Key enablers	Examples of quotes from primary care providers
Chronic disease diagnosis	"Sadly, when people have a chronic illness, it is much easier to talk about nutrition. I find the blood pressure helps, if there is an increase; I talk about weight, diet, and exercise." CHC, NP – participant 20
Patients showing interest	"I would say a lot of times patients actually bring up the topic if I am talking to them about their cholesterol, they will ask what they can do that is not medication. If I am talking about diabetes or cholesterol, I let them know about the non-medical management, which is obviously the preferred route because there are no side effects as opposed to medications that have side effects." CHC, FP– participant 17
Dietitian on site	"If somebody is coming in and they are here for a prescription renewal, it's hard to focus time but because I do have the option to refer them to the dietitian, it's a huge help." NPLC, NP – participant 1
Out of normal range blood test markers	"If cholesterol is elevated, glucose is elevated, fatty liver based on lab results, regardless of the age of the person. If none of these issues are there, it is possible that I would not bring it up." NPLC, FP – participant 9
Having access to handouts	"I like handouts because sometimes I know they are not necessarily listening and taking in the information as I am giving them. Let's say their blood pressure is out of whack and they don't want to come back to see the dietitian, I will print out the handout." NPLC, NP – participant 1
Trusting relationship with the patient	"A trusting relationship between the health professional and the patient is number one." CHC, NP – participant 19
The whole family has obesity	"When more than one family member has obesity, it is easier to bring up the topic of nutrition." FHT, NP – participant 12
Key barriers	**Examples of quotes from primary care providers**
Lack of time	"Time consuming and we only have 15-min appointments so sometimes there is no time." FHT, NP - participant 14
Patients not open to discussing it	"There are many clients who don't want to hear about it. They're unstably housed, they're in abusive relationships, they have a lot of priorities and talking about nutrition and weight management is not among them." CHC, NP – participant 18
Lack of rapport with the client	"Sometimes it's the rapport. Some patients don't care to interact." NPLC, NP – participant 1
Competing demands	"They just have so many complex issues, mostly psychosocial issues that are predominant in their daily lives that nutrition is not something I can bring up." CHC, NP – participant 19
Patient perceiving they already know what they need to change	"Some patients will say: yeah yeah, I've been told all this before, I know what to do, I just need to do it." NPLC, NP – Participant 3
Low comfort level of provider to address nutrition	"Some providers may not be as comfortable because they think it is a sensitive topic but really if you just open a dialogue about it often times it will be OK to talk about it (nutrition)." NPLC, NP – Participant 2
Patients not understanding the implications of excess body weight	"I think that some patients may not understand some of the health consequences that could occur due to excess weight and unhealthy lifestyle behaviours" NPLC, NP – Participant 7

> "I actually changed my technique when it comes to referring to the RD. If I give them the option, more often they are going to decline. I've actually changed how I bring it up. I say: I would like you to see the RD, I think she would be able to give you some good advice, I think she can give a good assessment of how your diet could be affecting your weight, cholesterol, blood pressure." NPLC, NP – participant 1

When asked if they believed their patients were convinced of the importance of dietetic referrals, some felt that most patients did not understand the importance of the referral. Some PCPs felt that the importance of making lifestyle changes is understood over time.

> "I feel that they understand the importance over time. So if they are coming in for back pain, and then another time for knee pain, or trouble sleeping. When they start complaining about different things then I can kind of rule out everything else and come back on the topic of nutrition and their weight. Sometimes the light goes off and they say: oh really, I didn't realize it was that important, I didn't realize how many aspects of my mental wellness or physical wellness that are contributed to that (nutrition and diet)." CHC, NP – participant 19

Instances in which a dietetic referral was provided

Most referrals seemed to be made when the patient was diagnosed with an obesity-related chronic disease rather than obesity alone. Table 3 outlines the instances in which dietetic referrals were made.

In addition, to get a better understanding of why PCPs made referrals to a RD, we asked about the enablers and barriers for providing such a referral (Table 4). Accessibility to a RD and cost-free service were the main enablers for providing a dietetic referral whereas wait times was mentioned to be a barrier.

Reinforcing the healthy eating advice

Working in a multidisciplinary clinic and having tools to communicate, such as EHRs, seemed to increase the likelihood of PCPs reinforcing healthy eating advice in follow-up visits with patients. However, this was dependent on PCPs having the time to do so.

> "If I have time we talk about what the RD suggested and I'll see her note in the file and I'll give a bit of positive reinforcement."
>
> FHT, FP – participant 14

> "And also, the next time I see the person I say, "How did it go with the dietitian?" And if they need a follow up on what was discussed I can look it up in the EHR and I will see that she [dietitian] also assessed their readiness to change and likeliness to make the change, so I think it's terrific for follow-up." CHC, NP – participant 18

Discussion

Summary of results

Questions on the screening process showed that most PCPs used objective measures, such as BMI and out of normal range blood test markers, for assessing which patients would benefit from further nutrition counselling. Some participants also seemed to ask subjective and non-validated questions to assess diet. The topic of nutrition was mostly brought up during physical examinations, which are infrequent now due to the shift towards episodic care. Similarly, due to competing demands and lack of time, nutrition care was provided when a patient was already diagnosed with a chronic disease or when the patients specifically asked diet-related questions. As for dietetic referral practices, some participants were aware that raising awareness before referring to a dietitian was important for patient adherence to nutrition counselling. However, they did not have adequate time to provide details regarding benefits of changing eating habits before providing a referral. Many enablers for providing a dietetic referral were listed, including the RD being on site and the service being cost-free for patients at point of access. While most participants felt that there were no barriers to providing a dietetic referral, some believed that the wait time to see the RD was an issue. PCPs felt that initiating nutrition counselling is time-sensitive and has to be done when patients are motivated. As such, some PCPs initiated the nutrition counselling themselves due to wait times. PCPs seemed to reinforce healthy eating advice in follow-up visits if time permitted. Reinforcing the dietitian's message was facilitated with EHRs as PCPs were aware of what was discussed in nutrition counselling sessions.

Comparison with existing literature

Although current screening practices are aligned with the recommended guidelines on the prevention and management of obesity (e.g., BMI and blood markers) [2], it can raise an issue when thinking of screening for nutrition-related diseases that are not linked to excess weight. Some PCPs mentioned that utilizing screening tools to assess diet might not be feasible due to time

Table 3 Instances in which a dietetic referral is provided by primary care providers

Themes	Examples of quotes from primary care providers
Patient asking for the dietetic referral	"If they are asking about weight loss I would then tell them that we have a RD for some counselling regarding weight." CHC, NP – participant 20
Patient was diagnosed with a chronic disease	"So any new diagnosis I automatically refer to the dietitian. For example, any of the triad of cardiac disease, renal failure disease, diabetes, the lipids; those types of patients I refer." NPLC, NP – participant 5 "There are only one and a half FTE {Full Time Equivalent} RDs so you want to prioritize people and so secondary and tertiary prevention usually takes a hold. Patients are more motivated when they're sick and in medicine we don't value prevention as much." FHT, FP – participant 10
Patient showing motivation or readiness to change	"Their readiness to change. I don't go on weight or BMI. It is their readiness. It is the same as smoking; I would never refer for smoking cessation if they are not ready. I bring up the topic but then they have to bring it back up to me and show me that they are ready and committed and want to change. If not the failure rates are close to 100%." FHT, FP – participant 15
Patient was at risk of developing a chronic disease	"I refer for weight management when it's related to a medical problem or when they are at risk for a disease to develop" CHC, FP – participant 17
Patient with an elevated BMI	"Everyone that has an elevated BMI, or that come in specifically asking to see the dietitian." NPLC, NP – participant 4
Patient experiencing pain related to obesity	"For people that are obese, it is something I will bring up, like those pain patients." NPLC, NP – participant 1

Table 4 Key enablers and barriers for providing a dietetic referral

Key enablers	Examples of quotes from primary care providers
Increasing access to a dietitian	"It's very easy here to make a referral since we have a dietitian on site and she is pretty quick to see patients." FHT, NP – Participant 12 "Access. How quickly they can be seen – not just location access, but also even how quickly they can get on the bandwagon. I find that sometimes if there are long delays – it wears off by the time they get in. Whereas if we have one (dietitian) on site and access is quick, I find it's received well because of that." NPLC, NP – participant 5
Increasing patient comfort	"Well it's on site and it's not a new environment where they have to meet strangers." NPLC, NP – participant 6
Cost-free dietitian service at point of care	"They (dietitians) are in the building and it is free for the patient." FHT, FP – Participant 15
Flexible schedule	"Being on site, free of charge, offered in the evenings so more availability for people working" FHT, FP – participant 14
Having a relationship with the dietitian	"Having a relationship with the dietitian. The more you know their abilities. I know the dietitian here is brilliant and I know that she is located in the clinic so that helps me sell it to the patient rather than saying 'you might get an appointment in 3 months across the city'." FHT, NP – participant 11
Key barriers	Examples of quotes from primary care providers
None	"None here but in general it would be cost and transportation, but they are already in to see us, we are ground floor, parking is free, easy access, senior access, wheelchair access. We worked hard to bring down the barriers." FHT, FP – participant 15
Wait times	"The wait time is 2 weeks so that is sometimes not soon enough because it gives patients time to change their mind but I think it is still good." CHC, NP – participant 19
Not thinking about making a dietetic referral	"Not thinking of it or making assumptions that the patient would not be interested. But it would still be good to offer it." NPLC, FP – participant 9
Patient not buying in	"Barriers include patient factors such as patients not buying in." CHC, FP – participant 21
Patients' negative perception of the session with the dietitian	"The lecture that people think they're going to get and the shame element about being overweight." NPLC, NP – participant 6
Requires the patient to come in again	"It would require another appointment." NPLC, NP – participant 4
Patients not showing interest	"Some people just aren't interested; they have hang-ups around weight and dieting and don't want to talk about it." CHC, NP – Participant 18
Patients' lack of time	"Those are typically the working group, that their time is fairly limited with family and work so they want a quick in and out, give me the information and I will do the work." CHC, NP – Participant 19

constraints. Some were unsure which time-effective and evidence-based questions to ask their patients for assessing their diet. As most PCPs seemed to ask subjective questions, it is important to increase awareness about validated tools such as the Rapid Eating Assessment for Patients (REAP). REAP has been suggested as a tool for health professionals to quickly assess who would benefit from further nutrition counselling [24, 25].

Since most participants mentioned that the topic of nutrition was discussed during physical examinations, the move towards episodic care may decrease health promotion opportunities in primary care. Expecting patients to initiate the topic of nutrition may be an issue if patients are unaware of the consequences of a poor diet and its link to chronic diseases. Moreover, patients have expectations from the primary care provider to ask about weight and to address their concerns by suggesting appropriate measures [26, 27]. Approaching the topic of nutrition only when patients were diagnosed with a chronic disease has been shown in this study and in the literature [28–30]. It also seemed that the discussion was more likely to occur as BMI increased, which is in line with previous findings [27, 31].

In contrast to what is suggested in the literature [32], some participants felt that raising awareness before referring patients to a dietitian had no influence on patient adherence to nutrition counselling. This may be due to the fact that some patients may already know the benefits of managing their weight but are unable to do so given the complexity of the condition and personal circumstances [26]. As highlighted in other studies, participating PCPs were more likely to bring up the topic if they had access to a free on-site dietetic referral option [15, 28]. As such, multidisciplinary clinics seemed to mitigate the barriers highlighted by PCPs working in non-multidisciplinary settings, and enabled PCPs to assist their patients with weight management [27, 33–35]. Wait times and lack of accessibility were also highlighted in previous studies [36, 37]. PCPs not thinking about the referral, patients not buying in, patients' negative perception of the RD session, and patients not wanting to come in were other barriers mentioned by PCPs. Some of these factors were also highlighted in previous studies [14, 38]. In contrast with previous international findings, none of these barriers included PCPs' unwillingness to collaborate with other health professionals [39].

After consulting the dietitian and setting out individualized goals, it is recommended that PCPs reinforce these goals in follow-up visits [7, 40]. Given the importance that patients attribute to their PCP's recommendations, it may help patients adhere to the nutrition care plan [41]. Having a dietitian on site and communication tools such as EHRs facilitated message reinforcement in follow-up visits. Studies have shown that not having a RD on site hinders communication, and in turn, prevents message reinforcement, [36, 37, 42] highlighting the importance of having support from allied health professionals to provide optimal care for obesity management [42, 43]. Although EHRs are perceived to play a role of a messenger [44], this study shows that message reinforcement occurs when PCPs have sufficient time during medical visits.

Strengths and limitations

This study provides important insights on how PCPs working in relatively new multidisciplinary primary care settings provide nutrition care to adult patients with obesity. Understanding how PCPs address nutrition and elucidating the enablers and barriers for providing nutrition care is crucial to inform the optimization of chronic disease prevention and management. Although the sample size may seem small, it did allow the researchers to reach data saturation indicating that future interviews may not have revealed new information. Moreover, the inclusion of different types of primary care settings allowed for diversity. Findings from this study can be transferred to other similar settings.

This study has some limitations. Although we tried to reach diversity in terms of gender, the sample mostly consisted of females. This may limit applicability to males as research has shown a difference in clinical practice based on gender. As well, this study only included multidisciplinary settings where primary care providers had access to other health professionals. Findings from this study may not be transferred to PCPs working in non-multidisciplinary based clinics.

Conclusions

Given that PCPs are the gatekeepers of the primary health care system, it is important to address the barriers they have highlighted in this study. Increasing awareness on evidence-based screening tools for diet assessment, providing training on how to discuss nutrition and weight, addressing barriers for providing a dietetic referral by reducing wait times, and encouraging message reinforcement are key for optimizing nutrition care. Importantly, as PCPs move towards providing episodic care, alternative solutions are required to ensure that patients are receiving appropriate preventive care.

Abbreviations

CHC: Community Health Centre; EHR: Electronic Health Record; FHT: Family Health Team; FP: Family physician; NP: Nurse practitioner; NPLC: Nurse Practitioner-Led Clinic; PCP: Primary care provider; RD: Registered Dietitian

Acknowledgements

The authors would like to thank the primary care providers who agreed to participate in this study, the Telfer School of Management for providing funding support, and Huda Shah, BSc (MSc candidate at the University of Waterloo) for editing the manuscript.

Funding

This study was funded by the University of Ottawa's Telfer School of Management (grant number: 147080).

Authors' contributions

SA, IG and IB developed the study design, carried out the data analysis and drafted the original manuscript. SA collected the data. IB and IG contributed to the conceptualization and design of the study. All authors contributed to the literature review and approved the final manuscript.

Competing interests

The authors declare that they have no competing interests.

Author details

[1]School of Public Health and Health Systems, Faculty of Applied Health Sciences, University of Waterloo, 200 University Avenue West, Waterloo, ON N2L 3G1, Canada. [2]Department of Health Systems, Telfer School of Management, University of Ottawa, 55 Laurier Avenue East, Ottawa, ON K1N6N5, Canada. [3]School of Nutrition Sciences, Faculty of Health Sciences, University of Ottawa, 25 University Private, Ottawa, ON K1N6N5, Canada.

References

1. World Health Organization. Obesity and overweight. 2017. http://www.who.int/mediacentre/factsheets/fs311/en/. Accessed 28 Aug 2017.
2. Brauer P, Gorber S, Shaw E, Singh H, Bell N, Shane AR, et al. Recommendations for prevention of weight gain and use of behavioural and pharmacologic interventions to manage overweight and obesity in adults in primary care. Can Med Assoc J. 2015;187(3):184–95.
3. Statistics Canada. Reported weight and height by age. 2015. https://www.statcan.gc.ca/pub/82-625-x/2015001/article/14185-eng.htm. Accessed 16 Aug 2017.
4. Canadian Medical Association. CMA recognizes obesity as a disease. 2017. https://www.cma.ca/En/Pages/cma-recognizes-obesity-as-a-disease.aspx. Accessed 11 Jan 2017.
5. Bray GA, Kim KK, Wilding JPH. And on behalf of the world obesity federation. Obesity: a chronic relapsing progressive disease process. Obes Rev. 2017;18:715–23.
6. Campbell-Scherer D, Sharma A. Improving obesity prevention and Management in Primary Care in Canada. Curr Obes Rep. 2016;5(3):327–32.
7. Lau DCW, Douketis JD, Morrison KM, Hramiak IM, Sharma AM, Ur E. 2006 Canadian clinical practice guidelines on the management and prevention of obesity in adults and children. Can Med Assoc J. 2007;176(8):S1–S13.
8. Rueda-Clausen CF, Benterud E, Bond T, Olszowka R, Vallis MT, Sharma AM. Effect of implementing the 5As of obesity management framework on provider-patient interactions in primary care: 5As of obesity management in primary care. Clin Obes. 2014;4(1):39–44.

9. Kirk SFL, Penney TL, McHugh T-L, Sharma AM. Effective weight management practice: a review of the lifestyle intervention evidence. Int J Obes. 2012;36(2):178–85.
10. Endevelt R, Gesser-Edelsburg A. A qualitative study of adherence to nutritional treatment: perspectives of patients and dietitians. Patient Prefer Adherence. 2014;4(8):147–54.
11. Flodgren G, Deane K, Dickinson HO, Kirk S, Alberti H, Beyer FR, et al. Interventions to change the behaviour of health professionals and the organisation of care to promote weight reduction in overweight and obese people. Cochrane Database Syst Rev. 2010;3:CD000984.
12. Tol J, Swinkels IC, Bakker DH, Seidell J, Veenhof C. Dietetic treatment lowers body mass index in overweight patients: an observational study in primary health care. J Hum Nutr Diet. 2014;27(5):426–33.
13. Willaing I, Ladelund S, Jørgensen T, Simonsen T, Nielsen LM. Nutritional counselling in primary health care: a randomized comparison of an intervention by general practitioner or dietician. Eur J Cardiovasc Prev Rehabil. 2004;11:513–20.
14. Padwal RS, Damjanovic S, Schulze KM, Lewanczuk RZ, Lau DCW, Sharma AM. Canadian Physicians' use of Antiobesity drugs and their referral patterns to weight management programs or providers: the SOCCER study. J Obes. 2011; https://doi.org/10.1155/2011/686521
15. Wynn K, Trudeau JD, Taunton K, Gowans M, Scott I. Nutrition in primary care, current practices, attitudes and barriers. Can Fam Physician. 2010;56:3e109–16.
16. Nicholas L, Dck R, Pond D. The role of the general practitioner and the dietitian in patient nutrition management. Asia Pacific J Clin Nutr. 2003;12(1):3–8.
17. Coombs J, Barrocas A, White J. Nutrition Care of Older Adults with chronic disease: attitudes and practices of physicians and patients. South Med J. 2004;97(6):560–5.
18. Dolor RJ, Østbye T, Lyna P, Coffman CJ, Alexander SC, Tulsky JA, et al. What are physicians' and patients' beliefs about diet, weight, exercise, and smoking cessation counseling? Prev Med. 2010;51(5):440–2.
19. Brauer PM, Sergeant LA, Davidson B, Goy R, Dietrich L. Patient reports of lifestyle advice in primary care. Can J Diet Pract Res. 2012;73(3):122–7.
20. Government of Canada. Primary health care transition fund. 2007. https://www.canada.ca/en/health-canada/services/primary-health-care/primary-health-care-transition-fund.html. Accessed 15 Aug 2017.
21. Patton MQ. Qualitative research and evaluation methods. 2nd ed. Newbury Park: Sage; 2002.
22. Myers MD. Qualitative research in business and management. 2nd ed. Thousand Oaks: Sage; 2013.
23. Johnson B. Examining the validity structure of qualitative research. Education. 1997;118(3):282–92.
24. Plourde G, Prudhomme D. Managing obesity in adults in primary care. Can Med Assoc J. 2012;184(9):1039.
25. Gans KM, Ross E, Barner CW, Wylie-Rosett J, McMurray J, Eaton C. REAP and WAVE: new tools to rapidly assess/discuss nutrition with patients. J Nutr. 2003;133(2):556S.
26. Torti J, Luig T, Borowitz M, Johnson J, Sharma A, Campbell-Scherer D. The 5As team patient study: patient perspectives on the role of primary care in obesity management. BMC Fam Pract. 2017;18:19.
27. Ferrante JM, Piasecki AK, Ohman-Strickland PA, Crabtree BF. Family Physicians' practices and attitudes regarding Care of Extremely Obese Patients. Obesity. 2009;17(9):1710–6.
28. Kloek CJ, Tol J, Veenhof C, Van der Wulp I, CS Swinkels I. Dutch General Practitioners' weight management policy for overweight and obese patients. BMC Obesity. 2014; 1(2).
29. Booth AO, Nowson CA. Patient recall of receiving lifestyle advice for overweight and hypertension from their general practitioner. BMC Fam Pract. 2010;11:8. https://doi.org/10.1186/1471-2296-11-8
30. Harris MF, et al. What predicts patient-reported GP management of smoking, nutrition, alcohol, physical activity and weight? Aust J Prim Health. 2011;18:123–8.
31. Asselin J, Osunlana AM, Ogunleye AA, Sharma AM, Campbell-Scherer D. Challenges in interdisciplinary weight management in primary care: lessons learned from the 5As team study. Clin Obes. 2016;6(2):124–32.
32. Public Health Agency of Canada. Weight management experiences of overweight and obese Canadian adults: findings from a national survey. 2017. http://www.phac-aspc.gc.ca/publicat/hpcdp-pspmc/32-2/ar-01-eng.php#footnote8. Accessed 10 Aug 2017.
33. Lebrun LA, Chowdhury J, Sripipatana A, Nair S, Tomoyasu N, Ngo-Metzger Q. Overweight/obesity and weight-related treatment among patients in U.S. federally supported health centers. Obes Res Clin Pract. 2013;7:5.
34. Claridge R, Gray L, Stubbe M, Macdonald L, Tester R, Dowell AC. General practitioner opinion of weight management interventions in New Zealand. J Prim Health Care. 2014;6(3):212–20.
35. Howatson A, Wall C, Turner-Benny P. The contribution of dietitians to the primary health care workforce. J Prim Health Care. 2015;7(4):324–32.
36. Harvey EL, Glenny A-M, Kirk SFL, Summerbell CD. An updated systematic review of interventions to improve health professionals' management of obesity. Obes Rev. 2002;3(1):45–55.
37. Campbell K, Engel H, Timperio A, Cooper C, Crawford D. Obesity management: Australian general practitioners' attitudes and practices. Obes Res. 2000;8:459–66.
38. Teixeira FV, Pais-Ribeiro JL, Maia A. A qualitative study of GPs' views towards obesity: are they fighting or giving up? Public Health. 2015;129:218–25.
39. Thuan J-F, Avignon A. Obesity management: attitudes and practices of French general practitioners in a region of France. Int J Obes. 2005;29:1100–6.
40. Dietz WH, Baur LA, Hall K, Puhl RM, Taveras EM, Uauy R, et al. Management of obesity: improvement of health-care training and systems for prevention and care. Lancet. 2015;385(9986):2521–33.
41. Post R, Mainous A, Gregorie S, Knoll M, Diaz V, Saxena S. The influence of physician acknowledgment of Patients' weight status on patient perceptions of overweight and obesity in the United States. Arch Intern Med. 2011;171:4.
42. Brown I, Stride C, Psarou A, Brewins L, Thompson J. Management of obesity in primary care: nurses' practices, beliefs, and attitudes. J Adv Nurs. 2007;59(4):329–41.
43. Cass S, Ball L, Leveritt M. Australian practice nurses' perceptions of their role and competency to provide nutrition care to patients living with chronic disease. Aust J Prim Health. 2014;20(2):203–8.
44. Chase DA, Ash JS, Cohen DJ, Hall J, Olson GM, Dorr DA. The EHR's roles in collaboration between providers: a qualitative study. AMIA Annu Symp Proc. 2014;2014:1718–27.

14

Primary care provider perceptions of enablers and barriers to following guideline-recommended laboratory tests to confirm chronic kidney disease

Danielle M. Nash[1,2*], Amit X. Garg[1,2,3,4], K. Scott Brimble[4,5] and Maureen Markle-Reid[2,6]

Abstract

Background: Patients should receive follow-up serum creatinine tests after an initial abnormal result to diagnose chronic kidney disease. However, half of the time this fails to occur in primary care. We interviewed primary care providers to better understand their perceptions of enablers and barriers to following this guideline-recommended care.

Methods: We performed a qualitative descriptive study guided by the Theoretical Domains Framework (TDF), a framework for behavioural change. We used purposeful sampling to recruit primary care providers (physicians and nurse practitioners) based on provider and practice characteristics (rural, solo versus team practice, etc.) from Ontario, Canada. We completed one-on-one interviews with providers using a semi-structured and open-ended interview guide based on the 14 TDF domains. We alternated between data collection and analysis, where we used directed content analysis to identify frequent, important, and conflicting enablers and barriers.

Results: We completed 13 interviews with nine primary care physicians and four nurse practitioners. Nine themes related to the TDF emerged from the data: 1) environmental context and resources, 2) knowledge, 3) memory, attention, and decision processes, 4) beliefs about consequences, 5) goals, 6) social or professional role, 7) behavioural regulation, 8) skills, and 9) optimism. Within these themes, we identified 16 enablers and five barriers. Some enablers included, providers' knowledge on appropriate testing, their motivation to order these tests, and their use of tools and resources to help order follow-up serum creatinine tests. However, providers perceived some barriers including that ordering confirmatory laboratory tests for chronic kidney disease was not always a priority in regards to other care they wish to provide. Providers also noted that a perceived barrier is patients not going to the laboratory to complete the test.

Conclusions: We identified novel enablers and barriers to primary care providers completing guideline recommended repeat testing for the diagnosis of chronic kidney disease. Similar research is needed to understand the views of patients. These research findings can be used to inform strategies to improve the quality of care.

Keywords: Chronic kidney disease, Laboratory tests, Qualitative research, Primary care, Family medicine, Theoretical domains framework

* Correspondence: danielle.nash@lhsc.on.ca

[1]ICES, London, Ontario, Canada

[2]Department of Health Research Methods, Evidence, and Impact, McMaster University, Hamilton, Ontario, Canada

Full list of author information is available at the end of the article

Background

Approximately 12.5% of all Canadians live with chronic kidney disease [1], which is characterized by a sustained reduction in kidney function and may include significant levels of protein in the urine. Early detection of chronic kidney disease allows healthcare providers to initiate appropriate management to help prevent or slow the patient's progression to kidney failure. Most patients with early stage chronic kidney disease are managed in the primary care setting and are only referred to nephrologists if they have advanced disease or are at increased risk of progression.

International guidelines published in 2013 from Kidney Disease Improving Global Outcomes (KDIGO) recommend that chronic kidney disease should be classified based on estimated glomerular filtration rate (eGFR) and level of albuminuria [2]. These guidelines recommend that patients with an initial eGFR < 60 mL/min/ 1.73 m^2 should have a repeat serum creatinine test within three months to diagnose chronic kidney disease [2]. Although these guidelines are well recognized by nephrologists, primary care providers are generally not aware of them. Additional efforts have been made in several jurisdictions to bridge this gap in primary care. For example, the Ontario Renal Network (ORN), the provincial agency responsible for the delivery of kidney care services in Ontario, Canada, released a flow diagram based on these clinical guidelines to aid primary care providers with appropriate screening, monitoring, management, and referral for chronic kidney disease (the KidneyWise toolkit) [3]. This toolkit provides specific advice for ordering follow-up serum creatinine tests. The ORN has attempted wide dissemination of this toolkit through national primary care conferences, social media, and integration into electronic medical records (EMRs).

Based on a previous population-based study among Ontario primary care providers, only 49% of patients with initial abnormal eGFR values received a repeat serum creatinine test in the following six months [4]. These findings are consistent with another Ontario study among primary care providers using an EMR [5]. Similarly, studies in other countries have shown that only 14 to 28% of patients with an initial eGFR < 60 mL/min/ 1.73 m^2 have a documented diagnosis for chronic kidney disease [6–9]. It is not clear why this guideline recommendation is not being followed in practice for half of the patients.

Previous literature on evidence-practice gaps in primary care have demonstrated that guideline-based recommendations are generally not being followed in practice due to lack of time and resources, limited relevance of research to practice, and patient-related factors [10–16]. Based on our detailed literature review, we did not find any previous studies on primary care providers' perspectives on the enablers and barriers to completing follow-up serum creatinine tests to confirm chronic kidney disease (Additional file 1). It is not clear if previously identified evidence-practice gaps are relevant to this practice.

There are many different frameworks and theories on clinical practice change and implementation of guidelines [17–19]. We used a robust framework of behavioural change, referred to as the Theoretical Domains Framework (TDF), in our study to shape our research questions, interview guide, and analysis [17, 20]. The TDF was developed to help understand why evidence-based guidelines may not be followed in practice and to help develop strategies to improve implementation of evidence into practice. It is a consensus framework based on 33 behaviour change theories and 128 theoretical constructs to inform implementation research [17]. Based on a validation study of the original TDF, the refined framework includes 14 domains and 84 theoretical constructs [20].

The purpose of this qualitative descriptive study was to use the TDF as a framework to elicit and describe the perceived enablers and barriers to following recommendations for ordering a repeat serum creatinine test after an initial abnormal kidney function test result by Ontario primary care providers.

Methods

Study design

We completed a qualitative descriptive study of primary care providers' perceived enablers and barriers guided by the TDF. This study design was used to provide an in-depth description of enablers and barriers with minimal interpretation of the data [21–23]. We followed the reporting guidelines from the COnsolidated criteria for Reporting Qualitative Research (COREQ) (Additional file 2) [24].

Ethics

In accordance with the Helsinki Declaration, we received research ethics approval from the Hamilton Integrated Research Ethics Board (# 2017–2286). We followed the Tri-Council Policy Statement 2 (TCPS2) guidelines on ethical conduct of qualitative research [25]. After sharing information about the study, we obtained verbal consent from providers for study participation. We sent the information and consent form by email to the participants if they preferred a copy. Participants received $25 compensation for their time, which was provided after each interview.

Sampling & Recruitment

We used purposeful sampling strategies of maximum variation and snowball sampling to identify information-rich participants. Eligible participants included primary care providers practicing in Ontario who are responsible for ordering laboratory tests (physicians and nurse practitioners).

We used a multi-faceted recruitment strategy. First, we contacted the four main Ontario primary care organizations, which circulated information about our study to their members: 1) Association of Family Health Teams of Ontario, 2) Nurse Practitioners Association of Ontario, 3) Ontario College of Family Physicians, and 4) Association of Ontario Health Centres. These organizations provided our study information to their members either through a regular newsletter, by posting the information on their website, or through an online bulletin. The information provided included a brief explanation of the study and directed people to contact the research team for further information.

Second, we compiled a list of potential participants from the College of Physicians and Surgeons of Ontario and Nurse Practitioners' Association of Ontario websites based on maximum variation selection criteria including rural versus urban clinics, provider sex, number of years practicing, family physician versus nurse practitioner, size of practice, and team versus individual practices. We contacted these individuals by calling or visiting primary care clinics in the province and briefly explaining the study to the healthcare providers or their administrative staff. We then provided practices with the study information flyer either by email, fax, or in person.

Third, we used snowball sampling by asking individuals to pass along our study information to potential participants to see if they would be interested in our study.

We decided a priori that we would recruit at least 13 participants. After the first 10 interviews, we planned on interviewing at least three more participants and completed recruitment when data saturation was reached and no new themes emerged with subsequent interviews [26, 27].

Data collection

One author (DMN; Doctoral student) conducted all one-on-one, semi-structured, open-ended interviews either in person (at the physician office) or by telephone. We developed the interview guide based on the TDF and piloted it prior to the study with two physicians (see Additional file 3). We used the results of the pilot to modify and reframe questions. Example questions included, "How easy or difficult is it for you to regularly order confirmatory tests for chronic kidney disease?" and "What do you think will happen if you do not order confirmatory tests for chronic kidney disease?". We revised questions slightly throughout the study as the data were analyzed. Based on the semi-structured format of the interviews, we used additional questions and probes to elicit further information or to ask participants to clarify answers. The interviews were audio recorded and transcribed verbatim. We uploaded the transcripts to NVivo 11 software for assistance with data management when performing the analysis.

We collected demographic and practice information, including provider's age and number of years in practice, to provide some aggregate descriptive information on study participants.

Analysis

We used directed content analysis by using the TDF as a framework to identify and describe the enablers and barriers derived from the data. Content analysis is a qualitative analytic technique where investigators systematically review and describe textual data using codes and themes [28]. Directed content analysis is both a deductive and an inductive analytic approach where an existing theory or framework is used to help guide the analysis and to generate initial concepts and themes [28]. Using this approach, we mapped the data to the 14 TDF constructs to help us identify enablers and barriers to guideline adherence for repeat serum creatinine testing to diagnose chronic kidney disease [17, 20]. We also identified any emerging themes from the data that did not fit into any of the TDF constructs.

The analysis was an iterative process, where we alternated between data collection and analysis. This allowed interview questions for subsequent data collection to be revised and also allowed us to determine when data saturation was reached.

We listened to the audio-recordings shortly after each interview and read through the transcripts to correct any errors in transcription and to fully immerse ourselves in the data.

The coding and broader themes were based on the TDF domains. We practiced investigator triangulation to increase credibility in research findings, where both DMN and MMR independently coded the first two interview transcripts, and compared coding to discuss agreement or disagreement. DMN completed the coding of the remaining transcripts independently, but with regular meetings with MMR to review coding progress. Any disagreements were resolved by consensus. We reviewed the transcripts from each interview and assigned initial codes based on the TDF domains to each data item, which typically included one to three sentences.

In the next phase of the analysis, we created sub themes within each broader domain. We then defined, refined and named these sub themes within the codebook, which was used to guide the remaining analysis, and revised throughout the study to reflect emerging themes. Finally, we identified the relevant TDF domains and sub themes by focussing only on the frequent, conflicting, or important themes (i.e. strong beliefs even if they were not as common across the participants).

Throughout the study, we practiced bracketing, which is the ability to separate our own values and opinions from influencing the participants' responses or our interpretation of the results. This is especially important in qualitative research, since the findings are subjective and based on interpretation by the researchers. To ensure credibility and confirmability of findings, DMN kept a reflective journal throughout the research process to recognize, document, and try to separate any assumptions that may have influenced the research. To ensure credibility of research findings, we also used peer debriefing by meeting with other experienced qualitative researchers from the Ottawa Hospital Research Institute who are familiar with the TDF, but who were not involved in our study. We discussed and confirmed preliminary findings that emerged from the data after completing nine interviews. Finally, we kept a detailed audit trail including the initial study protocol, DMN's reflective journal, audio recordings of the interviews, transcription files of the interviews, and minutes from research team meetings.

Results

Characteristics of the study participants

In total, we completed 13 interviews with 13 individual participants. We reached data saturation after the 10th interview, since no new themes emerged from interviews with participants 11 to 13. Nine out of 13 participants were female and the average age was 46 years. Nine participants were primary care physicians and the remaining four participants were nurse practitioners (see Table 1).

Relevant TDF domains

Themes emerging from the data reflected nine of the TDF domains: 1) environmental context and resources, 2) knowledge, 3) memory, attention and decision processes, 4) beliefs about consequences, 5) goals, 6) social or professional role, 7) behavioural regulation, 8) skills, and 9) optimism (see Table 2). In addition to these TDF themes, another theme emerged on completing laboratory tests/ patient factors.

Identified TDF enablers

Among the nine TDF themes, we identified 16 enablers perceived by primary care providers to ordering repeat serum creatinine tests (see Table 2). The majority of providers were aware of guidelines for ordering a repeat serum creatinine test and most had a positive opinion about using clinical guidelines to inform behaviour and decision-making (*knowledge*). For example: *"I don't think [guidelines] should determine [behaviour], but they should definitely guide it and direct it because it's, again, research based and trying to follow that."* The most commonly used clinical guidelines were for diabetes or the implementation of KDIGO chronic kidney disease guidelines in the ORN's KidneyWise toolkit (*environmental context and resources*). For example:

> *"I think that the algorithm approach is actually relatively simple as opposed to a lot of the other guidelines out there that have algorithms that are about three hundred things on a diagram and then having an application for it is useful. The KidneyWise application is actually quite useful."*

Although not all providers were aware of guidelines for ordering repeat serum creatinine tests, the majority still had the knowledge of when they should be ordering these tests (*knowledge*). For example:

> *"Let's just say I don't know anything about any guidelines. I have a practice that I do, that I believe is correct, so we'll see what happens there."* and *"Actually there's one today that just popped up that his glomerular filtration rate dropped like from 70 to 50 which is below normal, so I'm going to repeat it in three months."*

Furthermore, providers described that they would refer to guidelines when needed and then tailor the recommendations to the specific patient and their clinical presentation in order to decide when they should order confirmatory tests for chronic kidney disease

Table 1 Demographic and Practice Characteristics for the 13 Study Participants

Characteristics	Percentage/ Mean	Standard Deviation	Range (min – max)
Gender (% female)	69.2%		
Age (years)	45.8	9.2	29–59
Primary care physician or nurse practitioner (% primary care physician)	69.2%		
Number of years practicing	15.3	9.9	1–32
Medical school/ nurse practitioner program location (% Canada)	92.3%		
Practice location (% urban)	69.2%		
Practice type (% family health team/ family health group)	92.3%		
Approximate number of patients rostered/ in the practice	2248	3219	200–12,500

Table 2 Relevant Theoretical Domains Framework (TDF) Themes and Sub-themes Identified as Enablers or Barriers

Domain/ Theme	Sub-theme	Relevance	Enabler/ Barrier
Environmental context and resources	Using EMR tools	Frequent	Enabler
	Referring to guidelines	Frequent	Enabler
	Depending on support staff	Frequent	Enabler
Knowledge	Being aware of guidelines	Conflicting	Enabler
	Having a positive attitude toward guidelines	Conflicting	Enabler & Barrier
	Knowing what to do	Frequent	Enabler
Memory, attention and decision processes	Making a deliberate decision	Frequent	Enabler
	Forgetting	Important	Barrier
Beliefs about consequences	Being aware of clinical consequences	Frequent	Enabler
	Perceived low risk in delaying confirmatory test	Important	Barrier
	Weighing the costs and benefits	Frequent	Enabler
Goals	Prioritizing care goals	Conflicting	Enabler & Barrier
	Recognizing the importance	Frequent	Enabler
Social or professional role	Claiming responsibility	Frequent	Enabler
	Identifying practice type or role influences	Frequent	Enabler & Barrier
Behavioural regulation	Taking ownership of action	Frequent	Enabler
Skills	Demonstrating communication skills	Important	Enabler
Optimism	Having a positive attitude	Frequent	Enabler
N/A[a]	Completing laboratory tests/ patient factors	Frequent	Barrier

[a]This was not one of the TDF domains but was considered a relevant theme

(*environmental context and resources; memory, attention and decision processes*). For example:

> *"So usually the first thing if I get an abnormal creatinine or estimated glomerular filtration rate or positive albumin-to-creatinine ratio then it's to, kind of, look and see, okay, is this something new for this person or is this long-standing, is it getting worse, is it stable, is there something else going on, do they have a urinary tract infection... like, something that may account for the finding. If it's something that's completely new then, absolutely, it's repeated."*

Besides using clinical guidelines, providers frequently described the use of internal clinic resources to help decide when or if to order a repeat serum creatinine test (*environmental context and resources*). Many providers described the use of support staff (i.e. clerical staff or nurses) to follow up with patients about a repeat serum creatinine test. For example: *"I can just send tasks to certain nurses or support staff just to follow back up with them and ask them to order whatever I need to be done."* Even though providers agreed that having support staff would be helpful, not all providers had available support staff to assist with ordering laboratory tests or to follow-up with patients (*environmental context and resources*). For example:

> *"If the world was a perfect place some of this stuff could be off loaded to either a nurse or a nurse practitioner that I work with but the world is not a perfect place and we're all just too busy."*

Providers frequently described using different features in their EMRs to help decide whether or not to order laboratory tests or to remind themselves to order a follow-up test (*environmental context and resources; memory, attention and decision processes*). For example: *"The electronic medical record that allows me to kind of track... laboratory results of creatinines over time, is something that helps me determine whether or not I need to do a confirmatory test."* A couple providers also mentioned that having chronic disease registries (mostly for diabetes) could be used to help keep track of patients who may require a follow-up serum creatinine test. However, they mentioned that these registries generally require the help of support staff (who may or may not be available) to manage and track when patients need certain laboratory tests.

Many providers agreed that ordering a repeat serum creatinine test is a priority and helps to prevent potential adverse consequences for the patients (*goals; beliefs about consequences*). For example:

> *"You've just got to focus in on one or two different things, and sometimes the chronic kidney disease could get lost*

in transition. But usually it's incorporated, but that would be the most likely." and *"One [consequence] is that it continues to go up, and I miss that they're going into much worse renal failure. Another is that I give them things that are more toxic, or that are toxic to an already compromised kidney. Those would be the biggest ones."*

Providers also agreed that the benefits of ordering these tests outweigh the costs to the healthcare system (*beliefs about consequences*). For example: *"Yes, because it'll cost a lot more if [their kidney function] declines because we didn't check it."*

Overall, providers were generally optimistic about ordering follow-up laboratory tests for chronic kidney disease and were motivated to do so (*optimism; goals*). For example: *"Like there are no concerns about ordering any of these tests."* and *"... I try very hard, because I mean, kidneys are pretty important, right?"*

All participants agreed that ordering a follow-up serum creatinine test to confirm chronic kidney disease is part of their role as primary care providers (*social or professional role*). For example: *"Physicians have to be the ones in Ontario signing blood work requisitions, nurse practitioners and physicians."* Some participants described components of their professional role that enable them to order a repeat serum creatinine test. For example:

> *"As a nurse practitioner I'm allowed a little bit more time so it makes it a little easier, so I try and provide as much health teaching to the patient and write it on the lab slip when I want them to check it."*

Identified TDF barriers

We identified five barriers perceived by primary care providers to ordering a repeat serum creatinine test to diagnose chronic kidney disease (see Table 2). There were some conflicting perspectives on views of clinical guidelines where some providers had more pessimistic views (*knowledge*). For example:

> *"I'm going to assume that [guidelines] are evidence based or at least partially evidence based as much as guidelines can be because if you look at those guidelines in general they're about maximally 14% evidence based and the rest is opinion, so I assume that they are approximately the same as every other guideline."*

Some providers did not perceive that it was a priority to order a repeat serum creatinine test relative to other competing priorities in primary care (*goals*). For example:

> *"So I'll tell you what, we have 49 diseases that we deal with in family medicine. Kidneys are one small one, and there's very little to do with that repeat creatinine. There's nothing that changes. So is it a priority? No. There are many other things that are higher priority."*

Providers also described that sometimes they forget to order the repeat testing (*memory, attention and decision processes*), but many mentioned that using the EMR as a resource generally helps to prevent forgetting (*environmental context and resources*). For example:

> *"I think cognitive overload probably plays a part in everything that we do every day and it's a matter of sometimes things just get forgotten."* and *"...I guess once upon a time for me it would have been remembering when it was due. But electronic medical records make it that much easier because you can send yourself little reminders."*

Even though the majority of providers agreed that there are significant clinical consequences for the patients if follow-up laboratory tests are not ordered, a few providers perceived that waiting longer to confirm the initial test result would not change the care they provide for the patient (*beliefs about consequences*). For example:

> *"You know, it's nice to initiate in the workup once they are confirmed [chronic kidney disease] a little bit earlier, but if it has to wait until a year, I don't know that it makes a significant difference, 'cause patients usually present on an annual basis for blood work. Or that's their expectation. So sometimes you only have the chance to repeat it a year later."*

Some providers described components of their professional role that prohibit them from always ordering follow-up laboratory tests (*social or professional role*). For example, providers who work in a family health team described the following: *"...because they're multiple providers... it may be something that someone else has already investigated."*

Other factors influencing laboratory test completion

The providers in our study had perceived some patient barriers to completing repeat serum creatinine testing that did not fit within any of the TDF domains. For example, the most prevalent barrier identified was patient compliance (*completing laboratory tests/ patient factors*). Some providers described using communication skills with the patients to explain the importance of getting the laboratory test done, which they perceived helps to improve patient compliance (*skills*). For example: *"So, you know, we usually tell them that, no, we need to repeat this because your renal function, we need to make sure your kidneys are good. And then ... they're on board."*

In addition, providers described other actions that they take to help improve patient compliance in completing laboratory tests when ordered (*behavioural regulation*). For example:

> *"Providing more follow-up and making sure, again, tests are being done as asked of the patient just to make sure they are. So having maybe more tasks sent to myself reminding myself that things have been ordered, to recheck that."* and *"Well, one thing that I will tell you is that I do not file the abnormal test into the patient's chart until I am sure that the patient actually is aware of the abnormal result."*

Providers also mention laboratory factors which may influence whether or not the test is ordered, and ultimately if the patients complete the test (*completing laboratory tests/ patient factors*). For example: *"We used to have a lab in our family practice unit, right in the same building and that really was helpful for our patients in terms of any sort of laboratory investigations, but yeah."*

Discussion

Using a comprehensive framework of behaviour change to guide our analysis, we identified 16 enablers and five barriers perceived by providers for ordering repeat serum creatinine tests to diagnose chronic kidney disease. We found that there was an interaction between many of the TDF domains. For example, healthcare providers generally know what they should be doing (*knowledge*), are motivated to do so (*goals*), have the tools and resources required to perform the behaviour (*environmental context and resources*), and use both the information and tools to make an informed decision on whether or not to order a repeat serum creatinine test (*memory, attention and decision processes*). However, ordering follow-up serum creatinine tests was not always perceived as a priority (*goals*) or as directly influencing patient outcomes (*beliefs about consequences*), and might sometimes be forgotten (*memory, attention and decision processes*).

Based on our comprehensive literature search, this is the first qualitative study to assess the enablers and barriers perceived by primary care providers for the behaviour of ordering repeat serum creatinine tests to confirm a chronic kidney disease diagnosis. We found novel enablers and barriers that have not been reported in previous studies related to chronic kidney disease care or laboratory ordering in general, including the following enablers: making a deliberate decision and being aware of clinical consequences; and barriers: forgetting to order tests and prioritizing care goals.

Unlike other studies on guideline adherence for chronic kidney disease care, we found that providers are generally aware of guidelines or at least know that they should be ordering repeat serum creatinine tests to confirm chronic kidney disease [29–32]. Previous studies have shown low awareness of national (U.S.) and international guidelines specifically for chronic kidney disease. In contrast, we were interested in participants' awareness of any guidelines for confirming chronic kidney disease with repeat serum creatinine testing [2, 33]. As such, our participants were generally more aware of diabetes guidelines and a provincial kidney algorithm.

Although the majority of participants in our study had positive attitudes towards clinical guidelines for ordering follow-up serum creatinine tests, there were some dissenting views perceiving that these guidelines lacked clinical evidence. Estrella et al. (2003) conducted a survey with healthcare providers and also found that many participants did not perceive chronic kidney disease guidelines to be evidence-based [34].

Consistent with our study findings, previous studies have found that primary care providers perceive laboratory tests to be useful in assessing kidney function [31, 35]. However, we found that even though providers were generally motivated to order a repeat serum creatinine test and perceived this to be important, it was not always a priority. Furthermore, we identified another barrier where some participants perceived that the care they provide for the patient will not change if they do not order follow-up serum creatinine tests in a timely manner. This result is consistent with findings from Crinson et al. (2010), who performed focus groups with primary care providers on their perceptions of chronic kidney disease management [35].

Similar to our findings, previous studies have also shown that the use of internal resources are enablers to caring for patients with chronic kidney disease and ordering laboratory tests. For example, providers generally rely on support staff and use electronic medical records to provide better patient care [36–39].

Finally, previous studies on primary care providers' perceived enablers and barriers to ordering laboratory tests in general have also identified that a barrier is patients not completing the laboratory test [37, 40]. A mixed methods study on patient perceived barriers to not completing a laboratory test after initiating a new medication that required monitoring included barriers of forgetting or competing demands [41]. Since our study only included the primary care provider perspective, we cannot make any conclusions about the applicability of these patient-specified barriers to completing a repeat serum creatinine test. Additional research is needed to further investigate these findings.

Strengths and limitations

We used strategies suggested by Guba (1981) as outlined in our methods section to ensure rigour in our qualitative study [42]. This helps to increase the credibility, dependability, confirmability, and transferability of our study findings.

Another strength of our study is using the TDF to help frame our research, since it is comprehensive, validated, and has been successfully used in previous research on guideline implementation [17, 20]. Furthermore, the TDF also includes clearly defined domains that were applicable to our setting. A limitation of using a framework to guide our study is that we may have missed themes that were not captured through the TDF.

The findings from our study are transferable to other settings, for instance, primary care providers who work in similar primary healthcare settings across Canada. Based on the maximum variation sampling criteria that we applied, and our multi-faceted recruitment strategies, our findings likely apply to primary care physicians and nurse practitioners, female and male providers, urban and rural clinic settings (including Northern Ontario), practices of varying sizes, different types of practice models, and providers who have been practicing for different lengths of time. Even though we included both urban and rural primary care providers in our study, the majority of rural providers were nurse practitioners. This may have limited the perception specifically of rural primary care physicians. Furthermore, the majority of the participants in our study practiced in a family health team or a family health organization, thereby limiting the perceptions captured by solo-practicing providers. Previous literature has shown that providers perceive lack of effective reminders or tools to track laboratory tests in the EMRs is a barrier to ordering tests [37–39]. All participants in our study described that they used an EMR to order tests and most described this as an enabler. Therefore, our findings may not apply to primary care providers who do not use an EMR in practice.

Study implications

This research has implications on the care of patients with chronic kidney disease in the primary care setting. The results of our study can be used to inform future interventions to help improve care regarding repeat serum creatinine tests to diagnose chronic kidney disease.

Future strategies to improve confirmatory laboratory test ordering for chronic kidney disease need to be multi-factorial since many components of the TDF apply to this behaviour. By mapping the relevant TDF domains to the Behaviour Change Wheel, we can identify interventions that may help to improve adherence to this behaviour [20, 43]. For example, since we showed that an enabler is use of tools within EMRs, we could use an environmental restructuring intervention to improve reminders or prompts within the EMRs to order follow-up laboratory tests. As another example, we could use a persuasion intervention such as presenting convincing yet factual information on the importance of ordering confirmatory tests to delay disease progression. This would help overcome the perceived barriers of ordering repeat serum creatinine tests being a low priority and that there is little harm in delaying confirmatory testing.

The findings from this research can potentially be generalized to guideline-recommendations in primary care beyond chronic kidney disease. For instance, some of the enablers and barriers identified in this study might be applicable to confirmatory testing for hypothyroidism [44]. However, future research is needed to explore the applicability of these factors to the implementation of other guidelines in primary care.

Conclusions

Overall, we identified some novel enablers and barriers perceived by primary care providers in regards to ordering repeat serum creatinine tests to diagnose chronic kidney disease. The majority of participants know that they should be ordering these tests, and are generally motivated, and have the required resources to do so. However, some providers perceived that ordering a repeat serum creatinine test would not change the care they provide and it may not always be a priority to the provider or the patient. Providers also perceived that there may be other contributing factors beyond their control, such as patients not going to the laboratory to complete these tests. Future qualitative research with patients as the participants is needed to confirm and further investigate this finding.

Abbreviations

eGFR: Estimated Glomerular Filtration Rate; EMR: Electronic Medical Record; KDIGO: Kidney Disease Improving Global Outcomes; ORN: Ontario Renal Network; TCPS2: Tri-Council Policy Statement 2; TDF: Theoretical Domains Framework

Acknowledgements

We would like to thank Dr. Justin Presseau from the Ottawa Hospital Research Institute for his insightful feedback on the analysis.

Funding

Dr. Danielle Nash's training is supported by a Canadian Institutes of Health Research Doctoral award. Dr. Amit Garg was supported by the Dr. Adam Linton Chair in Kidney Health Analytics and a Clinician Investigator Award from the Canadian Institutes for Health Research. Dr. Maureen Markle-Reid was supported by the Canada Research Chairs Program.

Authors' contributions
DMN and AXG were responsible for study conception. DMN and MMR were responsible for the study design, analysis and interpretation of the results. DMN, MMR, AXG and KSB provided feedback on the study design and findings. DMN, MMR, AXG and KSB reviewed and approved of the manuscript.

Authors' information
DMN is a female doctoral student with qualitative research course experience but no previous qualitative interview experience. MMR is a nurse with training in qualitative research (PhD). AXG and KSB are nephrologists and clinician investigators.

Consent for publication
Not applicable.

Competing interests
The authors declare that they have no competing interests.

Author details
[1]ICES, London, Ontario, Canada. [2]Department of Health Research Methods, Evidence, and Impact, McMaster University, Hamilton, Ontario, Canada. [3]Department of Medicine, University of Western Ontario, London, Ontario, Canada. [4]The Ontario Renal Network, Toronto, Ontario, Canada. [5]Department of Medicine, McMaster University, Hamilton, Ontario, Canada. [6]School of Nursing, McMaster University, Hamilton, Ontario, Canada.

References

1. Arora P, Vasa P, Brenner D, Iglar K, McFarlane P, Morrison H, et al. Prevalence estimates of chronic kidney disease in Canada: results of a nationally representative survey. CMAJ. 2013;185:E417–23.
2. Kidney Disease. Improving global outcomes (KDIGO) CKD work group. KDIGO 2012 clinical practice guideline for the evaluation and Management of Chronic Kidney Disease. Kidney Int Suppl. 2013;3:1–150.
3. Ontario Renal Network. Referral Guidance: KidneyWise Clinical Toolkit [Internet]. 2015. Available from: kidneywise.ca. [cited 2016 May 26]
4. Nash DM, Brimble S, Markle-Reid M, McArthur E, Tu K, Nesrallah GE, et al. Quality of Care for Patients with Chronic Kidney Disease in the primary care setting: a retrospective cohort study from Ontario, Canada. Can J Kidney Heal Dis. 2017;4:1–14.
5. Tu K, Ba LB, Hunter K, Ba JR. Quality indicators for the detection and management of chronic kidney disease in primary care in Canada derived from a modified Delphi panel approach. C Open. 2017;5:E74–81.
6. LA S, Stewart RC, Su H-L, DeLoskey RJ, Astor BC, Fox CH, et al. Primary care detection of chronic kidney disease in adults with type-2 diabetes: the ADD-CKD study (awareness, detection and drug therapy in type 2 diabetes and chronic kidney disease). PLoS One. 2014;9:e110535.
7. Fraser SDS, Parkes J, Culliford D, Santer M, Roderick PJ. Timeliness in chronic kidney disease and albuminuria identification: a retrospective cohort study. BMC Fam Pract. 2015;16:18.
8. Ravera M, Noberasco G, Weiss U, Re M, Gallina AM, Filippi A, et al. CKD awareness and blood pressure control in the primary care hypertensive population. Am J Kidney Dis. 2011;57:71–7.
9. Razavian M, Heeley EL, Perkovic V, Zoungas S, Weekes A, Patel AA, et al. Cardiovascular risk management in chronic kidney disease in general practice (the AusHEART study). Nephrol Dial Transplant. 2012;27:1396–402.
10. Cabana MD, Rand CS, Powe NR, Wu AW, Wilson MH, Abboud P-AC, et al. Why Don't physicians follow a framework for improvement. JAMA. 1999;282: 1458–65.
11. Langley C, Faulkner A, Watkins C, Gray S, Harvey I. Use of guidelines in primary care--practitioners' perspectives. Fam Pract. 1998;15(2):105–11.
12. McKenna HP, Ashton S, Keeney S. Barriers to evidence-based practice in primary care. J Adv Nurs. 2004;45:178–89.
13. Calderon C, Sola I, Rotaeche R, Marzo-Castillejo M, Louro-Gonzalez A, Carrillo R, et al. EBM in primary care: a qualitative multicenter study in Spain. BMC Fam Pract. 2011;12:84.
14. O'Donnell CA. Attitudes and knowledge of primary care professionals towards evidence-based practice: a postal survey. J Eval Clin Pract. 2004;10:197–205.
15. Gerrish K, Guillaume L, Kirshbaum M, Mcdonnell A, Tod A, Nolan M. Factors influencing the contribution of advanced practice nurses to promoting evidence-based practice among front-line nurses: findings from a cross-sectional survey. J Adv Nurs. 2011;67:1079–90.
16. Quinlan E, Robertson S. The communicative power of nurse practitioners in multidisciplinary primary healthcare teams. J Am Acad Nurse Pract. 2013;25: 91–102.
17. Michie S, Johnston M, Abraham C, Lawton R, Parker D, Walker A. Making psychological theory useful for implementing evidence based practice: a consensus approach. Qual Saf Health Care. 2005;14:26–33.
18. May C, Rapley T, Mair F, Treweek S, Murray E, Ballini L, et al. Normalization Process Theory On-line Users' Manual, Toolkit and NoMAD instrument [Internet]. 2015. Available from: http://www.normalizationprocess.org. [cited 2016 Jun 9]
19. Damschroder LJ, Aron DC, Keith RE, Kirsh SR, J a A, Lowery JC. Fostering implementation of health services research findings into practice: a consolidated framework for advancing implementation science. Implement Sci. 2009;4:40–55.
20. Cane J, O'Connor D, Michie S. Validation of the theoretical domains framework for use in behaviour change and implementation research. Implement Sci. 2012;7:37.
21. Neergaard MA, Olesen F, Andersen RS, Sondergaard J. Qualitative description - the poor cousin of health research? BMC Med Res Methodol. 2009;9:52.
22. Sandelowski M, Sandelowski M. Focus on research methods: whatever happened to qualitative description? Res Nurs Health. 2000;23:334–40.
23. Sandelowski M. What's in a name? Qualitative description revisited. Res Nurs Health. 2010;33:77–84.
24. Tong A, Sainsbury P, Craig J. Consolidated criterio for reporting qualitative research (COREQ): a 32- item checklist for interviews and focus group. Int J Qual Heal Care. 2007;19:349–57.
25. Government of Canada. Tri-Council Policy Statement 2 - Chapter 10: Qualitative Research [Internet]. 2015. Available from: http://www.pre.ethics.gc.ca/eng/policy-politique/initiatives/tcps2-eptc2/chapter10-chapitre10/. [cited 2016 Mar 26]
26. Francis JJ, Johnston M, Robertson C, Glidewell L, Entwistle V, Eccles MP, et al. What is an adequate sample size? Operationalising data saturation for theory-based interview studies. Psychol Health. 2010;25:1229–45.
27. Creswell JW. Qualitative inquiry and research design choosing among five approaches. 3rd ed. California: SAGE Publications Inc.; 2013.
28. Hsieh H-F, Shannon SE. Three approaches to qualitative content analysis. Qual Health Res. 2005;15:1277–88.
29. Fox CH, Brooks A, Zayas LE, McClellan W, Murray B. Primary care physicians' knowledge and practice patterns in the treatment of chronic kidney disease: an upstate New York practice-based research network (UNYNET) study. J Am Board Fam Med. 2006;19:54–61.
30. Boulware LE, Troll MU, Jaar BG, Myers DI, Powe NR. Identification and referral of patients with progressive CKD: a national study. Am J Kidney Dis. 2006;48:192–204.
31. Abdel-Kader K, Greer RC, Boulware LE, Unruh ML. Primary care physicians' familiarity, beliefs, and perceived barriers to practice guidelines in non-diabetic CKD: a survey study. BMC Nephrol. 2014;15:64.
32. Vest BM, York TRM, Sand J, Fox CH, Kahn LS. Chronic kidney disease guideline implementation in primary care: a qualitative report from the TRANSLATE CKD study. J Am Board Fam Med. 2015;28:624–31.
33. Levey AS, Coresh J, Balk E, Kausz AT, Levin A, Steffes MW, et al. National Kidney Foundation practice guidelines for chronic kidney disease: evaluation, classification, and stratification. Ann Intern Med. 2003;139:137–47.
34. Estrella MM, Jaar BG, Cavanaugh KL, Fox CH, Perazella MA, Soman SS, et al. Perceptions and use of the national kidney foundation KDOQI guidelines: a survey of U.S. renal healthcare providers. BMC Nephrol. 2013;14:230.
35. Crinson I, Gallagher H, Thomas N, de Lusignan S. How ready is general practice to improve quality in chronic kidney disease? A diagnostic analysis. Br J Gen Pract. 2010;60:403–9.
36. Feldstein D, Baier Manwell L, Grasmick M. Primary care providers and chronic kidney disease management: a qualitative study. Soc Gen Intern Med. 2010;33:S368.

37. Goldman RE, Soran CS, Hayward GL, Simon SR. Doctors' perceptions of laboratory monitoring in office practice. J Eval Clin Pract. 2010;16:1136–41.
38. Elder NC, McEwan TR, Flach JM, Gallimore JJ. Management of Test Results in family medicine offices. Ann Fam Med. 2009;7:343–51.
39. Parker DR, Gramling R, Goldman RE, Eaton CB, Ahern D, Cover RT, et al. Physicians' perceptions of barriers and facilitators regarding adoption of the National Cholesterol Education Program Guidelines. Prev Cardiol. 2008;11(1):29–35.
40. West DR, James KA, Fernald DH, Zelie C, Smith ML, Raab SS. Laboratory medicine handoff gaps experienced by primary care Practices : a report from the shared networks of collaborative ambulatory practices and partners (SNOCAP). J Am Board Fam Med. 2014;27:796–803.
41. Fischer SH, Field TS, Gagne SJ, Mazor KM, Preusse P, Reed G, et al. Patient completion of laboratory tests to monitor medication therapy: a mixed-methods study. J Gen Intern Med. 2012;28:513–21.
42. Guba EG. Criteria for assessing the trustworthiness of naturalistic inquiries. JSTOR. 1981;29:75–91.
43. Michie S, van Stralen MM, West R. The behaviour change wheel: a new method for characterising and designing behaviour change interventions. Implement Sci IS. 2011;6:42.
44. Garber JR, Cobin RH, Gharib H, Hennessey JV, Klein I, Mechanick JI, et al. Clinical practice guidelines for hypothyroidism in adults: cosponsored by the American Association of Clinical Endocrinologists and the American Thyroid Association. Endocr Pract. 2012;18:988–1028.

Keys to success of a community of clinical practice in primary care: a qualitative evaluation of the ECOPIH project

David Lacasta Tintorer[1,2,3], Josep Maria Manresa Domínguez[2,3], Enriqueta Pujol-Rivera[4], Souhel Flayeh Beneyto[1], Xavier Mundet Tuduri[3,5] and Francesc Saigí-Rubió[6*]

Abstract

Background: The current reality of primary care (PC) makes it essential to have telemedicine systems available to facilitate communication between care levels. Communities of practice have great potential in terms of care and education, and that is why the Online Communication Tool between Primary and Hospital Care was created. This tool enables PC and non-GP specialist care (SC) professionals to raise clinical cases for consultation and to share information. The objective of this article is to explore healthcare professionals' views on communities of clinical practice (CoCPs) and the changes that need to be made in an uncontrolled real-life setting after more than two years of use.

Methods: A descriptive-interpretative qualitative study was conducted on a total of 29 healthcare professionals who were users and non-users of a CoCP using 2 focus groups, 3 triangular groups and 5 individual interviews. There were 18 women, 21 physicians and 8 nurses. Of the interviewees, 21 were PC professionals, 24 were users of a CoCP and 7 held managerial positions.

Results: For a system of communication between PC and SC to become a tool that is habitually used and very useful, the interviewees considered that it would have to be able to find quick, effective solutions to the queries raised, based on up-to-date information that is directly applicable to daily clinical practice. Contact should be virtual – and probably collaborative – via a platform integrated into their habitual workstations and led by PC professionals. Organisational changes should be implemented to enable users to have more time in their working day to spend on the tool, and professionals should have a proactive attitude in order to make the most if its potential. It is also important to make certain technological changes, basically aimed at improving the tool's accessibility, by integrating it into habitual clinical workstations.

Conclusions: The collaborative tool that provides reliable, up-to-date information that is highly transferrable to clinical practice is valued for its effectiveness, efficiency and educational capacity. In order to make the most of its potential in terms of care and education, organisational changes and techniques are required to foster greater use.

Keywords: Primary health care, Problem solving, Telemedicine, Referral and consultation, Education medical continuing

Background

A characteristic feature of primary (PC) surgeries is that they have to attend to a high number of patients suffering from many different health problems, whose clinical complexity is considerable [1, 2]. This means that physicians have to deal with several aspects at once, which may raise a multitude of issues in day-to-day clinical practice [3–6]. That is why such professionals require an effective system to search for and find information that enables them not only to update their knowledge, but also to solve problems efficiently and effectively [7–9].

Clinical sessions and individual conversations (in person and over the phone) with non-GP specialist care (SC) professionals are options that allow them to resolve such issues. However, given that the health system is at saturation point, communication between PC and SC is not easy, quick or effective, and it leads to many referrals

* Correspondence: fsaigi@uoc.edu
[6]Faculty of Health Sciences, Universitat Oberta de Catalunya, Barcelona. Av. Tibidabo, 39-43, 08035 Barcelona, Spain
Full list of author information is available at the end of the article

to SC (hospitalisation or specialist outpatient clinics) that generally entail excessive delays for appointments [2, 10].

Despite the increase in access to electronic sources of information, PC physicians usually raise their queries with other colleagues in the first instance, resorting to the Internet as the second option [8, 11–13]. Several experiences that make the most of the advantages that telemedicine offers with respect to improving communication between PC and SC have proved to be beneficial in terms of efficiency, cost-effectiveness and improved medical care [14], with a high degree of satisfaction [15–17].

One of the latest approaches is the creation of communities of practice (CoPs) [18]. Applied to the field of healthcare, communities of clinical practice (CoCPs) are online platforms that draw on the advantages of Web 2. 0 for the creation, dissemination and management of clinical knowledge by and among healthcare professionals working at different levels of care [19]. While evidence of their usefulness is still somewhat limited, these virtual communities have been shown to have not only a considerable capacity to transfer knowledge acquired in daily clinical practice [20–22], but also great educational potential [23–28].

While most studies have focused on analysing the results of CoCP use [29–31], on the promotion of evidence-based clinical practice [32, 33] and on final decision-making [34], it is crucial to consider the determinants of the use of CoCPs in order to fully understand the use thereof. In other words, it is necessary to perform an ex-ante analysis in the study of the determinants of COCP use instead of an ex-post analysis of the determinants of the results of CoCP use. Thus, this article presents an ex-ante analysis and aims to provide evidence of the determinants of CoCP use, beyond the study of the results thereof.

A CoCP called the ECOPIH was created in 2009. The abbreviation stands for *Eina de Comunicació Online entre Primària i Hospitalària* in the Catalan language, or Online Communication Tool between Primary and Hospital Care in English. It is a CoCP that uses a Web 2.0 platform for communication between PC and SC, bringing together healthcare professionals from PC centres and non-GP specialists from several hospitals in Badalona and Sant Adrià de Besòs (two cities in the Barcelona metropolitan area, Spain) [35]. The study of a CoCP after several years should enable an assessment to be made of whether it has met this need, by analysing the strengths and weakness that determine its use and identifying the changes that need to be made to ensure that it is used as standard in usual clinical practice.

The objective of this article is to explore healthcare professionals' views on CoCPs and the changes that need to be made in an uncontrolled real-life setting. Based on their experiences of ECOPIH and on their points of view, the characteristics that should contribute to the healthcare professionals' greater readiness to use the CoCP are analysed, as are the changes that need to be made for them to integrate it into their daily clinical practice.

Methods

Design

A descriptive-interpretative qualitative study was conducted through interviews of a group of key informants in order to learn about their perceptions of and opinions on the use and usefulness of the ECOPIH platform [36]. A qualitative methodology was appropriate for the purposes of achieving that objective because it enabled deeper knowledge to be gained of the context within which ECOPIH was used and, at the same time, it allowed the professionals' experiences and perceptions of and reasons for applying that tool to their daily practice to be evaluated [14, 37–39]. Taking into account the discourses of those professionals was essential in order to identify certain aspects that would otherwise be difficult to evaluate using other methodologies, such as social interaction between individuals and how it affects interprofessional collaboration and coordination, as well as the advantages stemming from the platform's use, and from technological and organisational changes.

Study setting

The study was conducted on the Barcelonès Nord-Maresme Primary Care Service (PCS) in Catalonia, Spain, which includes 10 PC centres and 3 SC centres (Metropolitana Nord International Health Centre in Santa Coloma de Gramenet, Barcelonès Nord i Maresme Occupational Health Unit in Badalona, and Germans Trias i Pujol University Hospital also in Badalona).

Participants and selection strategy

PC and SC professionals with communication skills were invited to take part in the study so that they could give comprehensive, in-depth opinions on the ECOPIH tool. They included a majority of users and a minority of non-users of the platform. The sampling method was theoretical, and it included professionals of different ages, professional disciplines (physicians/nurses), positions within the organisation (healthcare or managerial) and role within ECOPIH (participant or consultant). Pragmatic criteria of proximity, accessibility and ease of contact were also taken into account. Discursive representativeness was sought in order to ensure the most comprehensive breadth and depth of information and understanding of the phenomenon, and that is why a combined maximum variation sampling strategy was selected. The principal investigator approached the professionals in their workplace contexts by e-mail to request their participation in the study, looking for the predefined profiles mentioned above. This method offered the advantage of improving contact to request participation and, at the same time, it gave potential candidates greater autonomy to decide whether or not to participate in it. Moreover, we considered that, by having a closer relationship with the principal investigator, those candidates who accepted to participate would be more motivated to give their opinions. It could nevertheless be considered that this very factor might influence the sincerity with which criticism would be expressed. So, at the start of the interviews, special emphasis was placed on the importance of identifying the changes necessary to improve the tool and on the fact that the participants should express themselves with the greatest freedom. The study phenomenon is an innovative topic centred on a tool to facilitate communication between professionals working at different levels of care. Consequently, participation in the study meant that participants had to devote time to the interview in order to recount their experiences of and opinions on ECOPIH, showing critical capacity and interest in improving the tool. Informant selection was considered complete when the categories emerging from the analysis process were saturated. Under those circumstances, incorporating new informants into the study would have meant an unjustified burden for them and a greater analysis workload for the researchers, without providing any significant improvements to the findings [40–43]. A total of 30 professionals were invited to take part by e-mail. Those who accepted signed an informed consent form, which specified that the interviews would be audio recorded. Of those 30, only one person declined to take part because he/she did not want to be recorded. At the end of each session, the participants were offered the chance to receive a copy of the transcription for checking so that the research team could gather feedback from individual informants to assess the validity of findings and ensure that data were interpreted correctly.

Data-generating techniques

Data was obtained from focus groups, triangular groups and semi-structured individual interviews. These three types of interviews were used because they facilitated the informants' participation, given their geographical dispersion and other logistical aspects such as time availability for interviews. In addition, the triangular groups allowed topics to be covered in depth with less group pressure, thereby creating more interactive and productive dynamics.

The interviews were held at the centres where the professionals worked to make it easier for them. All the interviews were moderated by the study's principal investigator. Interview moderation was based on a pre-established topic script that the research team had agreed upon after a review of the literature and a pooling of their experience [see Additional file 1]. In addition, before the interviews started, the moderator stressed the need for the interviewees to express their opinions and experiences of ECOPIH in an honest manner, since the aim was not to obtain polite answers but instead to identify which elements of the tool could be improved. The participants' characteristics by interview technique type and length are shown in Table 1.

Data analysis

Verbatim transcriptions of the recordings were done by the principal investigator, and the informants' identifying data were anonymised [44]. To aid understanding in this article, quotations from the interviews have been translated into English by a professional academic translator and revised by the research team to verify that the meaning of the original discourse was maintained. The analysis procedures were done manually. A thematic interpretative content analysis [45, 46] was performed and the analysis procedures were done manually by the same

Table 1 Characteristics of the participants in the individual and group interviews

	Individual interviews	Triangular group	Focus group	TOTAL
Total number of participants	5	7	17	29
Number of interviews	5	3	2	10
Gender (M:F)	3:2	4:3	4:13	11:18
Age	< 35 years old: 0 35–50 years old: 4 > 50 years old: 1	< 35 years old: 0 35–50 years old: 4 > 50 years old: 3	< 35 years old: 2 35–50 years old: 10 > 50 years old: 5	< 35 years old: 2 35–50 years old: 18 > 50 years old: 9
PC:SC	2:3	2:5	17:0	21:8
Physician: Nurse	5:0	7:0	9:8	21:8
Number of directors	2	5	0	7
Use profile (NU:P:C)*	1:1:3	0:0:7	4:11:2	5:12:12
Length (minutes)	45–60	60–70	90–100	635

*Use profile. *NU* Non-user, *P* Participant, *C* Consultant

investigator. Firstly, the transcriptions were read carefully and repeatedly in order to get an in-depth knowledge and full understanding of them. Such reading enabled pre-analytical intuitions to be developed. In the analysis phase, quotations were identified and coded, and categories were created based on the script of topics explored in the interviews. These were then regrouped and, after analysing each category and establishing relationships, an explanatory framework was finally created. In the case of discourse polarisation (relating to the collaborative virtual environment and to non-access to health records, for example), it was described, analysed and interpreted because it was felt that it offered a relevant point of view. Data collection and analysis was performed in parallel. Thus, as the analysis progressed, the results suggested the acquisition of new data in order to expand and improve the phenomenon's interpretation, hence the incorporation of new key informants. In particular, an in-depth analysis of the tool's weaknesses and the proposals for increasing its use was performed. In the analysis phase, the analyst held regular meetings with the research team to discuss and agree on the analysis categories. In addition, the findings were discussed with a researcher outside the project, who was an expert in qualitative research. Quotations from discussions have been included to illustrate the process of interpretation based on data relevance and clarity. The research team remained conscious of their backgrounds and experiences, and how their positionality might influence the analysis and the interpretation of the data. Indeed, the research team was mindful of this throughout every stage of the study and was very clear that the priority was to identify what points could be improved and what changes were needed to ensure that the tool could be incorporated into the context of usual practice within primary care and to contribute to the expected improvements by means of its application, which may have partly controlled for its influence on the results. The research team tried, at all times, to have an ethnographic attitude and to delve into the meanings of the informants' opinions on and experiences of ECOPIH. In addition, the verbatim transcriptions – and translations thereof – illustrating the data were selected on the basis of criteria of clarity and relevance, and they show the participants' critical capacity.

Results

A total of 29 participants were recruited to the study, among whom were 18 women, 21 physicians and 8 nurses. Of the interviewees, 21 were PC professionals, 24 were users of ECOPIH and 7 held managerial positions. A total of 2 focus groups, 3 triangular groups and 5 individual interviews were conducted (Table 1). Additional file 2 shows the profile of each participant.

Overview

For a system of communication between PC and SC to become a tool that is habitually used and very useful, the interviewees considered that it should have a series of specific characteristics. Table 2 summarises the key points identified in the interviews and focus groups. The analysis of each of the topics and the relationships among them led to the creation of an explanatory framework of the key points for the platform's success (Fig. 1).

PC query handling

Many aspects of ECOPIH were valued positively. A considerable number of the interviewees highlighted the effectiveness and speed of responses, as well as the ease of accessing the platform and contacting a non-GP specialist. This speed (responses within 24–48 h) might not be quick enough for some members of the nursing group, who are used to the immediacy of consulting with colleagues nearest to them as a way of resolving queries (Table 2).

Type of information that people want to find

The information obtained from the ECOPIH query was valued positively by the interviewees because they considered it comprehensive, reliable and up to date.

On the other hand, some professionals mentioned the common difficulty of finding information that is directly applicable to real PC patients, because such patients are often under-represented in clinical practice guides or training courses. Clinical cases specific to PC patients were found in ECOPIH, thus facilitating the transfer of advice given by the non-GP specialists to clinical practice.

Several participants (INT. 9, 16, 26) mentioned that this aspect improved when the consultant non-GP specialist was a professional who had an understanding of PC and was close to it, since there were greater similarities in patient focus. In addition, a more personal relationship could be established, thus increasing trust in the answer (Table 2).

Knowledge management

In the interviews, the professionals identified the need to establish an approach that would bring different areas of care closer together in order to achieve a collaborative working culture that would benefit patients.

Different communication mechanisms between care levels have traditionally been set up. Despite that, the participants in our study stated that contact via these channels of a more classic nature had major limitations. Thus, the telephone channel presented the difficulty of locating the non-GP specialist and, when located, he/she did not often show the necessary predisposition, or perhaps the moment was not right for such interaction, which he/she experienced as an interruption. Classic face-to-face consultation also had physical and temporal

Table 2 What characteristics should a PC-SC communication tool have?

Topic	Key points identified
PC query handling	*"You search for the specialty, you click and then you send it. You don't need to have any personal contact to get someone to resolve it." INT. 16 (PC physician, female).* *"I tend to approach the people I work with more (…). I ask the people around me, I think it's more immediate. I'm quite impatient, so I need immediate answers." INT. 24 (PC nurse, female, non-user)*
Type of information	*"(The specialists) give you much more comprehensive information than they do when giving an immediate, off-the-cuff answer." INT. 15 (PC physician, female)* *"It is a reliable source because they are the go-to people." INT. 19 (PC nurse, female)* *"You may have the clinical practice guide and then you come across patients whose cases fall between the gaps in all of them. The fact that it's a real patient (in ECOPIH) helps a lot because courses focus mostly on the topic, so then it's quite hard to adapt it to specific cases that present in the surgery, such as patients with complex conditions. When it comes to providing care, they are real cases that you have to deal with and really need to consult on." INT. 15 (PC physician, female)*
Knowledge management	*"What we need is a forum where we can discuss things; that would be the ideal clinical session, where you can sit down with your colleagues… that doesn't happen, or happens very little in the teams. It was the type of tool I needed, that I'd been looking for, and it was good for me." INT. 4 (PC director, male)* *"When we call the hospital, they answer as fast as they can, as if you were bothering them." INT. 15 (PC physician, male)* *"Virtual consultation is convenient, provides an answer for that patient and is very powerful. But I still think that they are complementary tools for dealing with knowledge. If I put that query on ECOPIH, I'm asking a more generic question and will find a more generic answer that I can use for other patients too, and thousands of other colleagues of mine will also see it." INT. 4 (PC director, female)* *"ECOPIH is about building pillars for the future. The other system, virtual consultation, is about improving day-to-day management, the speed of action is much quicker at strategic management level. ECOPIH will give you that in the long term." INT. 28 (PC director, male)* *"We have quite a few clinical issues to resolve every day over the phone. If more people could see them, perhaps they wouldn't need to ask about them again. There are many duplicate consultations. That's the philosophy that needs to prevail." INT. 2 (SC physician, male)* *"It's more enriching when everyone can see it, it's much more enriching for me." INT. 13 (PC physician, female)* *"The larger the audience, the greater the fear of giving answers; some are undoubtedly a bit more defensive. It has an influence; it curbs the spontaneity that there would otherwise be in certain cases (…). I'm sure it has an influence, and a negative one in some cases." INT. 8 (SC physician, male)*
Cultural aspects	*"(If ECOPIH had come from the hospital), it would have been used less. Because, if it comes from opposition rather than joint work, it is the hospital that puts its stamp of authority on it, while in primary care they act like automatons within models that may not be the best because there's been no debate." INT. 28 (PC director, male)* *"If ECOPIH had come from the hospital, it would have been seen as something quite natural (by the specialists). Instead, it's something that comes from below, from family doctors. It has created an attitude of anticipation rather than enthusiasm. (…). ECOPIH balances things out, that's what technologies do, they are very democratic. Here, you treat specialists as equals, but that isn't understood in the hospital. (…) It's a change of role. (…) and there's resistance to change." INT. 3 (SC director, male)* *"Above all, I think it's an attitude of wanting to be more proactive, of shaking off your fears and wanting to do things differently." INT. 2 (SC physician, male)* *"I'd consult more often, but my feeling of embarrassment is quite intense. It's an insurmountable embarrassment." INT. 9 (PC physician, female)* *"There aren't enough nursing topics to consult on because, in nursing, you make your bed and you lie in it. Maybe the direction in nursing is the opposite. In medicine, questions are asked, and in nursing, maybe the experts should be the ones who present news so that people can be informed or debate can be generated." INT. 23 (PC nurse, female)* *"I find that some of the topics aren't very specific, there are many medical things." INT. 19 (PC nurse, female)*
Technological aspects	*"Access needs to be more direct. So that at the time when you have a query about a patient, when its fresh in your mind, you can make it more dynamic." INT. 15 (PC physician, female)* *"We did have some training, but when you start using it again, you forget what you've learned." INT. 22 (PC nurse, male)*
Organisational changes	*"It's something connected with work, but when you're at work you can't find the time to do it." INT. 19 (PC nurse, female)* *"It depends a lot on how you understand your profession. If you're curious and need to increase your knowledge, you'll use ECOPIH or you'll study at home, you have to read, you need time." INT. 4 (PC director, female)* *"If you link it to senior management, you might undermine the tool to some extent because it is perceived as a form of managerial control. When MBO ends, the tool ends because there hasn't been any personal motivation. It's risky, it might by counterproductive for the tool." INT. 28 (PC director, male)* *"Recognition of the tool itself by provider companies is what's missing; they need to integrate it into the initial visits. The two managers, of primary care and hospital care, need to sit down and decide what it means, how to recognise this work." INT. 3 (SC director, male)*
Legal liability	*"I understand that it's a secure tool. It doesn't worry me, I do things that are much more insecure than this, for example, replying by e-mail, a telephone call… The thing here, though, is that it's in writing, and it stays that way forever. The legal ramifications of this don't worry me, but the very lack of definition of project makes me wonder: 'Here, if I make a mistake and I receive a complaint about something I've said here, would the Catalan Health Institute consider it theirs?'." INT. 3 (SC director, male)*

constraints (limited timetables, a lack of recording for subsequent consultations, limited information conveyed to both professionals), which forced anyone who wished to raise a query with a non-GP specialist to do so through personal contacts in informal conversations ("cronyism") or by interrupting clinics.

Regarding the coexistence of ECOPIH alongside other SC communication systems, whether traditional (e.g., face-to-face consultations) are more innovative (e.g., virtual specialist consultations through access to patients' health records), several interviewees highlighted that, without underestimating the obvious advantages of such systems, the consultations of

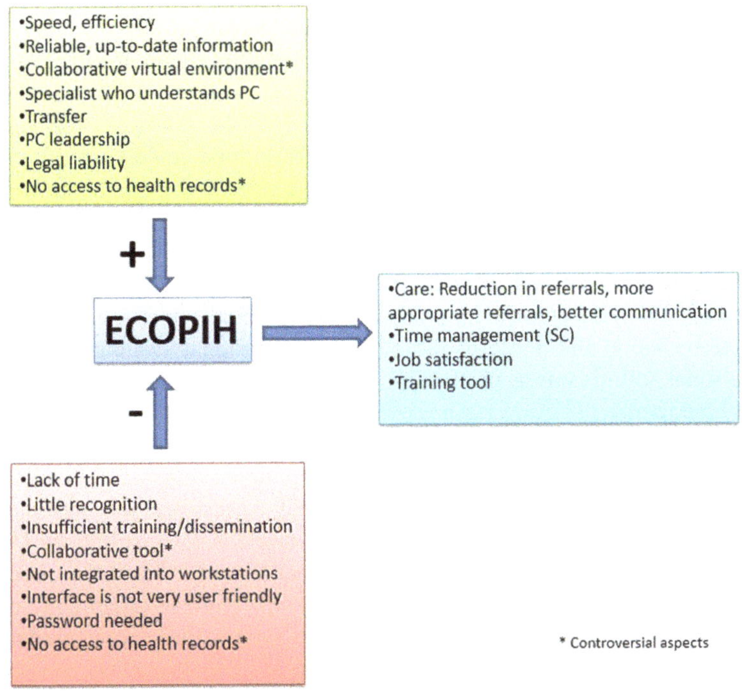

Fig. 1 ECOPIH explanatory framework

clinical cases raised via ECOPIH were more interesting and comprehensive, and that they added educational value for future cases. The tools were therefore complementary.

Several participants explained that such communication should ideally take place virtually. They also said that it would be positive if it became a common forum for sharing clinical cases. For most of the interviewees, the fact that content was visible to all users, who in turn could get involved in the discussion about the case, was an advantage. They also felt that it should be used more widely, so long as patient confidentiality was assured. This form of consultation was enriching because it allowed people to learn about other ways of working and helped to reassure professionals who could see that other colleagues had the same queries as they did. The transmitted knowledge was spread widely and learning was fostered. This was also highlighted by the non-GP specialists, who considered that many of the consultations they received via e-mail were similar. Thus, a public discussion forum would prevent duplicate consultations.

Despite that, a few professionals considered that creating debates on consultations was not positive and that they should stay within a question-answer system. They also felt that tense situations might be created if there was disagreement with the non-GP specialist. Some PC users believed that the collaborative aspect of the tool might represent a barrier because some professionals are reluctant to express themselves in public, because it might lead to doubts about who has access to the content (management, senior management, etc.) and because it might make the consultants' answers more defensive (Table 2).

Cultural aspects

The interviewees mentioned the effect of the tool's origin on predisposition towards its use. Thus, the PC professionals said that they would have been more receptive if the tool had been created within PC itself, which would have led to greater use. SC had remained expectant for the same reason.

On the other hand, some professionals interviewed considered that one of the main determining aspects of ECOPIH use was people's attitudes towards such tools. Thus, qualities like being receptive to new ideas, proactivity, enthusiasm and predisposition towards sharing doubts in a group situation were essential, and the lack thereof partly explained a low level of participation. They also highlighted the importance of shaking off one's fears of embarrassment when expressing one's doubts in public, though they also mentioned that this concern could be resolved in part if the consultations were anonymous.

On this point, it should be noted that, according to some of the interviewees, the nursing group was less accustomed to sharing their doubts and therefore adopted a passive attitude more often. Together with the fact that other users felt that few specific nursing-related topics were mentioned, this aspect meant that the nursing group's use of the tool was lower (Table 2).

Technological aspects

Regarding the technological aspects, the main problem that users referred to was the high number of platforms and workstations used in daily practice, each with its own particular characteristics: electronic health records, shared health records, e-mail, other consultation systems, etc. The use of ECOPIH via the e-Catalunya platform did not present any major difficulties other than the personal skills of each user of the technology. That said, it seemed to be a platform that was not sufficiently easy to use because it required too many clicks and intermediate steps to get to the consultations. Older users found the platform more difficult to handle, and personal attitude was again the key factor in overcoming that limitation.

Regarding the e-Catalunya platform, several professionals suggested the following improvements: making access easier by integrating it into habitual workstations or a mobile app; grouping information by topic given that a lot of content was building up over time; having an e-mail notification system containing the text of new contributions; and having the option to use filters or lists of the most frequent consultations.

Regarding the possibility of accessing the patients' health records, the participants felt that, while it would make the tool more formal, it could jeopardise its immediacy and ease of use, and would introduce conflicts with respect to confidentiality and disseminating knowledge among other users.

Although the e-Catalunya platform's operation was straightforward for most users, some professionals needed more ongoing support or training to maintain their skills in order to use the tool (Table 2).

Organisational changes

One of the main determining factors of ECOPIH non-use was the lack of available time during the working day, despite the fact that the tool was wholly connected with work. Most of the interviewees rejected the idea of spending their own time on this task, although some considered that learning and trying to resolve unclear cases in their own time was part and parcel of the profession.

On the other hand, the interviewees highlighted the little or zero recognition of the activities that they undertook in ECOPIH by the senior management of the various services or provider companies. As the platform evolved, someone suggested including its use as an evaluation indicator in the Management by Objectives (MBO) appraisal [47] in order to foster and recognise its use. It was a controversial topic because, while some people did consider it a good strategy to increase its use, most of the users were against that option because it might cause rejection due to it being interpreted as something connected with senior management.

In short, several users mentioned that the organisation should decide whether or not it wanted roll out a tool like ECOPIH, reflecting that commitment in a contract or agreement to enable the associated tasks to be included in the service portfolio of each specialty. Thus, the work done could be recognised by counting it as if it were a referral for consultation (Table 2).

Legal liability

Finally, all of the PC professionals interviewed were very clear about the fact that legal liability would fall to the PC professional dealing with the patient because that was how it was stated in the ECOPIH usage rules. The non-GP specialists taking part in this study were not concerned about this issue because they considered that the opinion expressed was advice, corresponding to the non-GP specialists' theoretical action as it would have been taken in a consultation. They highlighted that they habitually undertook other consultation activities as if they were referrals, such as telephone calls and e-mails, which were rather more insecure in legal terms. Nevertheless, a few interviewees did express certain doubts about the legality of these types of actions because the answers were recorded in writing, as was the reply from the institution in the event of a complaint (Table 2).

Benefits derived from using ECOPIH

According to the interviews conducted, the use of ECOPIH offered a series of professional and organisational benefits (Table 3). To begin with, most of the interviewees considered that ECOPIH reduced the number of referrals for two reasons. Firstly, it enabled the doubt that would

Table 3 Benefits derived from using ECOPIH

"Of course, it reduced referrals. You refer when you have doubts about how to handle a case and you want to seek the opinion of an expert in another topic. If you manage to get this information by other means and you end up handling the case while counting on the non-GP specialist's support at all times, ultimately you don't refer it." INT. 16 (PC physician, female).
"If you come across a case that has already been discussed, you don't refer it because you have the answer." INT. 13 (PC physician, female).
"It could prevent referrals that are sometimes unnecessary. (...) It should save on visits and that means saving money and duplicate tests, so it could be an efficient tool." INT. 26 (SC physician, female).
"It isn't a huge reduction in referrals, it's referring properly... and learning." INT. 9 (PC physician, female).
"It's efficient in the sense that the patient doesn't have to go from one place to another. It prevents silly consultations from getting onto the waiting list (...) and has the potential to improve the care offered to the patient. It's a good tool, it's useful and relevant, it's safe, it has the ability to resolve issues and is probably efficient, although I can't assure you of that. It's a new way of operating that, if it saves work, will ultimately make us more efficient." INT. 3 (SC director, male).
"I think ECOPIH improves the quality of care the patient gets. It helps me and my patient." INT. 4 (PC director, female).
"It does reduce referrals a little, and if it doesn't, it means they are made properly. Sometimes it isn't as much as saying 'refer it to me' as saying 'refer it to me, but do this' or 'refer it to me with this priority'. It provides clarification when it comes to having to refer or not." INT. 29 (SC physician, female).

usually have led to a referral to be resolved, and secondly, it allowed the professionals to read the cases raised beforehand, thus leading to a better handling of patients in PC and, therefore, a reduction in the number of referrals and visits to SC. Many of the participants explained that, besides referring fewer patients, any referrals that were made would be more appropriate. The professionals therefore considered ECOPIH an efficient tool.

Even those interviewees who occupied managerial positions felt that it was an efficient tool that could reduce waiting lists, especially when a referral could not be justified for any particular reason.

There was more consensus among the users about the fact that the tool improved the quality of the referrals, for several reasons. It prevented inappropriate referrals and increased higher quality referrals. In addition, they were clinical cases in which more thought and work had been invested, so much so that on a few occasions, the simple fact of preparing a case for consultation in ECOPIH had enabled it to be resolved. Finally, for those cases that were discussed and ultimately referred, a higher number of supplementary tests had already been done. In other words, even though the response to the cases raised was to refer them, such referral was done in a more appropriate and timely way.

Table 4 Overall appraisal of the tool

"You have a query and, before you know it, you find it (the solution) right there and you're really relieved, you resolve it straight away, you learn, you sort it out." INT. 15 (PC physician, female).
"It's a trustworthy tool for family doctors." INT. 14 (PC physician, male).
"Satisfaction with the profession itself because, apart from experience that gives you time, what we need to do is increase our own knowledge." INT. 4 (PC director, female).
"ECOPIH helps to manage time. It removes the urgency of demands. It's the best way to manage time, knowing what you've got in front of you and being able to decide on the right order of execution." INT. 8 (SC physician, male).
"For us, being in ECOPIH is a strength. It's a way of becoming visible. It has helped to break down barriers, to bring professionals closer together, and that will also have reinforced its use. It's a very positive tool for improving communication among the entire community of physicians." INT. 8 (SC physician, male).
"Creating feedback between primary and non-GP specialist care is unbeatable, I think the idea is really great." INT. 29 (SC physician, female).
"It has the educational aspect that a virtual visit doesn't have, and it has the care aspect too, depending on how you apply that to a particular case while working. For a physician, training and practice are one and the same thing. If you're well-trained, your practice is better, if you're practice is better, you work better with your patients, that means everything, referrals, etc." INT. 28 (PC director, male).
"People who regularly go into ECOPIH... after one or two years those people know a lot more, if they're active, than people who've done courses on goodness knows what. (...) It is a much more pragmatic, clear and practical kind of training because you can apply it straight away and can improve care." INT. 28 (PC director, male).
"It's expert learning, it's case-based learning because your learning from the case (...)." INT. 11 (PC physician, female).
"I can see a lot of advantages in it for learning, I'm surprised by how much I manage to learn. It would be an à la carte continuing medical education because you can choose the topic." INT. 12 (PC physician, female).

Overall appraisal of the tool

Several PC physicians stated that that they were happy when they had time to raise cases for consultation on the platform, were relieved when they obtained solutions to their queries, were confident about how to handle patients and, finally, were satisfied with the profession itself because they had managed to achieve optimum handling of particular cases in an independent manner.

Most of the non-GP specialists also referred to this increase in satisfaction, and they also considered that ECOPIH was a useful tool for improving time management because it led to less interference in daily activities at work than other consultation systems, e.g., the phone (Table 4).

From the SC point of view, participation in ECOPIH was valued positively in the majority of cases because it was considered a tool that enabled communication between care levels to be improved.

Most of the interviewees considered that ECOPIH fulfilled both the educational and the care functions. This was due in part to the fact that the knowledge acquired (education) became applicable to clinical practice (care), thus implying that they were two interrelated concepts.

Some participants clarified that raising cases for consultation would mostly have a care-related function because it generally enabled real clinical cases to be resolved so long as answers were given quickly. They nevertheless felt that it would also have an educational function for other members reading the consultations made. In contrast, they considered that sharing documents would basically have an educational function. In addition, the non-GP specialists saw other advantages, such as identifying training needs for PC and even the fact that the tool could become a means of accessing self-learning in SC.

Several interviewees highlighted that ECOPIH came across as a powerful training tool, mainly because learning was based on real cases, was much more pragmatic and was directly applicable to clinical practice or to similar future cases. A few participants added that having many specialities available for consultation made it a kind of à la carte continuing medical education. It should be noted that it was pointed out on several occasions that acting solely as an observer or reader of content could increase learning.

Discussion

The need for healthcare professionals to be able to access trustworthy sources of information is well known, as is the fact that scientific literature may not be able to give direct answers to clinical questions arising in daily practice [7, 11, 48]. Having a tool that provides quick, practical and reliable information is essential for PC professionals given the multitude of queries arising in daily clinical practice [2, 6, 8, 49–51]. The opinions of ECOPIH users showed that the tool managed to meet that need. The fact that consultant non-GP specialists knew about the context within which AP physicians worked made a definitive contribution to that, and even more so if they were the go-to professionals for the PC area from which patients were referred.

According to the participating professionals, the gap between PC and SC could be bridged by implementing virtual communication tools [52–54]. ECOPIH includes the Web 2.0 concept in communication among professionals, and it does so via a CoCP, thereby triggering a change in how knowledge is managed. CoPs provide a useful model for knowledge management as well as a mechanism that facilitates and promotes a new way of working and learning based on collaborative working and the use of collective intelligence [55]. They can be especially useful in PC, where flexibility and constant coordination are key aspects of caring for patients with significant multimorbidity [56, 57].

Not surprisingly, the ECOPIH tool has a very powerful educational component that combines four aspects that, in our opinion, are essential: peer learning with the presence of an expert [32–34, 58]; learning based on real clinical cases that is directly applicable to clinical practice [20, 21]; the dissemination of knowledge to the entire community [59] (even without any active participation, i.e., lurkers); and social interaction, which is one of the main channels through which healthcare professionals create their own tacit knowledge [19, 60–64]. As in any CoP, recently qualified physicians learn by interacting with experts, who in turn may acquire new skills. In addition, collective knowledge is created and becomes available to the community over time [58, 65, 66]. They also learn together by focusing on problems that are directly connected with their work, and this is something that increases the participants' motivation, since their learning is linked to problematic situations that they can recognise or perceive as real and applicable to their work [20–22]. This is particularly relevant because the tool provides a framework for the professional development of individuals in the workplace through different forms of participation [67–69]. Hence, the ECOPIH platform offers advantages from the points of view of care and education because its use is not limited to resolving specific cases. The non-GP specialists' advice and the literature attached to it also enable other colleagues to resolve similar cases. The accumulation of experience increases not only the group's explicit knowledge, but also its tacit or practical knowledge, which emerges from reflective practice and from gathering and sharing cases among professionals [56].

On the other hand, it is also worth noting ECOPIH's considerable usefulness as time management tool for SC professionals, since it allows them to decide on how much time to spend on communicating with PC by avoiding interruptions and duplicate consultations. However, the participants often identified the lack of time as the main determining factor of ECOPIH use for resolving queries. The use of virtual communication tools like ECOPIH requires organisational changes to allow PC and SC professionals to have that time available regularly. Although participation in a CoP occurs partly because it has a certain value for the users, irrespective of whether or not it is an institutional directive [59, 70, 71], an institution must commit to the tool by incorporating it into its service portfolio [72] and by giving recognition to participants in general and to consultants in particular [20]. However, the latter issue must be addressed with care because certain incentives to use it, such as MBOs, may represent a barrier to its use. In fact, despite the implementation of networked clinical structures aimed at improving patient care and facilitating knowledge-sharing among healthcare professionals beyond the boundaries of organisations, certain bureaucratic, hierarchical and intra-professional barriers may still exist [73]. On the other hand, the time barrier could be overcome through training [74, 75], the promotion of the tool's potential usefulness, high-value content and improved technological aspects [24, 58]. More research in this field is required [76].

This point ties in with the technological issues. Ideally, the platform should be integrated into habitual workstations without the need to enter a new password [74, 77–79] and the interface should be user friendly [80]. The platform should also have a series of technical features that make it easy to use (information search and filter functions, a mobile app, etc.) [11, 48, 49, 81]. While there is some controversy surrounding the issue, it is generally considered unnecessary to have access to the patients' health records, mainly to ensure that ECOPIH's ease of use is not compromised. Nevertheless, if it were technically possible, it might be interesting to have an optional link to access patients' health records in specific instances, so long as such access is password protected and contained within a secure environment.

Concerns about legal liability stemming from advice given by a non-GP specialist via an online app have been identified in several studies, especially among SC members [15, 80, 82–86]. While virtual consultations are often considered informal, a number of peculiarities make the legalities surrounding them somewhat complex, so this is something that must be reviewed before the implementation of an online CoCP. In the case of ECOPIH, this was not a contentious issue because it was made very clear, in writing and right from the start, that the responsibility for the patients' care fell to the PC professionals; this was made explicit during the training and was visibly very prominent on the tool itself.

According to the scientific literature, a key factor for the success of a telemedicine project is that clinical professionals should be responsible for its leadership [38, 80, 87]. In our case, the experience was led by a PC professional who had a perfect understanding of the reality of professionals in that sphere and of their needs. This enabled him to adapt the tool technically and organisationally. All of this entails a series of intangible benefits, which were identified on numerous occasions in the interviews conducted, as well as in previous studies [55, 88, 89]. By improving communication between care levels, greater peace of mind and confidence when handling patients is achieved [90, 91]. This leads to improved job satisfaction for PC and SC professionals [67, 92]. According to the users of this CoCP, ECOPIH helped them reduce the number of referrals and make them more appropriate [84, 93]. However, in order to evaluate every dimension of the tool, further research should be done from a qualitative perspective on the impact of CoCPs in financial terms (a reduction in referrals and visits, and cost analysis) and clinical terms.

The rigorous procedures used (a detailed description of the context and the participants, the reflexivity of the research team and the theoretical sample to achieve discourse saturation) ensure the validity of the findings in our setting. However, caution is needed before transferring these results to other settings. In this respect, the sample selected in our study also took into account pragmatic criteria such as access to the interviewees, hence the discourses of professionals working in a rural setting were not taken into consideration. Nor was the possible effect of the population's socioeconomic position, which might have an influence on professional practice, on workload and on the information requested by citizens, thereby modifying ECOPIH use.

Conclusions

In the healthcare sphere, inter- and intra-organisational networks are crucial to the creation and dissemination of clinical knowledge because such knowledge is experiential, implicit or tacit [93]. The ECOPIH platform has proved to be a useful, satisfactory tool for improving the healthcare provided by PC professionals. It stands out as a collaborative tool that provides reliable, up-to-date information that is highly transferrable to clinical practice. The users valued its effectiveness, efficiency and educational capacity, and they considered that it improved job satisfaction. In order to make the most of its potential in terms of care and education, organisational changes are required to free up sufficient time for participants to access the tool habitually (whenever needed), as well as cultural changes for knowledge-sharing and networking, and technological changes linked to the platform and to its integration into the healthcare professionals' habitual workstations.

Abbreviations

CoCP: Community of clinical practice; CoP: Community of practice; ECOPIH: Eina de Comunicació entre Primària i Hospitalària (Online Communication Tool between Primary and Hospital Care); ICT: Information and communication technologies; PC: Primary care; PCS: Primary Care Service; SC: Non-GP specialist care; UOC: Open University of Catalonia

Acknowledgements

This project has received a grant from the 7th 2011 Award on Primary Health Research of the Barcelona Health Region, Government of Catalonia.
This study was also supported with funding from Chair UAB–Novartis of the Universitat Autònoma of Barcelona. It did not play any role in the study design.
The English version of this work has been reviewed by Steven Norris thanks to the support of the eLearn Center at the Open University of Catalonia.

Authors' contributions

All the authors have made substantive intellectual contributions to a published study. DLT (ECOPIH Community Manager) contributed to formulating research question, literature search, study design, analysis and interpretation of results, and drafting the article. JMD has participated in the conception and design, acquisition of data, analysis and interpretation of data, and helped to draft the manuscript. EPR has participated in the design, analysis, interpretation of the data and results and made a critical review of the manuscript. SFB (ECOPIH Community Manager) has participated in the data collection, interpretation and dissemination of results, and helped to draft the manuscript. XMT has participated in the protocol design, interpretation of results and drafting the article. FSR has contributed to the formulating the research question, coordination study design, literature search, design of the study, interpretation of results and drafting the article. He is the guarantor of the article. All the authors have read, revised and approved the final manuscript.

Competing interests

The authors declare that they have no competing interests

Author details

[1]Centre d'Atenció Primària Gran Sol, Gerència d'Àmbit d'Atenció Primària Metropolitana Nord, Institut Català de la Salut, Avinguda del Doctor Bassols, 112 - 130, 08914 Badalona, Spain. [2]Unitat de Suport a la Recerca Metropolitana Nord, IDIAP Jordi Gol. CAP El Maresme, Camí del Mig, 36 planta 4a, 08303 Mataró, Spain. [3]Universitat Autònoma de Barcelona, Plaça Cívica, s/n, 08193 Bellaterra, Cerdanyola del Vallès, Spain. [4]Institut Universitari d'Investigació en Atenció Primària (IDIAP Jordi Gol), Gran Via Corts Catalanes, 587, àtic, 08007 Barcelona, Spain. [5]Unitat de Suport a la Recerca Barcelona Ciutat, IDIAP Jordi Gol, Carrer Sardenya 375, 08025 Barcelona, Spain. [6]Faculty of Health Sciences, Universitat Oberta de Catalunya, Barcelona. Av. Tibidabo, 39-43, 08035 Barcelona, Spain.

References

1. Rothman AA, Wagner EH. Chronic illness management: what is the role of primary care? Ann Intern Med. 2003;138:256–61.
2. Louro González A, Fernández Obanza E, Fernández López E, Vázquez Millán P, Villegas González L, Casariego Vales E. Análisis de las dudas de los médicos de atención primaria. Atención Primaria. 2009;41:592–7. https://doi.org/10.1016/j.aprim.2009.05.005.
3. Davidoff F, Miglus J. Delivering clinical evidence where it's needed: building an information system worthy of the profession. JAMA. 2011;305:1906–7. https://doi.org/10.1001/jama.2011.619.
4. Smith R. Strategies for coping with information overload. BMJ. 2010;341: c7126.
5. Grant RW, Ashburner JM, Hong CS, Hong CC, Chang Y, Barry MJ, et al. Defining patient complexity from the primary care physician's perspective: a cohort study. Ann Intern Med. 2011;155:797–804. https://doi.org/10.7326/0003-4819-155-12-201112200-00001.

6. Del Fiol G, Workman TE, Gorman PN. Clinical questions raised by clinicians at the point of care: a systematic review. JAMA Intern Med. 2014;174:710–8. https://doi.org/10.1001/jamainternmed.2014.368.
7. Davies K, Harrison J. The information-seeking behaviour of doctors: a review of the evidence. Health Inf Libr J. 2007;24:78–94. https://doi.org/10.1111/j.1471-1842.2007.00713.x.
8. Coumou HCH, Meijman FJ. How do primary care physicians seek answers to clinical questions? A literature review. J Med Libr Assoc. 2006;94:55–60.
9. González-González AI, Dawes M, Sánchez-Mateos J, Riesgo-Fuertes R, Escortell-Mayor E, Sanz-Cuesta T, et al. Information needs and information-seeking behavior of primary care physicians. Ann Fam Med. 2007;5:345–52. https://doi.org/10.1370/afm.681.
10. Montero Ruiz E, López-Álvarez J. La interconsulta médica: problemas y soluciones. Med Clin (Barc). 2011;136:488–90. https://doi.org/10.1016/j.medcli.2009.06.039.
11. Wilson P, Glanville J, Watt I. Access to the online evidence base in general practice: a survey of the northern and Yorkshire region. Health Inf Libr J. 2003;20:172–8.
12. Magin P, Morgan S, Wearne S, Tapley A, Henderson K, Oldmeadow C, et al. GP trainees' in-consultation information-seeking: associations with human, paper and electronic sources. Fam Pract. 2015;32:525–32. https://doi.org/10.1093/fampra/cmv047.
13. Norris A. Origins and Development. Essentials Telemed. Telecare, Chichester, UK: John Wiley & Sons, Ltd; 2001, p. 1–18. https://doi.org/10.1002/0470846348.ch1.
14. Zwarenstein M, Goldman J, Reeves S. Interprofessional collaboration: effects of practice-based interventions on professional practice and healthcare outcomes. Cochrane Database Syst Rev. 2009:CD000072. https://doi.org/10.1002/14651858.CD000072.pub2.
15. Angstman KB, Adamson SC, Furst JW, Houston MS, Rohrer JE. Provider satisfaction with virtual specialist consultations in a family medicine department. Health Care Manag (Frederick). 2009;28:14–8. https://doi.org/10.1097/HCM.0b013e318196def8.
16. Stoves J, Connolly J, Cheung CK, Grange A, Rhodes P, O'Donoghue D, et al. Electronic consultation as an alternative to hospital referral for patients with chronic kidney disease: a novel application for networked electronic health records to improve the accessibility and efficiency of healthcare. Qual Saf Health Care. 2010;19:e54. https://doi.org/10.1136/qshc.2009.038984.
17. Zanaboni P, Scalvini S, Bernocchi P, Borghi G, Tridico C, Masella C. Teleconsultation service to improve healthcare in rural areas: acceptance, organizational impact and appropriateness. BMC Health Serv Res. 2009;9:238. https://doi.org/10.1186/1472-6963-9-238.
18. Wenger E. Communities of practice: learning, meaning, and identity: Cambridge University Press; 1999.
19. Gabbay J, le May A. Evidence based guidelines or collectively constructed "mindlines?" ethnographic study of knowledge management in primary care. BMJ. 2004;329:1013. https://doi.org/10.1136/bmj.329.7473.1013.
20. Wenger E, Snyder W. Communities of Practice: The Organizational Frontier. Harv Bus Rev 2000;January-Fe:139–45.
21. Norman GR, Schmidt HG. Effectiveness of problem-based learning curricula: theory, practice and paper darts. Med Educ. 2000;34:721–8. https://doi.org/10.1046/j.1365-2923.2000.00749.x.
22. OSMA Legal Services Group. Social networking and the medical practice. J Okla State Med Assoc. 2010;103:517–26.
23. Maloney EJ. What web 2.0 can teach us about learning. Chron High Educ. 2007;53:B26.
24. McGowan BS, Wasko M, Vartabedian BS, Miller RS, Freiherr DD, Abdolrasulnia M. Understanding the factors that influence the adoption and meaningful use of social media by physicians to share medical information. J Med Internet Res. 2012;14:e117. https://doi.org/10.2196/jmir.2138.
25. Cain J, Policastri A. Using Facebook as an informal learning environment. Am J Pharm Educ. 2011;75:207. https://doi.org/10.5688/ajpe7510207.
26. Yamout SZ, Glick ZA, Lind DS, Monson RAZ, Glick PL. Using social media to enhance surgeon and patient education and communication. Bull Am Coll Surg. 2011;96:7–15.
27. Paton C, Bamidis PD, Eysenbach G, Hansen M, Cabrer M. Experience in the use of social media in medical and health education. Contribution of the IMIA social media working group. Yearb Med Inform. 2011;6:21–9.
28. Richardson B, Cooper N. Developing a virtual interdisciplinary research community in higher education. J Interprof Care. 2003;17:173–82. https://doi.org/10.1080/1356182031000081777.
29. Eysenbach G, Powell J, Englesakis M, Rizo C, Stern A. Health related virtual communities and electronic support groups: systematic review of the effects of online peer to peer interactions. BMJ. 2004;328:1166–0. https://doi.org/10.1136/bmj.328.7449.1166.
30. Li LC, Grimshaw JM, Nielsen C, Judd M, Coyte PC, Graham ID. Evolution of Wenger's concept of community of practice. Implement Sci IS. 2009;4:11. https://doi.org/10.1186/1748-5908-4-11.
31. Endslay S, Kirkegaar M, Linares A. Working together: communities of practice in family medicine. Fam Pract Manag. 2005;12:28–32.
32. Thompson GN, Estabrooks CA, Degner LF. Clarifying the concepts in knowledge transfer: a literature review. J Adv Nurs. 2006;53:691–701. https://doi.org/10.1111/j.1365-2648.2006.03775.x.
33. Doumit G, Gattellari M, Grimshaw J, O'Brien MA. Local opinion leaders: effects on professional practice and health care outcomes. Cochrane Database Syst Rev. 2007:CD000125.
34. Locock L, Dopson S, Chambers D, Gabbay J. Understanding the role of opinion leaders in improving clinical effectiveness. Soc Sci Med. 2001;53:745–57.
35. Lacasta Tintorer D, Flayeh Beneyto S, Alzaga Reig X, Torán Monserrat P, Manresa JM, Saigí Rubió F, Proyecto ECOPIH. Aprendizaje colaborativo en las consultas de atención primaria aplicado a la asistencia sanitaria. In: Xarxa d'Innovació Docent sobre Aprenentatge Cooperatiu (XIDAC) de la Universitat de Girona, editor. Jorn. sobre Aprendiz. Coop. 2013 (JAC-13). Nuevas Perspect. del Aprendiz. Coop. asistido por Ordenad., Girona; 2014. p. 112–23.
36. Lacasta Tintorer D, Flayeh Beneyto S, Manresa JM, Torán-Monserrat P, Jiménez-Zarco A, Torrent-Sellens J, et al. Understanding the discriminant factors that influence the adoption and use of clinical communities of practice: the ECOPIH case. BMC Health Serv Res. 2015;15:373. https://doi.org/10.1186/s12913-015-1036-4.
37. Greenhalgh T, Russell J. Why do evaluations of eHealth programs fail? An alternative set of guiding principles. PLoS Med. 2010;7:e1000360. https://doi.org/10.1371/journal.pmed.1000360.
38. May C, Harrison R, Finch T, MacFarlane A, Mair F, Wallace P, et al. Understanding the normalization of telemedicine services through qualitative evaluation. J Am Med Inf Assoc 2003;10:596–604. https://doi.org/10.1197/jamia.M1145.
39. Li LC, Grimshaw JM, Nielsen C, Judd M, Coyte PC, Graham ID. Use of communities of practice in business and health care sectors: a systematic review. Implement Sci. 2009;4:27. https://doi.org/10.1186/1748-5908-4-27.
40. Tuckett AG. Qualitative research sampling: the very real complexities. Nurse Res. 2004;12:47–61. https://doi.org/10.7748/nr2004.07.12.1.47.c5930.
41. Carlsen B, Glenton C. What about N? A methodological study of sample-size reporting in focus group studies. BMC Med Res Methodol. 2011;11:26. https://doi.org/10.1186/1471-2288-11-26.
42. Denzin NK. Interpretive biography: Sage; 1989.
43. Hennink MM, Kaiser BN, Marconi VC. Code saturation versus meaning saturation: how many interviews are enough? Qual Health Res. 2017;27:591–608. https://doi.org/10.1177/1049732316665344.
44. MacLean LM, Meyer M, Estable A. Improving accuracy of transcripts in qualitative research. Qual Health Res. 2004;14:113–23. https://doi.org/10.1177/1049732303259804.
45. Richards L, Morse JM. Readme first for a user's guide to qualitative methods. 1st ed. Oaks, California: Sage; 2013.
46. Pope C, Ziebland S, Mays N. Qualitative research in health care. Analysing qualitative data. BMJ. 2000;320:114–6.
47. Drucker P. Management: tasks, responsibilities and practices. New York: Harper & Row; 1993.
48. Isabel González-González A, Sánchez Mateos JF, Sanz Cuesta T, Riesgo Fuertes R, Escortell Mayor E, Hernández Fernández T. Estudio de las necesidades de información generadas por los médicos de atención primaria (proyecto ENIGMA). Atención Primaria. 2006;38:219–24. https://doi.org/10.1157/13092344.
49. Cook DA, Sorensen KJ, Wilkinson JM, Berger RA. Barriers and decisions when answering clinical questions at the point of care: a grounded theory study. JAMA Intern Med. 2013;173:1962–9. https://doi.org/10.1001/jamainternmed.2013.10103.
50. Ely JW, Osheroff JA, Chambliss ML, Ebell MH, Rosenbaum ME. Answering physicians' clinical questions: obstacles and potential solutions. J Am Med Inf Assoc. 2005;12:217–24. https://doi.org/10.1197/jamia.M1608.
51. Boulware DR, Dekarske AS, G a F. Physician preferences for elements of

effective consultations. J Gen Intern Med. 2010;25:25–30. https://doi.org/10.1007/s11606-009-1142-2.
52. Terraza Núñez R, Vargas Lorenzo I, Vázquez Navarrete ML. Coordination among healthcare levels: systematization of tools and measures. Gac Sanit. 2006;20:485–95.
53. O'Malley AS, Reschovsky JD. Referral and consultation communication between primary care and specialist physicians: finding common ground. Arch Intern Med. 2011;171:56–65. https://doi.org/10.1001/archinternmed.2010.480.
54. Bodenheimer T. Coordinating care–a perilous journey through the health care system. N Engl J Med. 2008;358:1064–71. https://doi.org/10.1056/NEJMhpr0706165.
55. Saigí-Rubió F, González-González I. Cooperative learning environments: virtual communities of practice in the healthcare sector. eLC Res Pap Ser. 2014;9:15–25.
56. Soubhi H, Bayliss EA, Fortin M, Hudon C, van den Akker M, Thivierge R, et al. Learning and caring in communities of practice: using relationships and collective learning to improve primary care for patients with multimorbidity. Ann Fam Med. 2010;8:170–7. https://doi.org/10.1370/afm.1056.
57. de Jong CC, Ros WJ, van Leeuwen M, Schrijvers G. How professionals share an E-care plan for the elderly in primary care: evaluating the use of an E-communication tool by different combinations of professionals. J Med Internet Res. 2016;18:e304. https://doi.org/10.2196/jmir.6332.
58. Barnett S, Jones SC, Caton T, Iverson D, Bennett S, Robinson L. Implementing a virtual community of practice for family physician training: a mixed-methods case study. J Med Internet Res. 2014;16:e83. https://doi.org/10.2196/jmir.3083.
59. Gray B. Informal learning in an online Community of Practice. J Distance Educ. 2004;19:20–35.
60. Saigí RF. Social networks for teaching and learning: the case of the telemedicine laboratory. Gac Sanit. 2011;25:254–6. https://doi.org/10.1016/j.gaceta.2010.11.008.
61. Pereles L, Lockyer J, Fidler H. Permanent small groups: group dynamics, learning, and change. J Contin Educ Heal Prof. 2002;22:205–13. https://doi.org/10.1002/chp.1340220404.
62. Donaldson A, Lank E, Maher J. Making the invisible visible: how a voluntary organization is learning from its work with groups and communities. J Chang Manag. 2005;5:191–206. https://doi.org/10.1080/14697010500119993.
63. Soubhi H, Colet NR, Gilbert JHV, Lebel P, Thivierge RL, Hudon C, et al. Interprofessional learning in the trenches: fostering collective capability. J Interprof Care. 2009;23:52–7. https://doi.org/10.1080/13561820802565619.
64. Lombardo MM, Eichinger RW. The career architect development planner. 1st editio. Lominger: Minneapolis; 1996.
65. Lave J, Wenger E. Situated Learning: Legitimate Peripheral Participation. 1st ed. Cambridge, UK: Cambridge University Press; 1991. doi:978–0521423748.
66. Wenger E. Communities of practice and social learning systems. Organization. 2000;7:225–46. https://doi.org/10.1177/135050840072002.
67. Hara N, Foon Hew K. Knowledge-sharing in an online community of health-care professionals. Inf Technol People. 2007;20:235–61. https://doi.org/10.1108/09593840710822859.
68. Widemark E. Community and learning: a virtual community of practice for nurse practitioners: Capella University; 2008.
69. Brown J, Duguid P. Organizational learning and communities-of-practice: toward a unified view of working, learning, and innovation. Organ Sci. 1991; 2:40–57. https://doi.org/10.1287/orsc.2.1.40.
70. Wenger E. McDermott RA, Snyder W. Cultivating Communities of Practice: A Guide to Managing Knowledge. Harvard Business School Press; 2002.
71. Curran JA, Murphy AL, Abidi SSR, Sinclair D, McGrath PJ. Bridging the gap: knowledge seeking and sharing in a virtual community of emergency practice. Eval Health Prof. 2009;32:312–25. https://doi.org/10.1177/0163278709338570.
72. Telemedicina: situació actual a Catalunya i altres regions. 2011.
73. Braithwaite J. Between-group behaviour in health care: gaps, edges, boundaries, disconnections, weak ties, spaces and holes. A systematic review. BMC Health Serv Res. 2010;10:330. https://doi.org/10.1186/1472-6963-10-330.
74. Straus SG, Chen AH, Yee H, Kushel MB, Bell DS. Implementation of an electronic referral system for outpatient specialty care. AMIA Annu Symp Proc. 2011;2011:1337–46.
75. Mair FS, May C, Finch T, Murray E, Anderson G, Sullivan F, et al. Understanding the implementation and integration of e-health services. J Telemed Telecare. 2007;13:36–7. https://doi.org/10.1258/135763307781645112.
76. Gagnon M-P, Légaré F, Labrecque M, Frémont P, Pluye P, Gagnon J, et al. Interventions for promoting information and communication technologies adoption in healthcare professionals. Cochrane Database Syst Rev. 2009: CD006093. https://doi.org/10.1002/14651858.CD006093.pub2.
77. Barnett S, Jones SC, Bennett S, Iverson D, Bonney A. Perceptions of family physician trainees and trainers regarding the usefulness of a virtual community of practice. J Med Internet Res. 2013;15:e92. https://doi.org/10.2196/jmir.2555.
78. David I, Poissant L, Rochette A. Clinicians' expectations of web 2.0 as a mechanism for knowledge transfer of stroke best practices. J Med Internet Res. 2012;14:e121. https://doi.org/10.2196/jmir.2016.
79. Kim Y, Chen AH, Keith E, Yee HF, Kushel MB. Not perfect, but better: primary care providers' experiences with electronic referrals in a safety net health system. J Gen Intern Med. 2009;24:614–9. https://doi.org/10.1007/s11606-009-0955-3.
80. Tuot DS, Leeds K, Murphy EJ, Sarkar U, Lyles CR, Mekonnen T, et al. Facilitators and barriers to implementing electronic referral and/or consultation systems: a qualitative study of 16 health organizations. BMC Health Serv Res. 2015;15:568. https://doi.org/10.1186/s12913-015-1233-1.
81. de Prado Prieto L, García Olmos L, Rodríguez Salvanés F, Otero Puime A. Evaluation of referrals in primary care. Aten Primaria / Soc Española Med Fam Y Comunitaria 2005;35:146–151. https://doi.org/10.1157/13071940.
82. Vimalananda VG, Gupte G, Seraj SM, Orlander J, Berlowitz D, Fincke BG, et al. Electronic consultations (e-consults) to improve access to specialty care: a systematic review and narrative synthesis. J Telemed Telecare. 2015;21:323–30. https://doi.org/10.1177/1357633X15582108.
83. Mahtani Chugani V, Martín Fernández RL, Soto Pedre E, Yanes López V, Serrano Aguilar P. Implementation of telemedicine programs in Spain: experience of the main actors involved in the decision-making process. Gac Sanit 2009;23:223e223–9 doi:101016/jgaceta2008. 06:005.
84. Segura J, Roldán C, Galera J, Naval J. What do Spanish physicians believe and expect about telemedicine? Results of a Delphi-based survey. Telemed J E Health. 2008;14:42–8. https://doi.org/10.1089/tmj.2007.0018.
85. Kim-Hwang JE, Chen AH, Bell DS, Guzman D, Yee HF, Kushel MB. Evaluating electronic referrals for specialty care at a public hospital. J Gen Intern Med. 2010;25:1123–8. https://doi.org/10.1007/s11606-010-1402-1.
86. Grimshaw JM, Winkens RAG, Shirran L, Cunningham C, Mayhew A, Thomas R, et al. Interventions to improve outpatient referrals from primary care to secondary care. Cochrane Database Syst Rev. 2005:CD005471. https://doi.org/10.1002/14651858.CD005471.
87. Loscertales FR, Rubió FS. Facilitators in the implantation of telemedicine services. Perspective of professionals involved in its design and implementation. An Sist Sanit Navar. 2011;34:235–44.
88. Hildreth P, Knowledge Networks KC. Innovation through communities of practice. London, UK: IGI Global; 2004. https://doi.org/10.4018/978-1-59140-200-8.
89. Senge P. The fifth discipline: the art and practice of the learning organization. New York: DoubleDay; 1990.
90. Hsu M-H, Ju TL, Yen C-H, Chang C-M. Knowledge sharing behavior in virtual communities: the relationship between trust, self-efficacy, and outcome expectations. Int J Human-Computer Stud. 2007;65:153–69. https://doi.org/10.1016/j.ijhcs.2006.09.003.
91. Dopson S, FitzGerald L, Ferlie E, Gabbay J, Locock L. No magic targets! Changing clinical practice to become more evidence based. Health Care Manag Rev. 2002;27:35–47.
92. Rolls K, Kowal D, Elliott D, Burrell AR. Building a statewide knowledge network for clinicians in intensive care units: knowledge brokering and the NSW intensive care coordination and monitoring unit (ICCMU). Aust Crit Care. 2008;21:29–37. https://doi.org/10.1016/j.aucc.2007.10.003.
93. Newell S, Edelman L, Scarbrough H, Swan J, Bresnen M. "Best practice" development and transfer in the NHS: the importance of process as well as product knowledge. Heal Serv Manag Res. 2003;16:1–12. https://doi.org/10.1258/095148403762539095.

16

Promoting independence, health and well-being for older people: a feasibility study of computer-aided health and social risk appraisal system in primary care

Kate Walters[1*], Kalpa Kharicha[1], Claire Goodman[2], Melanie Handley[2], Jill Manthorpe[3], Mima Cattan[4], Steve Morris[5], Caroline S. Clarke[1], Jeff Round[5] and Steve Iliffe[1]

Abstract

Background: With population ageing, research is needed into new low-cost, scalable methods of effective promotion of health and wellbeing for older people. We aimed to assess feasibility, reach and costs of implementing a new tailored computer-aided health and social risk appraisal system in primary care.

Methods: Design: Feasibility study.
Setting: Five General Practices in London (Ealing) and Hertfordshire, United Kingdom (UK)
Participants: Random sample of patients aged 65 + years.
Intervention: The Multi-dimensional Risk Appraisal for Older people (MRA-O) system includes: 1) Postal questionnaire including health, lifestyle, social and environmental domains; 2) Software system generating a personalised feedback report with advice on health and wellbeing; 3) Follow-up of people with new concerning or complex needs by GPs or practice nurses.
Evaluation: Feasibility of implementation; participant wellbeing, functional ability and quality of life; social needs, health risks, potential lifestyle changes; and costs of implementation.

Results: Response rates to initial postal invitations were low (526/1550, 34%). Of these, 454/526 (86%) completed MRA-O assessments. Compared to local UK Census data on older people, participants were younger, more were owner-occupiers and fewer were from ethnic minority groups than expected. A range of problems was identified by participants, including pain in last week (269/438, 61.4%), low physical activity (173/453, 38.2%), sedentary lifestyle (174/447, 38.3%), falls (117/439, 26.7%), incontinence (111/441 25.2%), impaired vision 116/451 (25.7%), impaired hearing (145/431, 33.6%), depressed mood (71/451, 15.7%), impaired memory (44/444 9.9%), social isolation (46/449, 10.2%) and loneliness (31/442, 7.0%). Self-rated health was good/excellent in 312/437 (71.4%), and quality of life and well-being were slightly above age-specific population norms. Implementation costs were low. Practices reviewed medical records of 143/454 (31.5%) of participants as a consequence of their responses, and actively followed up 110/454 (24.2%) of their patients.
(Continued on next page)

* Correspondence: K.walters@ucl.ac.uk
[1]Department Primary Care & Population Health, University College London (UCL), Royal Free Campus, Rowland Hill St, London NW3 2PF, UK
Full list of author information is available at the end of the article

(Continued from previous page)

Conclusions: A computer-aided risk appraisal system was feasible for General Practices to implement, yields useful information about health and social problems, and identifies individual needs. Participation rates were however low, particularly for the oldest old, the poorest, and ethnic minority groups, and this type of intervention may increase inequalities in access. Widespread implementation of this approach would require work to address potential inequalities.

Keywords: Ageing, Elderly, Primary Care, Health Promotion

Background

With increasing life expectancy major challenges face governments internationally [1], and the care and support of older people are widely recognised as a public health imperative. Current policy emphasises the importance of personalised preventative approaches in community settings [2–4]. There is, however, a limited evidence base about the most appropriate approaches to meet these broad aims. Complex interventions designed to improve physical function and maintain independent living show potential to alter health behaviours, improve general health perception and self-efficacy, and promote independence in older people [5].

An ideal multi-faceted approach to promote healthy ageing in the general population of older people should be low cost, easy to implement using existing structures, and demonstrate effectiveness in improving wellbeing in later life. In the UK the majority of older people are registered with a General Practitioner (GP), and primary care is one of the few services that has the ability to reach the general population of older people. There is a lack of evidence for effective primary care led population approaches to improving health and wellbeing in later life, and initiatives such as an annual over 75 years health check, generally an invitation to a face to face assessment with a nurse or physician for all people aged 75 and over, have had limited effectiveness [6], with no evidence on whether they might be cost-effective. This approach is potentially burdensome for primary care, particularly in the context of a rising older-old population. It may also miss opportunities for health promotion in younger age groups, such as those aged 65 – 74 years around the retirement window.

The Health Risk Appraisal for Older people (HRA-O) system is a health risk assessment tool focussed on risk factors for functional decline [7–9]. In this system older people are invited to complete a comprehensive survey on their health and wellbeing across different domains, and then receive an individualised report generated from their answers by a dedicated computer programme. If this report is also shared with primary care practitioners, those with more complex or concerning needs can be actively followed up for further face to face assessments. This process can be automated, using editable software, and the report can include healthy ageing advice, signposting to local and national resources, and be tailored to individuals based on their responses. It can create opportunities for promoting self-care and wellbeing, and has the capacity to integrate social and health care information for older people. Aggregated data have the potential to contribute to the development of profiles of local populations and their needs, and so refine and inform commissioning of services [10].

The pilot and feasibility studies of the HRA-O system in primary care showed that the technology can be culturally adapted to the UK, is acceptable to older people and GPs, and can identify under-utilisation of preventive services [7, 8]. A Randomised Controlled Trial (RCT) of HRA-O in the UK confirmed its acceptablity and had high response rates, but, without any local embedding of its use or reinforcement of its messages by active follow-up through primary care, its impact on changing health behaviour was limited [9]. However in Switzerland an RCT of the HRA-O, linked to active telephone follow-up by nurses and primary care physicians, led to signficant improvements in healthy behaviours after 2 years, and reduced mortality over 8 years [11]. Further development work to expand the HRA-O system to include social, economic and environmental factors determining well-being was undertaken in the UK in the Smarter Working in Social & Health Care project (SWISH) [10, 12]. In this study older people prioritised and developed a series of supplementary questions and feedback on housing, transport, income maximisation, safety, social isolation, care responsibilities, recent life events, access to services and environmental concerns, to add to standard Heath Risk Appraisal (HRA). We have combined the standard HRA-O with the new questions from the SWISH study to create a new broader assessment tool, the Multi-dimensional Risk Appraisal for Older people (MRA-O) system.

This experience raised two questions: 1) Can a multi-faceted intervention with local embedding and re-enforcement of tailored recommendations be integrated into routine primary care? 2) Are there added benefits to broadening primary care based health risk appraisal to include social, economic and environmental domains? The aims of this study were to test the feasibility and costs of using HRA-O and SWISH tools combined into a Multi-dimensional Risk Appraisal system for Older people (MRA-O), including local embedding and re-enforcement of use in routine primary care.

Methods

The intervention

The complex intervention had 2 stages:

Stage 1) Locally adapting and embedding the MRA-O technology Research staff facilitated a working group at each of two sites (see below) including 10–14 local representatives of older people, Public Health, GPs, Community Nursing, Adult Social Care, Local Council, Private Sector Providers, Voluntary and Community Organisations, to tailor the MRA-O system to local needs, systems and services. The locality working groups identified local agencies and individuals who could support older people in meeting individual needs identified using the MRA-O system. Supplementary web-searches were conducted, and resources/services identified and contacted by telephone, to collect up to date information on local services for older people in each area. This information was incorporated into the MRA-O software.

Stage 2) Feasibility of implementing the MRA-O in primary care The locally adapted MRA-O system was tested by conducting assessments using postal questionnaires with a random sample of older people registered with participating General Practices. Data were entered and automated personalised feedback was provided to individuals including details of local and national resources to support self-care and promote wellbeing. A copy of the feedback report was scanned into participating patients' GP health records and reviewed by a lead clinician in each practice (practice nurse, nurse practitioner, or GP). Those with complex or concerning needs had, with consent, additional follow-up from clinicians in primary care (practice nurse, nurse practitioner or GP) to encourage them to engage with actions to promote wellbeing. Practices were advised that the lead clinician should review the MRA-O report on arrival as with any clinical report they receive about patients, and decide on action needed with reference to the medical records, taking into account prior knowledge of the patient. They were given a flow-chart with brief instructions on the process, advised to follow-up those with new, complex and/or concerning needs, and given examples of these (e.g. recent unintentional weight loss, depression, severe pain, loneliness or multiple problems across several domains).

Study setting

We conducted the study in two localities (London Borough of Ealing, and the County of Hertfordshire, UK) representing urban and semi-rural locations, with different proportions of black and minority ethnic (BME) populations and different socio-economic characteristics. Two General Practices participated in Hertfordshire, and three in Ealing.

Study sample

A random sample of up to 1 in 3 community dwelling older people (aged 65 years and over) registered with participating General Practices were approached to complete assessments as described in Stage 2 above. The sampling ratio was determined according to the numbers of older people on the practice list, in order to achieve a target sample of 150–200 older people per practice, with an estimated response rate of 40%. We excluded those: living in nursing or residential care settings; with severe incapacitating/life-threatening/terminal illness; unable to provide informed consent (e.g. with moderate to severe dementia/learning disability); where an assessment would be considered burdensome at the time of recruitment (e.g. very recent bereavement or life-threatening illness).

Data collection

GPs wrote to all randomly selected eligible older people, inviting them to participate in the study. Those consenting to participate were sent a comprehensive (28-page) postal questionnaire survey. One postal reminder was sent to non-responders. All materials were produced in large print versions. Translated versions of the study information sheet and consent forms were available for the main other languages at study sites. The main questionnaire was in English only, and participants were encouraged to seek support from friends or family in completion if needed. A researcher assisted (by telephone) anyone who was unable to complete the written questionnaire due to, for example, sight, language or literacy problems. Data from the questionnaires were entered into the dedicated software programme by the research team.

Measurements

Socio-demographic characteristics

We collected data on age, gender, housing tenure, housing type, age of completion of full-time education, country of birth, English as first language, self-reported ethnic group, receipt of pension, receipt of financial benefits, household composition, marital/civil partnership status, previous main employment and current employment/volunteering. We also asked about mobile telephone use (regular/occasional/none) and internet use (most days/1-3 days per week/< once weekly/never).

Feasibility

We collected data on uptake and compared the socio-demographic characteristics of those participating with

UK 2011 Census data for that local area [13], where available. We recorded data on actions from practices following MRA-O assessments, including review of medical records, and consequent follow-up and referrals under-taken.

Quality of life, health behaviours and well-being

The MRA-O includes: a combination of the HRA-O [14] and additional questions generated from the SWISH study [12]. The HRA-O covers domains of physical health, functioning/activities of daily living, disability, psychological distress, memory and lifestyle behaviours, eg physical activity, nutrition, smoking, use of alcohol and problem alcohol drinking (the CAGE questionnaire [15]) and the four Fried questions (Changed walking half a mile/Walk half a mile less often/Changed climbing 10 steps/Climb 10 steps less often), which predict disablement [16]. Questions from the SWISH study [12] included were on housing, transport, income maximisation, safety, social isolation, care responsibilities, recent life events, access to services, and environmental issues. A supplementary questionnaire included measures of quality of life (SF-12) [17], well-being (Warwick-Edinburgh Mental Well-being Scale 14-item) [18] and health, social care and voluntary sector service use.

Cost of the intervention

Data were collected on work required from practices to complete the screening of practice lists, invite patients to participate and to perform patient assessments. Unit costs were estimated for all activities using published unit costs of health and social care activity [19]. From this data we estimated the direct costs of the intervention.

Analysis

Data from the MRA-O software were generated as Excel files and transferred to SPSS. Other data were directly entered in SPSS. Data were double entered and discrepancies resolved. Data were cross-checked by tabulations and histograms identifying missing data and anomalies and cleaned with reference to the original questionnaires. Descriptive data analysis was undertaken only, as the primary purpose of this study was to determine the feasibility of implementing this process.

Results

Response rates

We approached 6 practices to participate and 5 agreed, 2 in Hertfordshire and 3 in Ealing, with an average list size of 8,142 (range 4,264 – 10,231) registered patients. Of the 5 practices, 3 had not previously participated in any research. Response rates to initial postal invitations to older people to participate were low (526/1550, 34%). Of those initially expressing an interest, 454/526 (86.3%) returned full completed questionnaires. There were differences across sites, with 283/770 (36.8%) returned in Hertfordshire and 171/780 (21.9%) in London. Two participants contacted us for support in completing the questionnaire, and for one person to our knowledge the questionnaire was translated by and completed with her son as the participant could not read English.

Socio-demographic characteristics of participants

Characteristics of participants by study site are shown in Table 1. Overall the median age of participants was 73.2 years (IQR 68.9-78.9 years), 53% were female, 385/447 (86.1%) were White British ethnicity, 403/447 (90.2%) lived in owner-occupied accommodation, 274/451 (60.8%) had no post-16 years education, 118/454 (26.0%) only received a state pension. Compared to local UK 2011 Census data, participants were younger, more were owner occupiers and fewer were from ethnic minority groups than expected. UK 2011 Census data [13] showed that in Ealing's older population (65 and over) 13% were aged 85 or more, 55% were female, 69% were home owners, 33% lived alone and 37% were from Black, Minority Ethnic (BME) groups. In Hertfordshire, census data showed that 14.7% were over 84, 51% were female, 71% home owners, 28% lived alone and 9% were from BME groups.

MRA-O findings

Health problems (physical and psychological), life style and functioning

Table 2 shows health problems identified by participants. Overall health was reported as poor or fair in more than a quarter (125/437, 28.6%). Pain in the last week was very high in this sample (269/438 61.4%), as was pain that limited activity or disturbed sleep (160/429, 37.3%). Sensory deficits (vision and hearing) affected a quarter to a third of the sample. Just over a third of participants reported sedentary behaviour, defined as self-reported sitting for 4 or more hours daily (not including sleep periods). A quarter to a third of participants reported a change in walking half a mile or climbing stairs in the last year. There was a low prevalence of smoking at 5.1%, but the majority (84%) reported a high fat diet. A small proportion (6.8%) screened positive for a possible alcohol problem using the CAGE questions [15].

Social problems

A range of social problems was identified by participants (see Table 3). One in five reported difficulties in maintaining the upkeep of their home, and many (179/422, 42.4%) stated they were unsure if they were claiming all the benefits to which they were entitled. A substantial minority (188/453, 41.5%) reported being badly affected

Table 1 Characteristics of participants, by setting

Characteristic[a]	Urban (Ealing) n (%) N = 171	Semi-rural (Hertfordshire) n (%) N = 283	Overall n (%) N = 454
Age group			
65-74 years	94 (55.0%)	178 (62.9%)	272 (59.9%)
75-84 years	63 (36.8%)	88 (31.1%)	151 (33.3%)
85+ yrs	14 (8.2%)	17 (6.0%)	31 (6.8%)
Female	108 (63.2%)	132 (46.6%)	240 (52.9%)
Born outside UK (missing = 4)	60 (35.7%)	12 (4.3%)	72 (16.0%)
Self-reported Black & Minority Ethnic Group (missing = 7)	53 (31.7%)	9 (3.2%)	62 (13.9%)
Living alone (missing = 5)	53 (31.6%)	60 (21.4%)	113 (25.2%)
Married or equivalent (missing = 8)	93 (56.4%)	209 (74.6%)	302 (67.9%)
Owner occupier (missing = 7)	148 (89.2%)	255 (90.8%)	403 (90.2%)
Age completed education (missing = 3)			
16 years or less	74 (44.1%)	200 (70.7%)	274 (60.8%)
17 years or more	94 (56.0%)	83 (29.3%)	177 (39.3%)
Currently employed (missing = 8)	20 (12.0%)	30 (10.7%)	50 (11.2%)
Volunteering (missing = 7)	54 (32.1%)	57 (20.4%)	111 (24.8%)
Mobile phone use (missing = 10)			
Never	19 (11.7%)	27 (9.6%)	46 (10.4%)
Occasional	79 (48.4%)	147 (52.3%)	226 (50.9%)
Regular	65 (39.9%)	107 (38.1%)	172 (38.7%)
Internet use (missing = 9)			
Never	59 (35.8%)	104 (37.1%)	163 (36.6%)
Occasionally (<once a week)	13 (7.9%)	22 (7.9%)	35 (7.9%)
Sometimes (1-3 days a week)	20 (12.1%)	31 (11.1%)	51 (11.5%)
Often (4 or more days a week)	73 (44.2%)	123 (43.9%)	196 (44.0%)

[a]Data missing for some participants as indicated

by a recent life event. Around 16% (73/443) had caring responsibilities for others. A relatively low number (31/442, 7.0%) reported that they were lonely much of the time. A few (39/446, 8.7%) were concerned that others might take advantage of them financially; this broad category included nuisance (scam) telephone calls.

Quality of life and wellbeing

The mean quality of life scores were 53.2 (n = 412, SD8.6) on the mental component of the SF-12 and 43.9 (n = 412, SD 12.4) on the physical component. This is slightly higher (better health) than normative population values reported for this age group in the UK [20]. The mean wellbeing score on the Warwick-Edinburgh Mental Wellbeing scale was 54.3 (n = 407, SD 9.2), slightly above age-specific population norms (mean 51.6, SD 8.71) [21].

Feasibility: Practice follow-up and workload

Practices developed systems for dealing with new needs identified by the MRA-O questionnaire using the guidance described in Stage 2 of the intervention above. Overall 110/454 (24%) of participants were followed up by their practice nurse or nurse practitioner (in four practices) or GP (in one practice) by telephone and/or face to face consultation. The numbers followed up varied considerably between practices (range 10%–83%). Figure 1 shows the practice follow-up process and its outcomes.

Costs of MRA-O use

The costs relate to central administrative tasks and costs for individual GP practices to deliver the intervention. The central administrative task was to locally adapt the MRA-O software to integrate information on local services for needs identified by the MRA-O. We estimate this took up to two days of a junior administrator's time to verify and update the local contact information for a local directory of services, then enter this in the software. This would need to be updated annually, however is likely to take less time in future years.

Table 2 Prevalence of health, impairment and lifestyle risks

Item[a]	n (%) N = 454
General health	
Fair or poor self-rated health (missing = 17)	125 (28.6%)
Experienced pain in last 7 days (missing = 16)	269 (61.4%)
Pain causing impairment to activities or sleep (missing = 25)	160 (37.3%)
Physical activity	
Low level of physical activity (missing = 1)	173 (38.2%)
Not able to walk 1 km/½ mile (missing = 10)	70 (15.8%)
In those able to walk 1 km/½ mile:	
Difficulty walking 1 km/½ mile due to health (missing = 46)	63 (16.8%)
Changed walking 1 km/½ mile in last year (missing = 45)	101 (27.0%)
Walk 1 km/½ mile less often in last year (missing = 43)	95 (25.4%)
Cannot climb up 10 steps (missing = 6)	18 (4.0%)
In those able to climb up 10 steps:	
Difficulty climbing up 10 steps due to health (missing = 45)	95 (22.1%)
Changed climbing 10 steps in last year (missing = 42)	165 (38.4%)
Climb 10 steps less often in last year (missing = 42)	104 (24.2%)
Sitting 4+ hours/day (missing = 7)	174 (38.9%)
Functional ability	
Poor self-rated eyesight (rated fair, poor, very poor or blind) (missing = 3)	116 (25.7%)
Poor self-rated hearing (rated fair, poor, very poor or deaf) (missing = 23)	145 (33.6%)
Need help with IADLs (missing = 12)	105 (23.8%)
Need help with BADLs (missing = 5)	31 (6.9%)
Fallen in last 12 months (missing = 15)	117 (26.7%)
Urinary incontinence in last year (missing = 13)	111 (25.2%)
Of these 111, those incontinent at least 6 days in last year	81 (73.0%)
Psychosocial impairment	
Depressed mood (missing = 3)	71 (15.7%)
Subjective memory problems (missing = 10)	44 (9.9%)
At risk of social isolation (missing = 5)	46 (10.2%)
Fear of falling (missing = 10)	105 (23.6%)
Lifestyle risks	
Current smoker (missing = 7)	23 (5.1%)
Alcohol problem screening (CAGE) score 2+ (missing = 13)	30 (6.8%)
High fat diet (missing = 9)	375 (84.3%)

[a]Data missing for some participants as indicated

The intervention costs of the study for individual GP practices comprised fixed and variable components. The fixed costs relate to the set-up of the intervention. This was £125 (196 USD) per practice in the first year, and then £70 (110 USD) per practice in subsequent years. This covered the cost of identifying patients, including manually reviewing lists generated from electronic searches of GP registers to remove people who were ineligible. The variable costs related to the number of questionnaires sent, returned and requiring following up. These estimates include the costs of the postal questionnaire, data entry, report generation and checking, the time needed to review reports and carry out follow-up by nurse or GP. Data entry was estimated as 11-12 min per questionnaire, which could be performed by a junior administrator, and could be undertaken centrally or within practices.

Table 3 Prevalence of reported social problems

Problem[a]	n, % sample size = 454
Badly affected by recent life event (missing = 1)	188 (41.5%)
Upkeep of home difficult (missing = 10)	99 (22.3%)
Transport difficulties limit activity (missing = 8)	58 (13.0%)
Environment reduces quality of life (missing = 13)	32 (7.3%)
Environment limits activity (missing = 10)	24 (5.4%)
Unsafe in home (missing = 17)	20 (4.6%)
Difficult to keep home warm (missing = 7)	20 (4.5%)
Difficulty paying bills (missing = 7)	29 (6.5%)
Difficulty managing money (missing = 8)	18 (4.0%)
Concerned others might take/have taken advantage financially (missing = 8)	39 (8.7%)
Unsure if getting all benefits (missing = 32)	179 (42.4%)
Caring for another (missing = 11)	73 (16.5%)
Lonely much of the time (missing = 12)	31 (7.0%)

[a]Data missing for some participants as indicated

This cost was £6.71 (10.50 USD) per patient for every 1,000 patients receiving the questionnaire, based on 300 returning the questionnaire (30% response rate) and 24% of those responding requiring follow-up by the GP practice. This cost estimate excludes local adaption of the MRA-O software (stage 1), and refers to costs for using the MRA-O in General Practices. Costs are estimated in 2013 values.

Discussion

What this study shows

The MRA-O system functions as a 'virtual health check' with the added advantage of measures of social well-being. Unlike other approaches to risk assessment, the provision of computer generated personalised feedback and identification of solutions and services to address identified problems can facilitate self-management of the changes that occur with ageing. Its use is greater amongst those who are owner-occupiers, from white ethnic groups, and the 'younger old' age groups (65–84 years). This is similar to previous research [22]. This self-selection bias is likely to underestimate the prevalence of health and social problems in the older population.

Participants nonetheless reported a wide range of health risks and social problems, suggesting that it was not just reaching the 'worried well'. On reviewing the

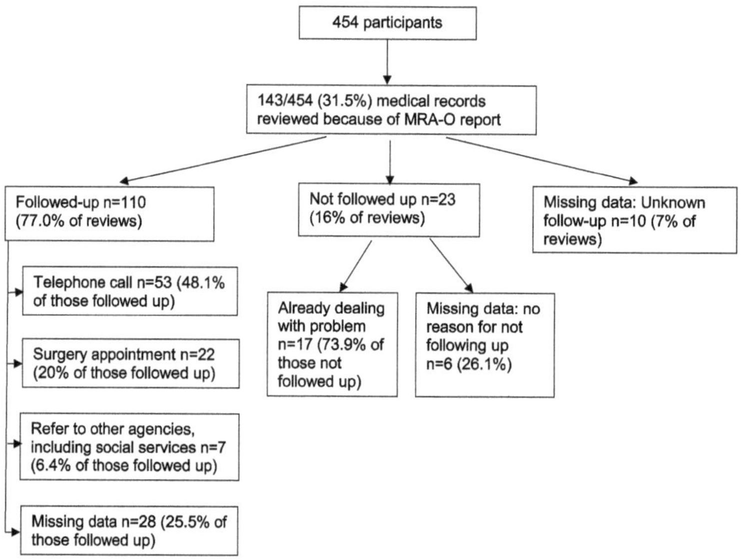

Fig. 1 Flow chart of practice follow-up of MRA-O reports

reports generated, the practice clinician (nurse or GP) needed to review the notes for just under a third of participants, and initiated further follow-up (generally a telephone call or appointment with the nurse or GP) in around a quarter of participants. This additional workload was feasible for practices to undertake as part of their usual care, without needing additional resources or support.

Comparison with other literature

A wide range of health and social problems was identified, a number of which were at similar levels to those expected, while others were more or less prevalent than in previous research. The proportion of participants who were sedentary is similar to the 40% in the ProAct65+ trial of a health promotion intervention (exercise) for older people in primary care [23]. Sedentary behaviour is associated with adverse physical and mental health outcomes [24], has deleterious health effects, even when physical activity recommendations are met [25], and sitting time is now recognised as a health risk factor independent of physical activity [26]. Older adults are most likely to be sedentary [27, 28]. Almost one in four participants aged 65 and over expressed fear of falling, again similar to other studies in similar populations [29].

In some domains very high prevalence rates were reported. The most striking of these was pain, where more than a third of the sample reported pain limiting their activity or sleep, and more than half had experienced pain during the last week. This is similar to the prevalence of pain identified using the same instrument in an earlier study [30]. Also notable was the salience of a high fat diet in more than 80% of those participating. This is significant given that the ageing process can be viewed as the cumulative effect of chronic health risks including hyperlipidemia, whilst among independently living older people low nutrient density of the diet and inadequate intakes of protein, vitamins, and minerals are the chief areas of nutritional concern [31]. A quarter to a third of respondents noted that their mobility had worsened in the last year. Self-reported preclinical disability (as captured by the Fried questions) predicts incident falls at 1-year follow-up, independent of other self-reported fall risk factors [32]. This is a group whose falls might be prevented, and whose disablement might be interrupted or delayed by intervention. Self-rated impairments in vision and hearing were higher than prevalence rates reported in other studies [33, 34], with nearly a third reporting hearing impairments and a quarter vision impairments.

Some domains were reported less frequently than expected, for example urinary incontinence was lower than shown in other community studies [35, 36] and subjective memory complaints which are reported to occur in 22 - 50% of those aged 65 and over, and increase with advancing age [37, 38]. Just under 7% of participants declared that they were lonely much of the time, compared with a population prevalence of around 16%; severe loneliness occurs in 7-10% of community dwelling people aged over 65 years [39, 40]. Rates of smoking were low, compared to published national statistics of 13% in those aged 60 and over [41], and risk of harmful drinking as measured by the CAGE questions [19] was lower than the published proportions drinking above the recommended limits (19% of men, and 9% of women, aged 65 and over) [42].

Strengths & limitations

This study reports the feasibility of the implementation of computer-aided health and social risk appraisal for the general population of older people (the MRA-O). This is a novel system that produces a personalised report on both health and social concerns, integrated into routine primary care. The MRA-O itself was developed using co-design methods with significant input from older people, and has undergone extensive and iterative field testing. The implementation study was undertaken in five UK General Practices across two contrasting neighbourhoods in urban London and semi-rural Hertfordshire, chosen to maximise diversity in setting, and in type of practice including those that do not typically take part in research. The findings may not, however, be generalizable to other settings or practices. There was good interest and engagement in participating in the study from General Practices, despite high workloads and the study being undertaken during a period of several changes to the organisation of healthcare in England.

There was a low response rate to the initial invitations to older people, but a high completion rate for those initially expressing an interest in participating, despite the need to complete a lengthy (28-page) questionnaire. We do not know if our findings on prevalence of health and social risks identified would apply to those not taking part. Comparison to local Census data suggests that the prevalence of health and social risks in participants in our study may be underestimates of true prevalence rates, and some groups are likely to be under-represented in those who took part (those over 85 years, those not owning their own home, and those from BME groups). Potential participants were aware that this was being conducted as part of a research study, and there were lengthy information sheets and consent forms regarding this; it is possible that response rates might be higher if this were part of routine clinical care.

Implications for research, policy and practice

The MRA-O system is feasible to implement in routine practice in primary care, as a case-finding tool that can identify individual health and social needs and risks in the general population of older people. However participation rates were low, particularly for older age people (85 years+), those of lower socio-economic status and older people from BME groups. Further work is needed to increase participation, addressing these inequalities [22, 43, 44]. Some approaches to increasing general participation, such as offering wider access through using web-based questionnaires, email and mobile applications, while attractive for this type of system and would increase operational efficiencies, may widen these inequalities still further. Our own findings confirm that, even in those participating, their use of the internet and regular use of mobile phone is low, particularly in older age groups, though this may change over time. Other potential options include use of a modified, shorter, more focussed questionnaire and/or distributing the initial questionnaire opportunistically, for example alongside annual influenza vaccination campaigns for older people, in routine consultations, or while waiting for appointments in clinics. It may be necessary to target specific audiences where uptake is lower, such as through social or religious groups for older people from BME groups or community centres and social activities for frailer older people over 85 years, where assistance can be given in person to complete the questionnaires.

We need a greater understanding of the best approaches to reach older people from these groups with lower participation rates to ensure any new general population based service does not introduce further inequalities of access. Our study demonstrates that using the MRA-O system can nonetheless identify a broad range of potential unmet needs and health/social risks in those that take part. Furthermore, busy practices were able to use their existing systems to follow up those that they considered had new, complex or concerning needs. We do not know however whether this leads to improvements in care or wellbeing and functioning for older people over time, or if this approach is cost-effective, and this would need to be tested, ideally in a substantive Randomised Controlled Trial. As needs in older people are dynamic and can accumulate over time, we would anticipate that the assessment process may need to be repeated with intervals. The optimum frequency of assessments still needs to be determined. This would balance potential benefit for patients against additional burden for the practices and what is feasible for them to deliver. In our study we asked practices to invite a random third of their older population, in order to reduce the burden on practices for those with large numbers of older people. On this basis one third could be invited annually to cover the whole population and then the process repeated three yearly.

Conclusions

A computer-aided health and social risk appraisal system is feasible to implement in General Practice settings and can identify a broad range of health, lifestyle and social concerns, provide tailored advice and sign-post older people participating to local services to meet their needs. However, response rates were not high, and there was some evidence that this type of approach may introduce inequalities in access for the older old (85 and over), those who are poorer and from BME groups. These issues should be addressed before implementation in practice.

Abbreviations

BME groups: Black and minority ethnic groups; CAGE: The CAGE alcohol screening questionnaire; HRA-O: Health risk appraisal for older people; MRA-O: Multi-dimensional risk appraisal for older people; SF-12: Short-form 12 item version – quality of life measure; UK: United Kingdom

Acknowledgements

We would like to thank Professor Andreas Stuck and Dr Stephan Born for their collaboration in the use of the Health Risk Appraisal for Older People (HRA-O) Software on which the MRA-O was based.

Funding

This study was funded by the Medical Research Council LLHW G1001822/1. The MRC had no role in the design, collection, analysis, and interpretation of data; in the writing of the manuscript; and in the decision to submit the manuscript for publication.

Authors' contributions

KW, SI, JM, CG, MC and SM designed the study, KK and MH collected the data, KK, CC and JR analysed the data, all authors contributed to the analysis and interpretation and approved the final version of the paper for publication.

Competing interests

The authors declare that they have no competing interests.

Consent for publication

Not applicable

Author details

[1]Department Primary Care & Population Health, University College London (UCL), Royal Free Campus, Rowland Hill St, London NW3 2PF, UK. [2]Centre for Research in Primary and Community Care, University of Hertfordshire, College Lane, Hatfield AL10 9AB, Hertfordshire, UK. [3]Social Care Workforce Research Unit, King's College London, Strand, London WC2B 4LL, UK. [4]University of Northumbria, Sutherland Building Newcastle-upon-Tyne, Newcastle NE1 8ST, UK. [5]Department of Applied Health Research, UCL, 1-19 Torrington Place, London WC1E 7HB, UK.

References

1. World Health Organisation. 10 facts on ageing and health 2015. http://www.who.int/features/factfiles/ageing/ageing_facts/en/. Accessed 22 Mar 2017.
2. World Health Organisation. World report on ageing and health. 2015. http://www.who.int/ageing/events/world-report-2015-launch/en/. Accessed 22 Mar 2017.
3. Centers for Disease Control and Prevention. Healthy Aging Program. http://www.cdc.gov/aging/services/index.htm. Accessed 15 Mar 2016.
4. Oliver D, Foot C, Humphries R. Making our health and social care systems fit for an ageing population. The King's Fund, March 2014. http://www.kingsfund.org.uk/publications/making-our-health-and-care-systems-fit-ageing-population. Accessed 15 Mar 2016.
5. Beswick AD, Rees K, Dieppe P, Ayis S, Gooberman-Hill R, Horwood J, et al. Complex interventions to improve physical function and maintain independent living in elderly people: a systematic review and meta-analysis. Lancet. 2008;371:725–35. doi:10.1016/S0140-6736(08)60342-6.
6. Frost H, Haw S, Frank J. Promoting health & well-being in later life: interventions in primary care and community settings. Edinburgh: Chief Scientist Office, Scottish Government; 2011 http://www.scphrp.ac.uk/promoting-health-wellbeing-in-later-life-interventions-in-primary-care-and-community-settings/. Accessed 15 Mar 2016.
7. Stuck AE, Elkuch P, Dapp U, Anders J, Iliffe S, Swift C, for the Pro-Age pilot study group. Feasibility and yield of a self-administered questionnaire for health risk appraisal in older people in three European countries. Age Ageing. 2002;31:463–7.
8. Iliffe S, Kharicha K, Harari D, Swift C, Stuck AE. A health risk appraisal for older people in general practice using an expert system: a pilot study. Health Soc Care Community. 2005;13:21–9.
9. Harari D, Iliffe S, Kharicha K, Egger M, Gillmann G, Von Renteln-Kruse W, et al. Promotion of health in older people: an RCT of health risk appraisal in British general practice. Age Ageing. 2008;37:565–71.
10. Manthorpe J, Kharicha K, Goodman C, Harari D, Swift C, Iliffe S. Smarter working in social and health care: professional perspectives on a new technology. Br J Soc Work. 2010;40(6):1829–46. doi:10.1093/bjsw/bcp100.
11. Stuck AE, Moser A, Morf U, Wirz U, Wyser J, Gillmann G, et al. Effect of health risk assessment and counselling on health behaviour and survival in older people: a pragmatic randomised trial. PLoS Med. 2015;12(10): e1001889. doi:10.1371/journal.pmed.1001889.
12. Iliffe S, Kharicha K, Harari D, Swift C, Goodman C, Manthorpe J. User involvement in the development of a health promotion technology for older people: findings from the SWISH project. Health Soc Care Community. 2010;18:147–59. doi:10.1111/j.1365-2524.2009.00882.x.
13. Office for National Statistics, UK 2011 Census http://www.ons.gov.uk/ons/guide-method/census/2011/index.html. Accessed 15 Mar 2016.
14. Stuck AE, Kharicha K, Dapp U, Anders J, von Renteln-Kruse W, Meier-Baumgartner HP, et al. Development, feasibility and performance of a Health Risk Appraisal questionnaire for older persons. BMC Med Res Methodol. 2007;7:1. doi:10.1186/1471-2288-7-1.
15. Dhalla S, Kopec J. The CAGE questionnaire for alcohol misuse: a review of reliability and validity studies. Clin Invest Med. 2007;30(1):33–41. http://cimonline.ca/index.php/cim/article/view/447.
16. Fried LP, Bandeen-Roche K, Chaves PHM, Johnson BR. Preclinical mobility disability predicts incident mobility disability in older women. J Gerontol. 2000;55A:M43–52.
17. Ware JE, Kosinski M, Keller SD. A 12-Item Short-Form Health Survey: construction of scales and preliminary tests of reliability and validity. Med Care. 1996;34(3):220–33.
18. Tennant R, Hiller L, Fishwick R, Platt S, Joseph S, Weich S, et al. The Warwick-Edinburgh Mental Well-being Scale (WEMWBS): development and UK validation. Health Qual Life Outcomes. 2007;14:63. doi:10.1186/1477-7525-5-63.
19. Curtis L. Unit Costs of Health and Social Care. Canterbury: Personal and Social Services Research Unit, University of Kent; 2012.
20. Pettit T, Livingston G, Manela M, Kitchen G, Katona C, Bowling A. Validation and normative data of health status measures in older people: The Islington study. Int J Geriatr Psychiatry. 2001;16(11):1061–70. doi:10.1002/GPS/479.
21. Warwick Edinburgh Mental Well-being Scale (WEMWBS). http://www2.warwick.ac.uk/fac/med/research/platform/wemwbs/. Accessed 15 Mar 2016.
22. Gaertner B, Seitz I, Fuchs J, Busch MA, Holzhausen M, Martus P, et al. Baseline participation in a health examination survey of the population 65 years and older: who is missed and why? BMC Geriatr. 2016;16:21. doi:10.1186/s12877-016-0185-6.
23. Iliffe S, Kendrick D, Morris R, Masud T, Gage H, Skelton D, et al. Multi-centre cluster randomised trial comparing a community group exercise programme with home based exercise with usual care for people aged 65 and over in primary care. Health Technol Assessment. 2014;18(49). doi:10.3310/hta18490.
24. de Rezende LFM, Rey-Lopez JP, Matsudo VKR, do Carmo Luiz O. Sedentary behavior and health outcomes among older adults: a systematic review. BMC Public Health. 2014;1:333. doi:10.1186/1471-2458-14-333.
25. Grontved A, Hu FB. Television viewing and risk of type 2 diabetes, cardiovascular disease, and all-cause mortality: a meta-analysis. JAMA. 2011; 305(23):2448–55. doi:10.1001/jama.2011.812.
26. Owen N, Healy GN, Matthews CE, Dunstan DW. Too much sitting: the population health science of sedentary behavior. Exerc Sport Sci Rev. 2010; 38(3):105–13. doi:10.1097/JES.0b013e3181e373a2.
27. Davis MG, Fox KR, Hillsdon M, Sharp DJ, Coulson JC, Thompson JL. Objectively measured physical activity in a diverse sample of older urban UK adults. Med Sci Sports Exerc. 2011;43(4):647–54. doi:10.1249/MSS.0b013e3181f36196.
28. Bennie JA, Chau JY, van der Ploeg HP, Stamatakis E, Do A, Bauman A. The prevalence and correlates of sitting in European adults-a comparison of 32 Eurobarometer-participating countries. Int J Behav Nutr Physical Activ. 2013; 10(1):1. doi:10.1186/1479-5868-10-107.
29. Kumar A, Carpenter H, Morris R, Iliffe S, Kendrick D. Which factors are associated with fear of falling in community dwelling older people? Age Ageing. 2014;43(1):76–84. doi:10.1093/ageing/aft154.
30. Carmaciu C, Iliffe S, Kharicha K, Harari D, Swift C, Gillman G, et al. Health risk appraisal in older people: 3. the experience, impact and context of pain & their implications for general practitioners. Br J Gen Pract. 2007;57:630–5.
31. Mithal A, Bonjour JP, Boonen S, Burckhardt P, Degens H, El Hajj FG, et al. Impact of nutrition on muscle mass, strength, and performance in older adults. Osteoporos Int. 2013;24:1555–66. doi:10.1007/s00198-012-2236-y.
32. Clough-Gorr K, Erpen T, Gillmann G, von Renteln-Kruse W, Iliffe S, Beck J, et al. Preclinical mobility disability as a risk factor for falls in community-dwelling older adults. J Gerontol A Biol Sci Med Sci. 2008;63(3):314–20.
33. Charles N. Estimates of the number of older people with a visual impairment in the UK. Br J Visual Impairment. 2007;25:199–215.
34. Akeroyd MA, Foreman K, Holman JA. Estimates of the number of adults in England, Wales, and Scotland with a hearing loss. Int J Audiol. 2014;53:60–1. doi:10.3109/14992027.2013.85053.
35. Sims J, Browning C, Lundgren-Lindquist B, Kendig H. Urinary incontinence in a community sample of older adults: prevalence and impact on quality of life. Disabil Rehabil. 2011;33(15-16):1389–98. doi:10.3109/09638288.2010.532284.
36. Wu JM, Vaughan CP, Goode PS, Redden DT, Burgio KL, Richter HE, et al. Prevalence and trends of symptomatic pelvic floor disorders in U.S. women. Obstet Gynecol. 2014;123(1):141–8. doi:10.1097/AOG.0000000000000057.
37. Larrabee GJ, Crook TH. Estimated prevalence of age-associated memory impairment derived from standardized tests of memory function. Int Psychogeriatr. 1994;6(01):95–104.
38. Genziani M, Stewart R, Béjot Y, Amieva H, Artero S, Ritchie K. Subjective memory impairment, objective cognitive functioning and social activity in French older people: Findings from the Three Cities study. Geriatr Gerontol Int. 2013;13:139–45. doi:10.1111/j.1447-0594.2012.00873.x.
39. Luanaigh CO, Lawler BA. Loneliness and the health of older people. Int J Geriatr Psychiatry. 2008;23:1213–21.
40. Victor CD, Scambler SJ, Bowling A, Bond J. The prevalence of and risk factors for loneliness in later life: a survey of older people in Great Britain. Ageing Society. 2005;25:357–75.
41. Health & Social Care Information Centre Statistics on Smoking England. 2014. http://www.hscic.gov.uk/catalogue/PUB14988/smok-eng-2014-rep.pdf. Accessed 15 Mar 2016.
42. Health & Social Care Information Centre Statistics on Alcohol England. 2014. http://www.hscic.gov.uk/catalogue/PUB15483. Accessed 15 Mar 2016.
43. Hussain-Gambles M, Atkin K, Leese B. Why ethnic minority groups are under-represented in clinical trials: a review of the literature. Health Soc Care Community. 2004;12(5):382–8.
44. Emmel N, Hughes K, Greenhalgh J, Sales A. Accessing socially excluded people – trust and the gatekeeper in the researcher-participant relationship. Sociological Research Online 2007;12(2): http://www.socresonline.org.uk/12/2/emmel.html. Accessed 24 July 2016.

17

Heart failure labelled patients with missing ejection fraction in primary care: prognosis and determinants

Miguel-Angel Muñoz[1,2,3], Xavier Mundet-Tuduri[1,2,3*], Jordi Real[2,6], José-Luis Del Val[1,2], Mar Domingo[1,2], Ernest Vinyoles[1,2,5], Ester Calero[1,2], Caterina Checa[2,4], Nuria Soldevila-Bacardit[1,2] and José-María Verdú-Rotellar[1,2,3]

Abstract

Background: It is common to find a high variability in the accuracy of heart failure (HF) diagnosis in electronic primary care medical records (EMR). Our aims were to ascertain (i) whether the prognosis of HF labelled patients whose ejection fraction (EF) was missing in their EMR differed from those that had it registered, and (ii) the causes contributing to the differences in the availability of EF in EMR.

Methods: Retrospective cohort analyses based on clinical records of HF and attended at 52 primary healthcare centres of Barcelona (Spain). Information of 8376 HF patients aged > 40 years followed during five years was analyzed.

Results: EF was available only in 8.5% of primary care medical records. Cumulate incidence for mortality and hospitalization from 1st January 2009 to 31th December 2012 was 37.6%. The highest rate was found in patients with missing EF (HR 1.84, 95% CI 1.68 -1.95) compared to those with preserved EF. Patients hospitalized the previous year and those requiring home healthcare (HR 1.81, 95% Confidence Interval 1.68-1.95 and HR 1.58, 95% CI 1.46-1.71, respectively) presented a higher risk of having an adverse outcome. Older patients, those more socio-economically disadvantaged, obese, requiring home healthcare, and taking loop diuretics were less likely to have an EF registered.

Conclusions: EF is poorly recorded in primary care. HF patients with EF missing at medical records had the worst prognosis. They tended to be older, socio-economically disadvantaged, and more fragile.

Keywords: Primary care, Heart failure, Echocardiography, Diagnosis

Background

It is well established that heart failure (HF) symptoms, especially during the early stages, are not specific. This is particularly evident in obese and elderly populations, and in patients suffering from chronic pulmonary diseases [1–3]. Up to 60% of HF patients are not properly diagnosed, and as many as 38% who are HF registered have not had an echocardiogram registered in their medical records [4, 5]. We are unaware of the causes related to this lack of information. Two studies have shown that some General Practitioners did not take in account EF to diagnose HF [6, 7]. It is, therefore, difficult to properly estimate the prognosis and evaluate the efficacy of evidence-based treatment in a large number of HF patients, especially since much of the data comes from clinical trials in which the population has been strictly selected.

Prior hospitalization as a consequence of HF has been considered a valid criterion to confirm diagnosis. Nevertheless, it is possible that gaps exist in sharing information between the hospital and primary care setting which may lead to under registration of HF cases in the primary care Electronic Medical Records (EMR).

Most HF patients, especially the oldest ones and those with multimorbidity, are mainly managed in the primary

* Correspondence: xmundet.bcn.ics@gencat.cat
[1]Institut Català de la Salut, Barcelona, Spain
[2]Primary Healthcare University Research Institute IDIAP-Jordi Gol, Barcelona, Spain
Full list of author information is available at the end of the article

care setting [8] and, especially those in terminal phases of their disease, are not eligible to be referred to a specialist for an echocardiography.

Regarding the validity of the diagnosis, Schultz et al., argued that if a physician is treating a patient as having HF it is reasonable to consider that this patient is properly labelled HF [9].

Considering the ejection fraction (EF) as a measure to estimate prognosis has proven controversial [10, 11] a recent meta-analysis found lower mortality in HF patients with preserved ejection fraction (HF-PEF) than in those with reduced ejection fraction (HF-REF) [12]. In addition, it has been reported that in patients with unknown EF (i.e. unrecorded) mortality is similar to those with HF-REF and higher in those with HF-PEF [13].

Our study is aimed at analysing the different prognoses of patients registered as HF in primary healthcare records, depending on whether they have HF-REF, HF-PEF, or Possible HF (HF labelled patients with missing ejection fraction), and, if possible, to ascertain the causes contributing to the differences in EF availability in the EMR.

Methods

The present study is a retrospective cohort analysis with four year follow-up. It is based on the clinical information included in the EMR of all HF patients labelled at the 52 primary healthcare centres of the Institut Català de la Salut in Barcelona (Spain).

Clinical information is centralized in the SIDIAP database (Information System for the Development of Research in Primary Care). This database has been shown to be a valid source for cardiovascular disease research [13] and is linked to the Catalan hospital discharge database CMBD-AH (Conjunto Mínimo Básico de Datos de Altas Hospitalarias) [14].

All adult patients >40 years living in Barcelona (Spain), who were labelled HF diagnosis (International Classification Diseases: I.50) registered in their primary EMR on December 31st, 2012, were included.

The registration date of the HF labelling in the EMR was considered as the date of study inclusion. The duration of the study was from the 1st January, 2009 to 31st December, 2012.

Prognosis was determined by hospital admission as a consequence of HF and the global mortality that occurred during the study period.

Event-free time was defined as the period between diagnosis registration and the first hospital admission as a consequence of HF, global mortality, or the last contact with the primary care services.

Ejection Fraction: in order to be able to compare our results with previously published studies, HF patients were classified into three categories according to the EF closest to the date of the inclusion: HF-REF (EF < 50%), HF-PEF (EF > = 50%), and Possible HF (when no information, either quantitative or qualitative, about EF was found in the medical records) (Fig. 1).

The following potentially confounding variables at baseline for EF effect were considered: age, gender, hospitalization for HF the year prior to inclusion in the study, smoking habit, cardiovascular risk factors (hypertension, diabetes, hypercholesterolemia, obesity), cardiovascular comorbidity (coronary heart disease, atrial fibrillation, stroke, peripheral arterial disease), other comorbidities (chronic obstructive pulmonary disease, chronic nephropathy), cardiovascular drug use (antiagregants, lipid lowering drugs, beta-blockers, angiotensin converting-enzyme inhibitors or angiotensin receptor blockers, and loop diuretics). We also recorded whether the patients required domiciliary healthcare. Socio-economic levels were measured by the MEDEA index which categorizes populations in quintiles, the first one representing the least disadvantaged. This index is based on several items (unemployment, percentage of manual and temporary workers and persons with insufficient education overall and in young people) [15].

The whole population registered as HF in the primary care EMR in Barcelona (Spain) was included in the analysis, resulting in a sample of 8376 HF patients. These sample reflects the whole population labelled as HF.

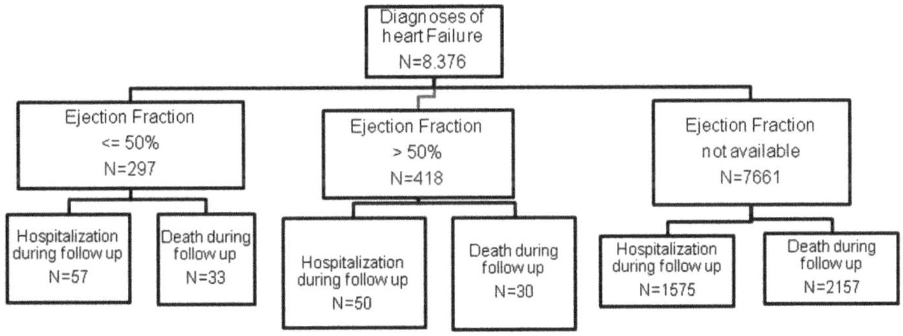

Fig. 1 Classification of heart failure patients according to ejection fraction in primary care electronic medical records

In 52 participating primary healthcare centres were registered more than one million subjects. Such a sample size reaches 94% statistical power (estimated power for Cox regression with Wald test; alpha = 0.05 two sides) with a minimum of 30% events observed. It thus ensures enough statistical power to answer the main questions of the study.

Data are expressed as frequencies and percentages for categorical variables, and means (standard deviation) for continuous ones. Baseline homogeneity of variables according to the EF was analysed. The one-way ANOVA, and Chi-square tests were used to evaluate differences amongst groups with different or missing EF.

Cumulate incidence of mortality, hospital admission or a combined variable of both events during the follow-up period was estimated for each group (HF-REF, HF-PEF, and Possible HF).

To evaluate the differences among groups according to the time from the inclusion date, Cox regression models crude and adjusted were made. The Hazard Ratio (HR) of each group with respect to the reference was calculated and 95% confidence intervals (95%CI) were estimated to compare the groups. The models were compiled using the Enter Method, including clinically relevant co-variables and those statistically associated with the previous EF (< or equal to 50%, > 50%, or not available). We evaluated goodness-of-fit and the Cox model's proportional risk assumption, as well as the interactions at different levels of exposure to each drug, using the Schoenfeld residual analysis. Furthermore, to evaluate the factors related to the probability of having an EF, multivariable logistic regression was performed. For all analyses, a two-tailed $p < 0.05$ was considered statistically significant. IBM-SPSS PC v21 package was used to perform statistical analysis.

Results

From 1st January, 2009 to 31st December 2012, a total of 8376 patients labelled with HF met study criteria,. Median follow-up to event or end of the study was 16.3 months. During the study period, 1608 (19.2%) patients died and 2264 (27.0%) were hospitalized.

Women represented 55.9% of patients and mean age of the population was 78.0 (SD 10.2) years.

Among the sample, 3013 patients (36%) had been admitted to hospital during the year prior to inclusion in the study as a consequence of HF. Ejection fraction was available only in 8.5% of the EMR.

The flow chart represents the distribution of outcomes according to EF (Fig. 1).

By comparing the three categories according to EF, patients in the group with HF-REF were predominantly men (67.0%), had been hospitalized as a consequence of HF the year prior to inclusion in the study (43.8%), and suffered more frequently from coronary heart disease (42.7%). These patients were more often treated with ACE inhibitors and beta-blockers (85.5 and 69.9%, respectively).

Patients with Possible HF were older, required home healthcare, obese, and more frequently treated with loop diuretics. With the exception of coronary disease, no differences were observed in the proportion of patients with atrial fibrillation, stroke history, peripheral artery disease, chronic pulmonary disease, and chronic renal failure according to the EF among the three categories.

The use of ACE inhibitors and beta- blockers was very similar in the group of HF-PEF and Possible HF. The highest proportion of hospitalized or died patients was in the group of Possible HF (39.1%) (Table 1).

Table 2 shows the crude and adjusted hazard ratios for hospitalization or death. Cumulate incidence was 37.6%, and the highest rate was found in patients with Possible HF.

The oldest patients presented 60% more risk (HR: 1.6; CI95%:1.40-1.83) of having an adverse event than the younger ones (≤71 years). Being hospitalized as a consequence of a decompensation the year prior to inclusion almost doubled the risk for re-hospitalization or death (HR: 1.81; CI95%:1.68-1.95). In addition, patients requiring home healthcare had 60% (HR:1.58; CI95:1.46-1.71) more risk than the others of having an adverse event. This risk was also higher among patients living in socio-economically disadvantaged neighborhoods (HR:1.13; CI95%:1.01-1.27).

Hypertension, diabetes, pulmonary and renal diseases, and cardiovascular comorbidity were also associated with a higher risk of having an adverse outcome. Medication for hypercholesterolemia and hypertension, however, worked as protective factors. In contrast, patients taking loop diuretics had a higher rate of adverse outcomes.

Patients hospitalized the year before and without an EF registered in the EMR presented an HR of 4.99, and a 95% Confidence Interval 3.67 to 6.78, for being hospitalized or dying during follow-up.

The adjusted analysis to identify the causes related to the higher probability of missing an EF in the medical records showed that among patients who were elderly, more socio-economically disadvantaged, obese, requiring home healthcare, and taking loop diuretics it was less common to have one registered (Table 3).

Discussion

Our study found that patients labelled with HF who did not have an EF registered in their primary care EMR presented the highest rates of death and hospital re-admissions with respect to those who did. Patients hospitalized as a consequence of HF decompensation the

Table 1 Characteristics, clinical profile, and treatment according to the ejection fraction of heart failure patients

	EF >50 *n*=418		EF <=50 *n*=297		No EF *n*=7661		EF>50 versus No EF	EF < =50 versus No EF
	n	%	N	%	n	%	*p* value	*p* value
Gender (women)	253	60,5	98	33,0	4331	56,5	0,109	<0.001
Age (Mean,SD)	77.1 (9.5)		74.2 (11.5)		78.3 (10.2)		0.053	<0.001
Socioeconomic deprivation index								
1 (less disadvantaged)	98	23.4	60	20.2	1486	19.4		
2	126	30.1	97	32.6	1377	17.9		
3	102	24.4	53	17.8	1533	20.0		
4	60	14.3	48	16.1	1544	20.1		
5 (more disadvantaged)	29	6.9	36	12.1	1586	20.7	<0.001	<0.001
Previous hospitalization for heart failure	91	21.8	130	43.8	2792	36.4	<0.001	0,010
Patients requiring home care	64	15.3	54	18.1	2124	27.7	<0.001	<0.001
Cardiovascular risk factors								
Hypertension	328	78.4	214	72.0	5823	76.0	0,250	0,118
Diabetes	129	30.8	108	36.3	2528	33.0	0,365	0,227
Hypercholesterolemia	145	34.6	97	32.6	2241	29.2	0,018	0,206
Obesity	71	16.9	42	14.1	1742	22.7	0,006	<0.001
Smoking habit	26	6.2	33	11.1	619	8.0	0,380	<0.001
Cardiovascular disease								
Coronary heart disease	94	22.4	127	42.7	2009	26.2	0,090	0,000
Atrial fibrillation	150	35.8	98	33.0	2794	36.4	0,809	0,222
Stroke	37	8.8	30	10.1	770	10.0	0,426	0,978
Peripheral artery disease	26	6.2	24	8.0	463	6.0	0,883	0,151
COPD	65	15.5	49	16.50	1240	16.19	0,731	0,886
Chronic renal failure	83	19.8	53	17.85	1397	18.24	0,404	0,864
Drug therapy								
ACE inhibitor or ARB	305	73.0	254	85.5	5736	74.9	0,382	<0.001
Beta-blocker	212	50.7	205	69.0	3729	48.7	0,416	<0.001
Loop diuretics	246	58.8	212	71.38	5889	76.8	<0.001	0,028
Outcomes								
Hospitalization	50	11,96	57	19,1	2157	28,1	0,000	0,001
Mortality	30	7,18	33	11,1	1545	20,1	0,000	0,000

EF Ejection Fraction, *SD* Standard deviation, *COPD* Chronic obstructive pulmonary disease, *ACE* angiotensin converting enzyme, *ARB* Angiotensin Receptor Blocker

year prior to study inclusion presented a higher probability of having an adverse outcome during follow- up.

The use of administrative databases could be a limitation to properly answer some research questions. The difficulty of having an accurate HF diagnosis registered is well known. Although it has been reported that most HF diagnoses registered in EMR correspond to authentic cases, about one-quarter are not recorded [16].

On the other hand, the use of a large primary care database allows us to have information about the whole population and confers a high external validity. This validity has been previously analyzed and found good for the study of cardiovascular diseases [13]. Although MEDEA deprivation index is not an individual measure but an ecological one, it is useful as a proxy to determine socioeconomic position of the population living in a geographical area.

The MAGGIC study had already reported higher mortality in Possible HF patients, but their proportion of missing EF was lower in our study and some questions were not completely answered, such as socioeconomic position and setting of care (ambulatory or home healthcare, and). In this way we found that patients requiring home care and those in more disadvantaged economic position had a higher probability of not having a EF registered at their EMR.

Table 2 Cumulate incidence and hazard ratio, crude and adjusted, for hospitalization or death, with respect to socio demographic characteristics, clinical profile, and treatment received for heart failure

	Cumulate Incidence		Crude Hazard Ratio		Adjusted Hazard Ratio	
	Rate (%)	95% Confidence interval	HR	95% Confidence interval	HR	95% Confidence interval
Goblal incidence	37.6	36.5-38.7				
Ejection Fraction						
Ejection Fraction>50	17.0	13.3-20.7	1		1	
Ejection Fraction <=50	27.3	22.1-32.4	1.81	1.31-2.49	1.36	0.99-1.88
Missing Ejection Fraction	39.1	38.0-40.2	2.33	1.84-2.95	1.84	1.45-2.33
Previous hospitalization for heart failure	51.3	49.5-53.1	2.18	2.03-2.34	1.81	1.68-1.95
Gender (Male)	39.8	38.2-41.4	1.15	1.07-1.23	1.24	1.14-1.34
Age (quintiles)						
(<=71 years; reference	29.0	26.8-31.1	1		1	
72 - 78	33.3	31.2-35.5	1.14	1.02-1.28	1.03	0.91-1.16
79 - 82	38.1	35.6-40.5	1.43	1.27-1.61	1.21	1.07-1.37
3 - 86	41.1	38.5-43.6	1.62	1.44-1.82	1.30	1.14-1.48
>=87	48.8	46.2-51.3	2.17	1.94-2.43	1.60	1.40-1.83
Socio economic deprivation index						
1 (less disadvantaged)	33.5	31.1-35.8	1		1	
2	36.7	34.3-39.1	1.08	0.96-1.21	1.10	0.98-1.24
3	37.3	34.9-39.6	1.06	0.95-1.19	1.01	0.90-1.13
4	38.6	36.2-41.0	1.11	0.99-1.25	1.03	0.92-1.16
5 (more disadvantaged)	42.8	40.4-45.3	1.28	1.14-1.43	1.13	1.01-1.27
Patients requiring home care	57.0	55.0-59.1	2.13	1.98-2.29	1.58	1.46-1.71
Cardiovascular risk factors						
Hypertension	38.3	37.1-39.5	1.13	1.04-1.22	1.08	0.99-1.19
Diabetes	41.6	39.7-43.5	1.25	1.16-1.34	1.17	1.08-1.26
Hypercholesterolemia	34.5	32.6-36.4	0.90	0.83-0.97	0.94	0.86-1.02
Obesity	37.7	35.5-40.0	0.99	0.91-1.08	1.00	0.92-1.10
Smoking habit	39.2	35.5-43.0	0.98	0.87-1.11	1.04	0.91-1.19
Cardiovascular diseases						
Coronary heart disease	41.5	39.4-43.6	1.21	1.12-1.31	1.11	1.02-1.21
Atrial fibrillation	42.4	40.6-44.2	1.31	1.22-1.41	1.05	0.96-1.15
Stroke	44.7	41.2-48.1	1.41	1.26-1.57	1.15	1.03-1.29
Peripheral artery disease	45.4	41.0-49.8	1.45	1.27-1.66	1.11	0.97-1.28
Other comorbidities						
Chronic obstructive pulmonary disease	45.1	42.3-47.8	1.39	1.28-1.52	1.25	1.14-1.37
Chronic renal failure	44.8	42.3-47.4	1.47	1.35-1.60	1.18	1.08-1.29
Drug therapy						
ACE inhibitor or ARB*	37.3	36.1-38.5	0.91	0.84-0.99	0.85	0.78-0.93
Beta-blocker	37.9	35.3-40.5	1.00	0.91-1.09	1.03	0.94-1.14
Loop diuretics	42.5	41.3-43.8	2.27	2.05-2.51	1.64	1.48-1.82
Statins	35.1	33.6-36.6	0.87	0.81-0.94	0.85	0.79-0.93

[a] *ACE* angiotensin converting enzyme, *ARB* Angiotensin Receptor Blocker

Table 3 Factors related to the probability of having an ejection fraction registered in electronic medical records

	OR[a]	95% Confidence interval
Age (quintiles)		
<=71 años (reference)	1	
72 - 78	0.86	0.68-1.08
79 - 82	0.71	0.55-0.92
83 - 86	0.81	0.63-1.05
87+	0.50	0.37-0.68
Socio economic deprivation index		
1 (less disadvantaged)	1	
2	1.55	1.24-1.94
3	0.99	0.78-1.25
4	0.68	0.52-0.88
5 (more disadvantaged)	0.41	0.30-0.56
Patients requiring home care	0.71	0.56-0.88
Obesity	0.68	0.55-0.85
Drug therapy for heart failure		
ACE inhibitor or ARB[b]	1.25	1.02-1.53
Beta-blockers	1.23	1.01-1.51
Loop diuretics	0.59	0.49-0.71

[a]Odds ratio adjusted by gender, hypertension, diabetes, hypercholesterolemia, smoking habit, coronary heart disease, atrial fibrillation, stroke, peripheral artery disease, and previous hospitalization for heart failure
[b] *ACE* angiotensin converting enzyme, *ARB* Angiotensin Receptor Blocker

On the other hand, Possible HF patients had up to 50% more probability of having adverse outcomes than those with HF-REF, and the risk doubled with respect to HF-PEF patients [13].

We have identified several factors which could help explain these findings. Firstly, patients who lacked information about EF were older, as has been reported by other authors in patients attended for acute heart failure at hospital emergency rooms [17]. In our population, the probability for the oldest patients of having an EF recorded in their EMR was less than 50% with respect to the others.

Socio-economic inequality regarding access to specialized care in newly diagnosed HF patients, and a lower probability of undergoing invasive cardiac procedures for the less disadvantaged populations, have been previously described [18, 19]. Nevertheless, most evidence comes from countries with differing healthcare systems where accessibility could vary. In contrast, the Spanish National Health System provides healthcare universal and free. Previous studies performed by our group did not find any inequality regarding therapeutic management in populations suffering from coronary heart disease [20] or at high cardiovascular risk [21, 22].

We, cannot, therefore, satisfactorily account for the fact that the more socio- economically deprived patients showed a lower probability of having an echocardiography performed.

Due to their deteriorated health, patients needing home care are not usually candidates to be referred to undergo tests and explorations, including EF measures. As a consequence, the probability of having an echocardiography is lower than in those with a better life expectancy. Home healthcare is generally oriented towards achieving a better quality of life rather than actually lengthening it. In addition, patients needing this service usually have a very limited quality of life and the hypothetical availability of their EF figures would probably not result in treatment changes. A recent experience in united Kingdom showed that a program of basic cardiac scans ('Quick scans') performed in highest risk population could reduce the demand of echocardiography and optimize the detection of structural disease [23].

In agreement with other authors, we found that previous history of HF hospitalization, especially in the previous year, is a powerful predictor for having recurrent events [24–26].

In addition, and again concurring with other publications, we observed that the use of loop diuretics was associated with a higher risk of mortality and hospitalization in HF patients. It has been argued that this effect occurs especially when doses are high and glomerular filtration declines [27].

Conclusions

EF is poorly recorded in primary care. HF patients with EF missing at medical records had the worst prognosis with regard to hospitalisation and survival. They tended to be older, socio-economically disadvantaged, and more fragile.

Abbreviations

CMBD-AH: Conjunto Mínimo Básico de Datos de Altas Hospitalarias; EF: Ejection fraction; EMR: Electronic Medical Record; HF: Heart failure; HF-PEF: Heart failure patients with preserved ejection fraction; HF-REF: Heart failure patients with reduced ejection fraction; HR: Hazard ratio; SIDIAP: Information System for the Development of Research in Primary Care

Acknowledgements

We would like to acknowledge the SIDIAP team for their accesibility and help.

Funding

This study has been granted by the Primary Healthcare University Research Institute IDIAP-Jordi Gol.

Authors' contributions

MAM, XM, J R, JLV, EV, MD and JMVR participated in the data management, analysis and interpretation of results, the elaboration and revision of the drafts of the manuscript and in the approval of the final version. CC, EC, and NS participated in the data management, elaboration of the last draft and the approval of the final version. All authors read and approved the final manuscript.

Competing interests
The authors declare that they have no competing interests.

Consent for publication
Not applicable.

Author details
[1]Institut Català de la Salut, Barcelona, Spain. [2]Primary Healthcare University Research Institute IDIAP-Jordi Gol, Barcelona, Spain. [3]Universitat Autònoma de Barcelona, Bellaterra, Spain. [4]EAP Dreta de l'Eixample, Barcelona, Spain. [5]Universitat de Barcelona, Barcelona, Spain. [6]Epidemiologia i Salut Pública, Universitat Internacional de Catalunya, Sant Cugat, Spain.

References
1. McMurray JJ, Adamopoulos S, Anker SD, et al. ESC Guidelines for the diagnosis and treatment of acute and chronic heart failure 2012: The Task Force for the Diagnosis and Treatment of Acute and Chronic Heart Failure 2012 of the European Society of Cardiology. Developed in collaboration with the Heart Failure Association (HFA) of the ESC. Eur Heart J. 2012;33(14): 1787–847.
2. Rutten FH, Moons KG, Cramer MJ, et al. Recognising heart failure in elderly patients with stable chronic obstructive pulmonary disease in primary care: cross sectional diagnostic study. BMJ. 2005;331(7529):1379.
3. Daniels LB, Clopton P, Bhalla V, et al. How obesity affects the cut-points for B-type natriuretic peptide in the diagnosis of acute heart failure. Results from the Breathing Not Properly Multinational Study. Am Heart J. 2006; 151(5):999–1005.
4. Otero-Raviña F, Grigorian-Shamagian L, Fransi-Galiana L, et al. Morbidity and mortality among heart failure patients in Galicia, N.W. Spain: the GALICAP Study. Int J Cardiol. 2009;136:56–63.
5. Hobbs F, Doust J, Mant J, et al. Diagnosis of heart failure in primary care. Heart. 2010;96:1773–7.
6. Skånér Y, Backlund L, Montgomery H, Bring J, Strender LE. General practitioners' reasoning when considering the diagnosis heart failure: athink-aloud study. BMC Fam Pract. 2005;6(1):4.
7. Hobbs FD, Jones MI, Allan TF, et al. European survey of primary care physician perceptions on heart failure diagnosis and management (Euro-HF). Eur Heart J. 2000;21:1877–87.
8. González-Juanatey JR, Alegría Ezquerra E, Bertomeu Martínez V, et al. Insuficiencia cardiaca en consultas ambulatorias: comorbilidades y actuaciones diagnóstico-terapéuticas por diferentes especialistas, Estudio EPISERVE. Rev Esp Cardiol. 2008;61:611–9.
9. Schultz SE, Rothwell DM, Chen Z, et al. Identifying cases of congestive heart failure from administrative data: a validation study using primary care patient records. Chronic Dis Inj Can. 2013;33(3):160–6.
10. Owan TE, Hodge DO, Herges RM, et al. Trends prevalence and outcome of heart failure with preserved ejection fraction. N Engl J Med. 2006;355:251–9.
11. Bhatia RS, Tu JV, Lee DS, et al. Outcome of heart failure with preserved ejection fraction in a population-based study. N Engl J Med. 2006;355:260–9.
12. Meta-analysis Global Group in Chronic Heart Failure (MAGGIC). The survival of patients with heart failure with preserved or reduced left ventricular ejection fraction: an individual patient data meta-analysis. Eur Heart J. 2012; 33:1750–7.
13. Poppe KK, Squire IB, Whalley GA, et al. Meta-Analysis Global Group in Chronic Heart Failure. Known and missing left ventricular ejection fraction and survival inpatients with heart failure: a MAGGIC meta-analysis report. Eur J Heart Fail. 2013;15(11):1220–7.
14. Ramos R, Balló E, Marrugat J, et al. Validity for use in research on vascular diseases of the SIDIAP(Information System for the Development of Research in Primary Care): the EMMA study. Rev Esp Cardiol. 2012;65(1):29–37.
15. Available on: http://catsalut.gencat.cat/ca/proveidors-professionals/registres-catalegs/registres/cmdb/
16. Domínguez-Berjón MF, Borrell C, Cano-Serral G, et al. Constructing a deprivation index based on census data in large Spanish cities (the MEDEA project). Gac Sanit. 2008;22(3):179–87.
17. McCormick N, Lacaille D, Bhole V, et al. Validity of heart failure diagnoses in administrative databases: a systematic review and meta-analysis. PLoS One. 2014;9(8):e104519.
18. Cleland JG, McDonagh T, Rigby AS, et al. The national heart failure audit for England and Wales 2008–2009. Heart. 2011;97(11):876–86.
19. Ehrmann Feldman D, Xiao Y, Bernatsky S, Haggerty J, Leffondré K, Tousignant P, Roy Y, Abrahamowicz M. Consultation with cardiologists for persons with new-onset chronic heart failure: a population-based study. Can J Cardiol. 2009;25(12):690–4.
20. Hetemaa T, Keskimäki I, Salomaa V, et al. Socioeconomic inequities in invasive cardiac procedures after first myocardial infarction in Finland in 1995. J Clin Epidemiol. 2004;57(3):301–8.
21. Munoz MA, Rohlfs I, Masuet S, et al. Analysis of inequalities in secondary prevention of coronary heart disease in a universal coverage health care system. Eur J Public Health. 2006;16(4):361–7.
22. Mejía-Lancheros C, Estruch R, Martínez-González MA, et al. Socioeconomic status and health inequalities for cardiovascular prevention among elderly Spaniards. Rev Esp Cardiol. 2013;66(10):803–11.
23. Chambers J, Kabir S, Cajeat E. Detection of heart disease by open access echocardiography: a retrospective analysis of general practice referrals. Br J Gen Pract. 2014;64(619):e105–11.
24. Senni M, Gavazzi A, Oliva F, et al. In-hospital and 1-year outcomes of acute heart failure patients according to presentation (de novo vs. worsening) and ejection fraction. Results from IN-HF Outcome Registry. Int J Cardiol. 2014;173:163–9.
25. Khazanie P, Heizer GM, Hasselblad V, et al. Predictors of clinical outcomes in acutedecompensated heart failure: Acute Study of Clinical Effectiveness of Nesiritide in Decompensated Heart Failure outcome models. Am Heart J. 2015;170(2):290–7.
26. Bello NA, Claggett B, Desai AS, et al. Influence of previous heart failure hospitalization on cardiovascular events in patients with reduced and preserved ejection fraction. Circ Heart Fail. 2014;7(4):590–5.
27. Damman K, Kjekshus J, Wikstrand J, et al. Loop diuretics, renal function and clinical outcome in patients with heart failure and reduced ejection fraction. Eur J Heart Fail. 2016;18(3):328–3.

18

A systematic review of primary care models for non-communicable disease interventions in Sub-Saharan Africa

Jennifer Kane[1*], Megan Landes[1,2], Christopher Carroll[3], Amy Nolen[1] and Sumeet Sodhi[1,2]

Abstract

Background: Chronic diseases, primarily cardiovascular disease, respiratory disease, diabetes and cancer, are the leading cause of death and disability worldwide. In sub-Saharan Africa (SSA), where communicable disease prevalence still outweighs that of non-communicable disease (NCDs), rates of NCDs are rapidly rising and evidence for primary healthcare approaches for these emerging NCDs is needed.

Methods: A systematic review and evidence synthesis of primary care approaches for chronic disease in SSA. Quantitative and qualitative primary research studies were included that focused on priority NCDs interventions. The method used was best-fit framework synthesis.

Results: Three conceptual models of care for NCDs in low- and middle-income countries were identified and used to develop an a priori framework for the synthesis. The literature search for relevant primary research studies generated 3759 unique citations of which 12 satisfied the inclusion criteria. Eleven studies were quantitative and one used mixed methods. Three higher-level themes of screening, prevention and management of disease were derived. This synthesis permitted the development of a new evidence-based conceptual model of care for priority NCDs in SSA.

Conclusions: For this review there was a near-consensus that passive rather than active case-finding approaches are suitable in resource-poor settings. Modifying risk factors among existing patients through advice on diet and lifestyle was a common element of healthcare approaches. The priorities for disease management in primary care were identified as: availability of essential diagnostic tools and medications at local primary healthcare clinics and the use of standardized protocols for diagnosis, treatment, monitoring and referral to specialist care.

Keywords: Non-communicable diseases, Sub-Saharan Africa, Primary healthcare, Prevention, Treatment, Systematic review

Background

Non-communicable diseases (NCDs), primarily cardiovascular disease (CVD), diabetes mellitus (DM), respiratory disease and cancer, are the leading cause of death and disability in the world [1]. In 2010, the Global Burden of Diseases Study estimated global mortality from 235 causes of death and demonstrated evidence of an epidemiological transition from infectious diseases to chronic non-infectious causes of mortality [2]. Underlying this transition in developing countries is a trend towards urbanization, widespread demographic shifts in populations with an increasingly elderly population, and lifestyle changes (such as unhealthy diets and physical inactivity) [3]. In Sub-Sahara Africa (SSA) it is projected that NCD deaths will be greater than communicable, maternal, perinatal and nutritional diseases deaths combined by 2030 [4, 5]. This emerging double burden of disease challenges SSA's struggling health infrastructure and demands an effective response while recognizing the context of scarce resources within the region [6].

Primary care is for most patients the gateway to the healthcare system, yet in resource-limited settings most primary health care is focused on acute episodic care [7] and chronic disease is often deferred to specialist care

* Correspondence: jjbkane@gmail.com
[1]Department of Family and Community Medicine, University of Toronto, Toronto, ON, Canada
Full list of author information is available at the end of the article

delivered at secondary and tertiary centers. Through lessons learned via the implementation of care models for HIV and TB (In the advent of delivering human immunodeficiency virus (HIV) and tuberculosis (TB) care in SSA), we have seen these chronic diseases treated effectively though primary care models for communicable diseases (CD) [8, 9]. Through these primary care models, decentralized clinics for chronic CD care has allowed for rapid and massive scaling up of HIV/TB services, allowing greater access to care primarily for patients in rural locations – by reducing travel time and costs [10]. Currently there is a lack of evidence and guidelines for primary care models focused on the prevention and management of priority NCDs (DM, CVD and respiratory disease) in the SSA context. This systematic review will focus on this knowledge gap and build upon build upon relevant models of disease management in SSA [11]. In this review our aim is to systematically review the literature for evidence to guide the development of primary care models for DM, CVD and respiratory disease.

We have chosen these three disease categories based on the existing literature. The emphasis from the World Health Organization (WHO) and many other steering groups for chronic NCD prevention and management is focused on CVD, DM, cancer and respiratory disease including asthma and chronic obstructive respiratory disease (COPD) [12]. This grouping is based on the common underlying behavioral risk factors of unhealthy diet, physical inactivity, smoking and excess alcohol consumption [4]. We do not focus on cancer diagnosis and management given the increased complexities involved, however we recognize that flexibility should be recognized as a key component of developing an NCD primary care model such that it could respond in future to include other cost-effective interventions such as mental health and cancer integration, which has shown some success in low-cost interventions being piloted and rolled-out [13, 14].

Methods

With both conceptual primary care models for NCDs in low-and middle-income countries (LMIC) and case studies in SSA of primary care models for NCDs available in the literature, a methodology to synthesize the relevant literature was needed. "Best fit" framework synthesis is a recently described methodology in the literature [15, 16]. It allows a generic conceptual model of care to be built upon via primary research data from a relevant but potentially different population. Best-fit" framework synthesis was the chosen method because it allowed the review to make use of existing primary care models for NCDs, developed for LMICs generally, as the framework against which to code evidence from primary studies specifically conducted in SSA contexts.

First, conceptual models of care for the particular diseases of interest were identified. These models were condensed to key themes to develop an a priori framework. Second, a further systematic review of the literature was undertaken to identify primary research studies focused on primary care interventions for NCDs in SSA, for inclusion in the review. Data from the primary studies are coded based on the a priori themes and any new themes from the primary studies were derived for evidence not included in the a priori framework already. Through the a priori framework and the addition of new themes, the generation of a synthesized new conceptual model of care, relevant to the context of interest, was created through a combination of framework and thematic approaches to synthesis.

A priori framework

The a priori framework was developed using an approach published by Carroll et al [15]. A systematic search was conducted to identify models and frameworks of primary care interventions in LMICs. Inclusion criteria are outlined in Table 1. A flowchart of the literature search for the a priori framework can be found in Additional file 1.

Three relevant papers were identified: two applied the directly observed treatment short course (DOTS) model of care approach for TB, previously applied to scaling up HIV care and now adapted for management of NCDs [8, 11, 17]. The remaining model of care adapted the chronic care model (CCM) framework specifically for LMIC to address priority NCDs [18]. Following thematic analysis, a process described elsewhere for developing an a priori framework from more than one relevant model [15] (see also Additional file 2), a framework with 13 distinct themes focusing on diagnosis, prevention and management of priority NCDs was developed from these three models of care. All 13 themes and their definitions are listed in Table 2.

Primary research studies

Four electronic database (MEDLINE, Embase, Global Health and CINAHL) were interrogated to identify primary research studies [15] relevant to primary care

Table 1 Inclusion criteria for the a priori framework models

Setting/Population	Low and middle income countries
Program or intervention focus	Packages of primary care interventions for priority NCDs
Research type/Study design	Publications describing or testing model or framework
Exclusions	•Markov or economic model •Animal model •Model solely focused on health promotion – model of care must include medical management of diseases

Table 2 A priori framework with definitions of themes for coding

Themes derived for coding	Definitions
Case finding	Passive screening for NCDs of patients presenting to local health facilities
Modify risk factors	Everyone seen in primary care should be assessed for common risk factors such as smoking, alcohol, obesity and counseled in lifestyle modifications
Standardized treatment	Algorithm protocol for which medications and dose for DM, asthma, COPD or HTN
Standardized diagnosis	Algorithm outlining protocol for making a diagnosis of DM, asthma, COPD or HTN
Standardized referral pathway	Algorithm with protocol for when to refer a patient needing more complex management to secondary or tertiary care
Standardized follow-up appointments	Guidelines outlining when patients should return for follow-up appointment, ensuring that pre-booked appointments are available at the clinic
Adherence support	Some form of support to patients for adherence to medication and follow up appointments at the clinic (i.e. text message reminder)
Task-shifting/Multidisciplinary clinic	NPC to have the primary role in screening, preventing and managing NCDs
Training of staff	Curriculum to train the health care staff delivering care for NCDs management
Decentralized care	Primary care clinics should be available and accessible to patients living in rural areas
Essential medicines	Consistent supply and access to medicines needed to treat NCDs, primarily drugs outlined in treatment algorithm so that treatment is not interrupted
Essential diagnostics	Essential equipment needed to follow diagnostic protocol for screening and follow-up of NCDs
Systematic monitoring and evaluation	Efficient system for data collection of NCDs (of key indicators such as number died, lost to follow-up, stopped treatment or referral)

NCD non-communicable diseases, *COPD* chronic obstructive pulmonary diseases, *HTN* hypertension, *NPC* non-physician clinician

models for NCDs in SSA. The following MeSH headings were used: non-communicable disease, chronic disease, cardiovascular disease, chronic obstructive lung disease, diabetes, primary care, preventive care and Africa of the South of the Sahara. Using the World Bank listing of countries in SSA, MeSH and key word search was developed to include all individual countries. An example of the full search strategy can be seen in Additional file 3. A grey literature search was conducted of Google Scholar, African Wide Info and Eldis using the same combination of key terms. Bibliographies of key articles were also searched for additional references. This iterative approach helped cast the net further to draw on relevant studies focused on primary health care approaches for the management of NCDs in SSA.

The inclusion criteria applied to primary research studies from the literature search are described in Table 3. Given the focus of this synthesis on models of care for NCD management, studies looking at both quantitative and qualitative outcomes were included, allowing an exploration of intervention descriptions and how the different models of care work in context in SSA. The synthesis is descriptive in nature and does not link models of care to intervention success.

Data extraction

A data extraction form for the primary research studies was developed that focused on study design, location, type of NCD, intervention and outcomes, along with the themes outlined in the a priori framework. The evidence coded against the thematic framework came from the description of the intervention itself, and the quantitative and qualitative outcomes in the results section of the paper. Two authors (JK, AN) independently extracted data from the studies using this deductive approach. The synthesis also involved the secondary thematic analysis of evidence not captured by the themes of the a priori framework, This inductive approach allowed the authors (JK, AN) to add to the known themes of the framework and thus to develop a the thematic framework specifically for NCDs in SSA.

Consideration of study quality

Two authors (JK, AN) undertook independent quality assessment of the included studies using tools adapted for critically appraising both qualitative, quantitative and mixed method studies [19, 20]. No sensitivity analysis based on study quality was performed because none of the studies was found to be of poor quality: the quality of the included studies was generally similar.

Generation of a new model of care framework

Following the systematic review, the authors (JK, AN) reviewed again the a priori concepts and the list of new themes generated from the primary studies. This resulted in a finalized list key to the model of care for NCDs in SSA. Revisions were also made to some of the a priori themes as a result of the synthesis. The synthesis then involved looking for relationships and common characteristics between themes to derive higher-level

Table 3 Inclusion criteria for the primary research studies

Setting/Population	Sub-Saharan Africa
Program or Intervention Focus	Packages of primary care interventions for priority NCDs
Research type /Study design	Quantitative and qualitative research studies describing intervention or development of package of care
Exclusions	•Interventions solely base on health promotion – intervention must include medical management of diseases •Children/pediatric •Not focused on 1 of 3 priority NCDs management (CVD, asthma/COPD, DM)

NCD non-communicable disease, *CVD* cardiovascular disease, *COPD* chronic obstructive pulmonary disease, *DM* diabetes mellitus

concepts. This allowed the analysis of the a priori framework and primary data to move beyond simply a description of a list of themes to a synthesized conceptual model of care for NCDs in SSA. A new finalized model of care from this synthesis was presented.

Results

Quantity and quality of included studies

The search generated 3759 unique citations from across four databases. Twenty-two full papers from theses results were screened of which 12 satisfied the inclusion criteria (Fig. 1). Results from the grey literature and bibliographic references of key articles did not generate any additional studies relevant to the selection criteria. All studies were appraised for quality using the relevant methodology [19, 20] and none was assessed as low quality. The results are summarized in Additional file 4.

A summary of the features of the primary research studies included is included in Table 4. The 12 primary research studies were conducted in Kenya [21, 22], Ethiopia [23, 24], Uganda [25], South Africa [26–28], Nigeria [29], Cameroon [30, 31] and Tanzania [32]. Eleven of these studies were quantitative [21–26, 28–33] one was mixed methods [27] and none was exclusively qualitative in methodology. Two of these studies were early in the development of the intervention and had limited evaluative component [21, 24]. Seven of the studies focused on care delivered solely in a rural setting [21, 22, 24–26, 28, 30] while two focused exclusively on urban primary care of services [23, 32]. Three of the studies included care delivery in both urban and rural settings where the package of care was delivered [27, 29, 31]. As per the inclusion criteria all of the interventions included a package of care for at least one of the priority NCDs - DM, CVD and asthma/COPD. Three of the studies focused on DM care alone [23, 24, 26] and two focused on hypertension (HTN) alone [29, 32]. Four of the studies focused on HTN and DM management together [22, 25, 27, 30] and two studies developed an

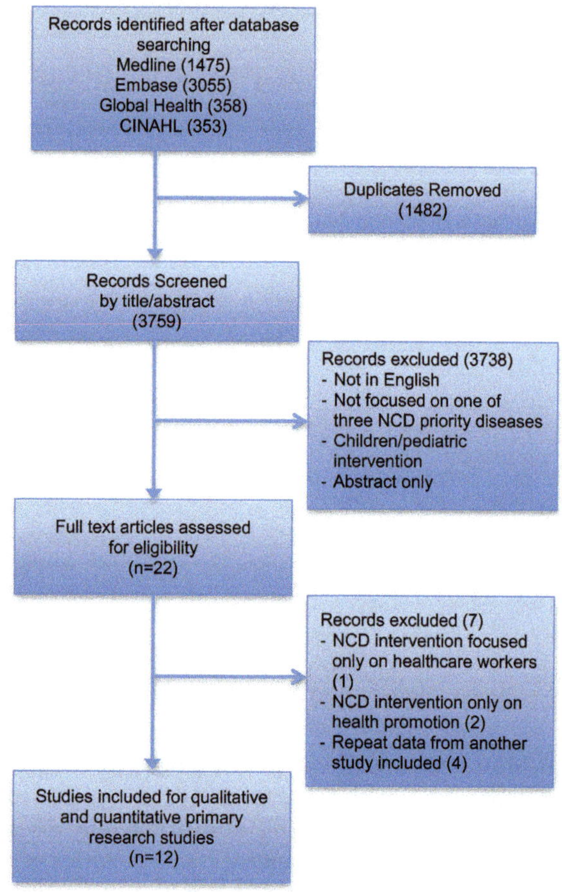

Fig. 1 PRISMA flowchart detailing results of literature search and study screening of Primary Research Studies

intervention focused on HTN, DM and asthma together [28, 31]. None of the interventions looked at a package of care for COPD.

Creation of a new conceptual framework

The data from these primary studies was used to help construct an evidence-based conceptual model of care for management of NCDs in SSA. The majority of the themes identified in the a priori model could be identified in and were supported by the primary data for this review. The results of this coding against the a priori concepts can be seen in Tables 5 and 6 (the full details of each theme in each study are provided in Supplementary material, Additional files 5 and 6).

The new conceptual model of care

In deriving the new conceptual model of care, the a priori theme of "training of staff" was slightly altered to "train and retrain staff" as this was more consistent with what was found in the primary studies. Although there was minimal data in the primary studies relevant to the theme of adherence, it was further revised to "adherence

Table 4 Description of primary research studies

Article	NCD Focus	Study Design	Location	Intervention	Outcome	Quality[a]
Pastakia 2013	DM & HTN	Feasibility study	Rural Kenya	Community vs. home based screening	Low follow up at health center, HTN 31%, DM 22–23% follow within 3 months	Adequate
Rabkin. 2012	DM	Pre/post intervention	Urban Ethiopia	Protocol of DM care implemented for HIV patients	Increase BP measurements, fundoscopy exams, booked next appointment after intervention	Adequate
Chamie 2011	DM & HTN	Feasibility study	Rural Uganda	POC testing for NCD screening alongside HIV testing campaign	Moderate follow up at health center, HTN 43% and DM 61% a health center	Adequate
Price 2011	DM	Observational cohort study	Rural South Africa	Empowerment based education about DM, clinical algorithm	Hba1c at baseline 10.8, decreased to 7.5 at 18 months, 9.7 at 4 years	Adequate
Bloomfield 2013	CVD & Pulmonary	Program description	Rural Kenya	Twining relationship for academic model for NCD clinical care	No evaluation phase yet, description of model for academic partnership	Adequate
Mendis 2010	HTN	Cluster Randomized trial	Urban/rural Nigeria	WHO CVD risk management package vs. standard care for HTN	SBP and DBP were lower in Nigerian group ($p = 0.0002$), 2% of patients referred to next level of care, decreased BMI, smoking, increased fruits and vegetables	Adequate
Labhart 2010	HTN & DM	Observational cohort study	Rural Cameroon	Implementation of package of care for HTN/DM for NPC (75 clinics)	Retention of patients at 1 year 18.1%, SBP decreased 22.8 mmHg/DBP decreased 12.4 mmHg/FPG decreased by 3.4 mmol/L ($p < 0.001$)	Adequate
Kengne 2009	HTN, DM & asthma	Feasibility study	Urban/rural Cameroon	Implementation of package of care for HTN/DM/asthma at PHC (5 clinics)	Decrease of SBP 11.7 and DBP 7.8 ($p < 0.001$), decrease 1.6 mmol/L ($p < 0.001$), decreased days with asthma attacks in follow up at 2 years	Adequate
Katz 2009	DM & HTN	Observational cohort study	Urban/rural South Africa	Chronic care model clinic for DM and HTN implemented	Half lost to follow up (49%), 55% of DM patient referred to specialist clinic (76% of these didn't need referral), 31% of DM controlled with hba1c <7%	Adequate
Bovet 2008	HTN	Prospective population based survey	Urban Tanzania	Health care services after positive screening test for HTN	34% sought health-care provider in 12-mth period, anti-HTN taken by 34% at some point, 3% at end of 12 month follow-up	Adequate
Mamo 2007	DM	Program description	Rural Ethiopia	Implementation of RN-led decentralized NCD clinics	75% of DM patients attended FU appointments, only 11.4% of DM patients could be transferred to PHC clinics because lack of insulin supply at PHC	Adequate
Coleman 1998	HTN, DM & Asthma	Observational cohort study	Rural South Africa	Implementation of RN-led NCD package of care intervention	RN's able to control 68% of HTN, 82% of DM (NIDDM), 84% of those with asthma	Adequate

[a]If a paper had >50% of the CASP and MMAT checklist then the study was deemed of adequate quality assessment

Table 5 A Priori themes in primary research studies for NCDs interventions in SSA

	Themes from a priori framework						
Article	**Screening**	**Prevention**	**Control: Decision Support**				
	Case Finding	*Modify Risk Factors*	*Standard diagnosis*	*Standard treatment*	*Referral pathway*	*Adherence*	*Follow-up*
Pastakia 2013							
Rabkin 2012							
Chamie 2012							
Price 2011							
Bloomfield 2011							
Mendis 2010							
Labhardt 2010							
Kengne 2009							
Katz 2009							
Bovet 2008							
Mamo 2007							
Coleman 1998							

Is framework theme present in the model in an included study? Grey = Yes, White = Unclear; Light Grey = No

Is framework theme present in the model in an included study? Grey = Yes, White = Unclear; Light Grey = No

Table 6 A Priori themes in primary research studies for NCDs interventions in SSA

	Themes from a priori framework					
Article	**Control: Human Resources**		**Control: Decision Support**			
	Task-shifting	Training of staff	Decentralized care	Essential diagnostics	Essential medicines	Systematic monitoring & evaluation
Pastakia 2013						
Rabkin 2012						
Chamie 2012						
Price 2011						
Bloomfield 2011						
Mendis 2010						
Labhardt 2010						
Kengne 2009						
Katz 2009						
Bovet 2008						
Mamo 2007						
Coleman 1998						

Is framework theme present in the model in an included study? Green=Yes; White=Unclear; Light Grey=No

Is framework theme present in the model in an included study? Green = Yes; White = Unclear; Light Grey = No

to medications" and "adherence to follow-up appointments" to echo the interventions and results in the data.

There were four new themes from the primary studies looking at NCD interventions in SSA. These themes were: "staff competence", "dedicated NCD staff", "review criteria" and "communication with MD/specialist". The a priori model failed to capture these themes, but because the included studies were principally conducted in rural settings in SSA, these new themes are relevant to the context and setting of implementing a model of care in SSA.

These revisions and additions to the a priori model helped to create, through a deductive and inductive approach, a synthesized evidence-based NCD model of care for SSA that can be seen in Table 7.

The new conceptual model of care is centered on three higher concepts: screening, prevention and control of NCDs. The majority of existing interventions found in this review fall within the control concept, which can be further broken down into four categories: quality improvement, human resources, decision support and health systems. These themes are further illustrated with evidence from the primary data.

Screening

The articles describing this element clearly articulate that screening of individuals with NCDs should take a *passive case finding* approach by opportunistically screening patients presenting to health centers. The authors of these models advocate not taking an active case finding approach as its felt to be too labor intensive in a resource poor setting. Eight of the interventions did have a screening component to the them [21, 22, 25, 27, 29–32], however three studies were discordant with this a priori theme by embracing an active case finding approach, either going door-to door or holding community fairs [22, 25, 32]. The common measured outcome of these studies was a very poor linkage to care for those identified to screen positive for the priority NCDs. Although the concept of active case finding can seem ideal to reach more individuals, in context these primary studies reinforce that passive case finding is a more cost-effective approach in SSA.

Prevention

All of the primary research studies described an element of *modifying risk factors* for NCDs through counseling of patients. The various topics for counseling included: dietary advice, physical activity, obesity, salt intake and smoking cessation. One study by Price et al. [26] reported on the impact of empowerment by education around risk factors and disease progression delivered monthly over the first 3 months of care. Education alone in this study showed a significant decrease in HbA1c at 18 months from 10.6 +/- 4.2% to 7.6 +/- 2.3% ($p < 0.001$).

Control

Quality improvement

Two of the primary studies incorporate *review criteria* of a minimum standard of care for primary care clinicians as an important element of a package of care for NCDs [27, 31]. Maher et al. [11] stresses in his conceptual framework for NCDs in LMIC that care must attain a minimal standard of quality to have improved patient outcomes and Kengne et al. [31] describe review criteria as "must do" criteria for clinics delivering the NCD package of interventions to ensure quality standards. For diabetes care delivered in Soweto, authors incorporated criterion-related validity of appropriate referrals to

Table 7 A priori including the new concepts and themes

A priori concepts	New concepts	A priori themes	Revised and new themes
Screening		Case finding	
Prevention		Modify risk factors	
Control	Quality improvement		Review criteria
			Staff competence
	Health systems	Essential medicines	
		Essential diagnostics	
		Systematic monitoring and evaluation	
		Decentralized care	
	Decision support	Standardized treatment	Adherence to medications
		Standardized diagnosis	Adherence to follow-up
		Standardized referral pathway	Communication with MD/specialist
		Standardized follow-up appointments	
	Human Resources	Task-shifting/Multidisciplinary clinic	Train and retrain staff
			Dedicated NCD staff

specialist [27]. This study demonstrated that very few of the patients referred to specialist care in fact needed to be referred (<20%); these patients instead could have been treated at the primary care level. This process of quality standards through review criteria ensures an intervention is implemented successfully and effectively for patients and the limited health care resources.

Similarly in ensuring quality of care, *competency* amongst health care workers must be included in a package of care for NCDs. Four of the primary studies mentioned protocols to ensure clinical competency amongst mainly non-physician clinicians (NPC) [22, 27, 30, 31]. This included pre and post questionnaires after training, observed patient encounters by senior staff and key informant interviews of physicians on NPC performance. Katz et al. [27] demonstrated through questionnaires that trained RN's for NCD care were more knowledgeable than untrained however only 31% were familiar with the current DM guidelines. Further qualitative data from this study showed physicians working with the RN's expressed concern of their lack of knowledge of targets to control DM or HTN. This evaluation of competency allowed the clinics to realize gaps in clinical knowledge amongst NPCs and refine teaching on certain topics to ensure a competent trained primary health care (PHC) team delivered care.

Health systems

Most of the primary studies for this review had *essential medications* available at the PHC [21, 23, 25–31]. At a minimum, a first line medication was available. Essential medications available at the local primary health care clinic is vital to controlling NCDs. This theme was made clear in the a priori and primary research articles, referring to lessons learned from ART for the HIV epidemic and the DOTS program for TB and how important uninterrupted access to medications for chronic disease control is. *Essential diagnostics* included a glucometer and a blood pressure machine available for all the interventions, as most focused on DM and HTN. *Systematic monitoring and evaluation* as described in the a priori model is a means of collecting data on patients in NCD clinics. Six interventions had a standard checklist or flow sheet that they collected patient's information on [21, 23, 27, 29–31], none of these were electronic health records. *Decentralized* primary health care for NCDs in SSA allows individuals living in rural and remote locations access care [34]. This concept was incorporated into all but two of the studies, looking at rural locations for implementation of their clinics [21, 22, 24–28, 30, 31].

Human resources

Task shifting has been an essential component of HIV care delivery in SSA [35, 36] and likewise will be a necessity to how NCD care is delivered in SSA given the health work force shortage. Task shifting gives clinical responsibilities typically done by physicians to less specialized health care workers to deliver care more effectively in resource-limited settings [36]. All of the primary studies had some element of task with eight of the primary research studies describing NPC led clinics, predominantly by RN's [21, 24, 26–31, 37].

Providing training for staff is indispensable when a large part of the workforce is transitioning to new roles and responsibilities and the theme of *train and retrain* is an important element to several of the interventions described in the primary literature [23, 24, 29–31]. This ongoing training allows, in this resource challenged health care system with high staff turnover, the ability of new staff to be educated and deliver NCD management on an ongoing basis. Katz el al [27]. described a mean staff turnover of 32 +/- 24% per clinic in South Africa, with some clinics as high as 75%. Retraining incorporated into interventions such as in Labhardt et al. [30] allowed staff already trained a refresher course on NCDs.

Integrating NCD clinics within CD can have several advantages for chronic disease management. As seen by the a priori framework, the models of care for NCD management in LMIC embrace the public health approach adapted for communicable disease control such as HIV and TB [8, 11, 17]. That integration however needs to be balanced with the NPC workload. What would seem as ideal, to have one NPC trained for HIV, TB and NCD primary care, can stretch RNs or health care workers. This theme was interpreted as *dedicated NCD staff*, meaning not simply asking staff to do more roles but either hiring more staff for NCD care or giving dedicated time to NPC already working in clinics to manage increase case load of NCD patients [27].

Decision support

Standardization of diagnosis and *treatment* help ensure quality of standards for clinical care. Ten of the studies had a standardized diagnostic algorithm to follow [21, 22, 25–32]. Treatment algorithms were also included in seven of the studies [21, 23, 26–30], with three studies providing step-by-step protocols for medication [28, 30, 31].

Standardized referrals ensure that primary care clinics have a specialist available for patient's management of disease when it is beyond their scope. Most studies supported when patients were on maximum therapy and their NCD was still not controlled would be referred to secondary or tertiary clinics [24, 27, 28, 30, 31]. Other standard reasons for referral were significant comorbidities (cardiovascular disease, chronic kidney failure) or requiring insulin [26, 27, 29].

As resource limited settings embrace task shifting, ease of access to consult physicians was an important theme to be integrated into the model of care. This theme was categorized as *communication with MD/specialist.* Having a referral pathway was indispensable but more immediate communication with a doctor or specialist could optimize patient management [27]. Two expressed examples of this from an RN led NCD intervention:

> *"No doctors help with up-scaling of medications (and) nurses hands (are) tied behind their back as they have responsibility without authority."* [27]

> *"We need to be able to communicate with specialists easily in case of problems we encounter about patients management."* [27]

Beaglehole et al. [18] point out in their conceptual primary care model that *standardized follow-up appointments* are needed for patients with chronic diseases. Health care predominantly lacks structure in SSA and tends to be focused on acute episodic care, without any planned follow up. This primary health care system redesign requires a different organizational structure in place. The vast majority of the studies had scheduled appointments but a more significant theme was lack of compliance with these scheduled follow-up appointments. Although none of the studies had implemented any reminders for *adherence to follow-up appointments,* this theme was interpreted as being very important given the high attrition rates across the studies. Labhardt et al. [30] retained 18% of patients at one year in their study and Katz et al. [27] lost 49% of NCD patients from their clinics by two years. Price et al. [26] started with 320 patients in their cohort, ending up with 80 at the end of four years in their study. Further planning needs to be centered on this important concept.

There was very little study data to code against the theme of *adherence to medications.* More research is needed to understand if adherence is a problem and if so, how to promote medication adherence amongst NCD patients. Coleman et al. [28] give some thought to this in their study as they had patients return to clinic for a monthly visit until their disease was controlled. Then they allowed a bi-annual clinic visit for their hypertension, diabetes or asthma that were well controlled. This allowed patients to be prescribed medication for 6 months without a clinical review. Overall their adherence to medication (self-reported) was 87%.

Discussion

By identifying several conceptual models for packages of care for NCDs and combining evidence from primary research studies, this review used a "best fit" framework synthesis to develop a new conceptual model of care for NCDs in SSA. This review aimed to assess what features characterize models of primary care for NCDs in SSA by focusing on the interventions themselves and the mechanisms behind these interventions. This was not with the goal of determining the most effective model of care. In identifying models of care for NCD in LMIC for the a priori framework, two of the three frameworks were already focused on SSA. Data from the primary research studies supplemented the a priori themes but likely less so than if these models were more generic for all LMICs.

The a priori themes emphasized an overall change in approach to NCDs in LMICs, moving from acute, episodic care focused on individuals to a public health programmatic structure focused on organized monitoring and evaluation of patient outcomes, standardized quality care and systematic follow up [8, 11, 17, 18]. Adapting disease guidelines in the face of extreme shortages of health care workers requires NPC to be delivering care [34] and to ensure effective implementation standardized protocols for diagnosis, treatment and monitoring need to be in place [38]. This simplification of management protocols builds upon the success of HIV service delivery in resource poor settings as demonstrated by the DOTs framework [8, 39]. Furthermore, this standardized public health approach to disease control goes beyond the individual clinic level and can inform population based interventions. For example, routine data collection via standardized protocols for NCDs at each clinic can inform on the national burden of disease and further contribute to accurate drug forecasting [8].

Further, this public health approach stresses opportunistic case finding as the most cost-effective intervention for screening in SSA [8, 11, 17, 18]. This was reemphasized in the primary studies demonstrating very poor linkage to care for active case finding [22, 25, 32]. However Beaglehole et al. point out some obstacles when opportunistic case finding is operationalized [18]. Patients will often be presenting with acute issues and providers will need to be proactive screening for asymptomatic NCDs within a limited consultation time. This may need further consideration and adaptation with more operational research in SSA.

New themes derived from the primary studies emphasize contextual factors unique to SSA. Health worker shortages are prevalent across all LMIC however it is the extreme case in SSA. The ratio of physician to patient is as low as 1 per 1000 in Tanzania and 2 per 1000 in Malawi [40]. As a result with the majority of care delivered via NPCs in SSA there needs to be appropriate quality assurance. Ensuring quality of care was mentioned in the conceptual models of care however specifics of how to operationalize this were more vague. The concept of quality improvement including both staff competence and review criteria were made clear through the operational primary research studies in SSA. This likely reflected that with NPCs being crucial to scaling up care in SSA there needs to be more regulation to address greater variability in the care delivered.

Aside from increasing the sheer number of NPCs via additional training and funding, incentives and creating a better work environment to retain health care workers is essential [18]. The new themes derived from primary research in SSA of communication with MD/specialist and dedicated NCD staff emphasizes this point. Given increasing responsibility, NPCs need more access to senior health care workers to manage patients and with an already large burden of workload with communicable disease management adding further patient load caring for NCDs will need to be done cautiously.

The emphasis of this review was to use the literature to develop a medical model of care for NCDs in SSA, focused specifically on CVD, DM, and respiratory diseases – chronic obstructive pulmonary disease (COPD) and asthma. This excluded studies solely focused on health promotion, education or other psychosocial interventions. Although the non-medical management of NCDs is essential to a package of care, this review aimed to summarize a model of care that could be implemented at decentralized primary care clinics in SSA.

How exactly this model of care would be implemented gives way to the Alma Ata discussion of selective versus comprehensive health care [34]. HIV care has typically been implemented as a vertical program in LMIC. The infrastructure already developed in SSA for the delivery of chronic care for HIV, could be leveraged for an integrated horizontal program for NCDs [9, 41–43]. A case example in Swaziland of an NCD clinic for DM and HTN not having booked appointments, standardize treatment protocol, referral system and patient counseling despite being in the same clinic delivering HIV care having these tools and strategies demonstrates missed opportunity of leveraging an already present infrastructure [44]. With an increasing number of individuals on ART in SSA, the increased risk of diabetes and hyperlipidemia associated with ART suggests potential synergies in a horizontally integrated HIV-NCD model of care [45].

Finally, it is worthy of note that this is the first instance of "best fit" framework synthesis being conducted on data from quantitative and mixed method studies [15, 16]. All previous published examples of the method have focused on the synthesis of qualitative evidence alone [15, 16]. This evidence synthesis has demonstrated that "best fit" is equally viable as an approach for synthesizing quantitative and/or mixed method studies: the method facilitates the identification and development of a relevant a priori framework, against which quantitative data can be coded equally as well as qualitative data. Given the relative lack of detailed guidance on how to conduct narrative synthesis in systematic reviews [46], "best fit" framework synthesis clearly offers a well-specified approach that can make sense of studies and evidence that cannot be readily combined using statistical or qualitative approaches.

Limitations of this review

The focus of this review was on SSA, to help build a relevant contextual model of care for this area. Of the forty-eight countries in SSA, only seven SSA countries had primary studies that fit the inclusion criteria. Although limited in numbers of countries that had operational data, the consistent themes derived from these studies suggest these could likely be generalizable to other parts of SSA.

Many different study designs were included in this review, looking at different outcomes (primary and secondary) and different interventions. It had been explored doing a more quantitative synthesis of certain outcomes such as Hba1c or BP improvement with packages of care in SSA, however the interventions and outcomes were too heterogeneous in the studies to summarize them in such a way. Through secondary thematic analysis common themes stemmed from the literature, however it is more difficult given the diversity of study design and focus to make generalizations.

Another limitation of the quantitative studies, predominantly cohorts, was the high attrition rate. Although the outcomes and results were used informally to feedback about the interventions contextual factors to build a model of care, the low retention rates of patients in the studies speaks to the interventions themselves and risk of bias in the outcomes. These studies need to be interpreted with caution.

Conclusions

Despite the limitations of the data, this review conducted a thematic analysis to develop a conceptual model of care for NCDs in SSA. This medical model of care emphasized three major concepts for the components of an intervention; screening, prevention and control. Furthermore, following synthesis, the control of NCD component could be further broken down into: health systems, quality improvement, decision support and human resources, each with more detailed themes that contextualized these concepts. The scarcity of data available for this important research topic emphasized the urgent need for more research. Specifically further research looking at the effectiveness of these models of care is essential to help roll out piloted research to then scale up for national programs. Political will and commitment must be combined with increasing public awareness to harness resources and global attention for addressing this growing epidemic of NCDs in SSA.

Additional files

Additional file 1: Literature results for the a priori framework.

Additional file 2: Models of care for NCDs in LMIC.

Additional file 3: Example of search terms for primary research studies.

Additional file 4: Quality assessment of primary research studies.

Additional file 5: A Priori themes in primary research studies for NCDs Interventions in SSA.

Additional file 6: A Priori themes in primary research studies for NCD interventions in SSA.

Abbreviations

CD: Communicable disease; COPD: Chronic Obstructive Pulmonary disease; CVD: Cardiovascular disease; DM: Diabetes mellitus; HTN: Hypertension; LMIC: Low-and middle-income countries; NCD: Non-communicable disease; NPC: Non-physician clinician; PHC: Primary health care; SSA: Sub-Saharan Africa

Funding

Not applicable.

Authors' contributions

JK contributed to study design, literature review and wrote the manuscript. ML contributed to study design, interpretation of data and manuscript editing. SS contributed to study design and interpretation of data. CC contributed to methodological design and manuscript editing. AN contributed to the literature review. All authors read and approved the final manuscript.

Competing interests

The authors declare that they have no competing interests.

Consent for publication

Not applicable.

Author details

[1]Department of Family and Community Medicine, University of Toronto, Toronto, ON, Canada. [2]Dignitas International, 2 Adelaide Street West, Suite 200, Toronto M5H 1L6, Canada. [3]Health Economics and Decision Science (HEDS), School of Health and Related Research (ScHARR), University of Sheffield Regent Court, Regent Street, Sheffield S1 4DA, UK.

References

1. Hunter DJ, Reddy KS. Noncommunicable diseases. N Engl J Med. 2013;369(14):1336–43.
2. Lozano R, Naghavi M, Foreman K, Lim S, Shibuya K, Aboyans V, et al. Global and regional mortality from 235 causes of death for 20 age groups in 1990 and 2010: a systematic analysis for the Global Burden of Disease Study 2010. Lancet. 2013;380(9859):2095–128.
3. Miranda JJ, Kinra S, Casas JP, Davey Smith G, Ebrahim S. Non-communicable diseases in low-and middle-income countries: context, determinants and health policy. Trop Med Int Health. 2008;13(10):1225–34.
4. World Health Organization. WHO global status report on non-communicable diseases 2010. Geneva: World Health Organization; 2011.
5. Mathers CD, Loncar D. Projections of global mortality and burden of disease from 2002 to 2030. PLoS Med. 2006;3(11):e442.
6. Maher D, Ford N, Unwin N. Priorities for developing countries in the global response to non-communicable diseases. Glob Health. 2012;11:8(14).
7. Walley J, Graham K, Wei X, Kain K, Weston R. Getting research into practice: primary care management of noncommunicable diseases in low- and middle-income countries. Bull World Health Organ. 2012;90(6):402.
8. Harries A, Jahn A. Adapting the DOTS framework for tuberculosis control to the management of non-communicable diseases in Sub-Saharan Africa. PLoS Med. 2008;10:5(6).
9. Nigatu T. Integration of HIV and noncommunicable diseases in health care delivery in low- and middle-income countries. Prev Chronic Dis. 2012;9:e93.
10. Houben RM, Van Boeckel TP, Mwinuka V, Mzumara P, Branson K, Linard C, et al. Monitoring the impact of decentralised chronic care services on patient travel time in rural Africa-methods and results in Northern Malawi. Int J Health Geogr. 2012;11(1):49.
11. Maher D, Smeeth L, Sekajugo J. Health transition in Africa: practical policy proposals for primary care. Bull World Health Organ. 2010;88(12):943–8.
12. World Health Organization. Sixty-fifth World Health Assembly. Second Report of Committee A, Agenda Item 13.1/2. Geneva: World Health Organization; 2012.
13. Sahasrabuddhe W, Parham GP, Mwanahamuntu MH, Vermund SH. Cervical cancer prevention in low-and middle-income countries: feasible, affordable, essential. Cancer Prev Res. 2012;5(1):11–7.
14. Gureje O, Chisholm D, Kola L, Lasebikan V, Saxena S. Cost-effectiveness of an essential mental health intervention package in Nigeria. World Psychiatry. 2007;6(1):42–8.
15. Carroll C, Booth A, Leaviss J, Rick J. "Best fit" framework synthesis: refining the method. BMC Med Res Methodol. 2013;13:13(37).
16. Carroll C, Booth A, Cooper K. A worked example of "best fit" framework synthesis: a systematic review of views concerning the taking of some potential chemopreventive agents. BMC Med Res Methodol. 2013;16:11(29).
17. Maher D, Harries A, Zachariah R, Enarson D. A global framework for action to improve the primary care response to chronic non-communicable diseases: a solution to a neglected problem. BMC Public Health. 2009;9(1):355.
18. Beaglehole R, Epping-Jordan J, Patel V, Chopra M, Ebrahim S, Kidd M, et al. Improving the prevention and management of chronic disease in low-income and middle-income countries: a priority for primary health care. Lancet. 2008;372(9642):940–9.
19. Critical Appraisal Skills Programme. Oxford, UK: CASP UK; 2013 [cited 13 Jan 2014]. Available from: http://www.casp-uk.net/.
20. Pace R, Pluye P, Bartlett G, Macaulay AC, Salsberg J, Jagosh J, et al. Testing the reliability and efficiency of the pilot Mixed Methods Appraisal Tool (MMAT) for systematic mixed studies review. Int J Nurs Stud. 2012;49(1):47–53.
21. Bloomfield GS, Kimaiyo S, Carter EJ, Binanay C, Corey GR, Einterz RM, et al. Chronic noncommunicable cardiovascular and pulmonary disease in sub-Saharan Africa: An academic model for countering the epidemic. Am Heart J. 2011;161(5):842–7.
22. Pastakia SD, Ali SM, Kamano JH, Akwanalo CO, Ndege SK, Buckwalter VL, et al. Screening for diabetes and hypertension in a rural low income setting in western Kenya utilizing home-based and community-based strategies. Glob Health. 2013;16:9(21).
23. Rabkin M, Zenebe M, Bruce K, Ahmed R, Koler A, Tadesse Y, et al. Strengthening health systems for chronic care: leveraging HIV programs to support diabetes services in Ethiopia and Swaziland. J Trop Med. 2012;137460:18.
24. Mamo Y, Seid E, Adams S, Gardiner A, Parry E. A primary healthcare approach to the management of chronic disease in Ethiopia: an example for other countries. Clin Med. 2007;7(3):228–31.
25. Chamie G, Kwarisiima D, Clark TD, Kabami J, Jain V, Geng E, et al. Leveraging rapid community-based HIV testing campaigns for non-communicable diseases in rural Uganda. PLoS One. 2012;7(8):e43400.
26. Price C, Shandu D, Dedicoat M, Wilkinson D, Gill GV. Long-term glycaemic outcome of structured nurse-led diabetes care in rural Africa. QJM. 2011;104(7):571–4.
27. Katz I, Schneider H, Shezi Z, Mdleleni G, Gerntholtz T, Butler O, et al. Managing type 2 diabetes in Soweto - The South African Chronic Disease Outreach Program experience. Prim Care Diabetes. 2009;3(3):157–64.
28. Coleman R, Gill G, Wilkinson D. Noncommunicable disease management in resource-poor settings: a primary care model from rural South Africa. Bull World Health Organ. 1998;76(6):633–40.
29. Mendis S, Johnston SC, Fan W, Oladapo O, Cameron A, Faramawi MF. Cardiovascular risk management and its impact on hypertension control in primary care in low-resource settings: a cluster-randomized trial. Bull World Health Organ. 2010;88(6):412–9.
30. Labhardt ND, Balo J-R, Ndam M, Grimm J-J, Manga E. Task shifting to non-physician clinicians for integrated management of hypertension and diabetes in rural Cameroon: a programme assessment at two years. BMC

Health Serv Res. 2010;10:339.
31. Kengne A, Pascal E, Sobngwi L, Fezeu PA, Dongmo S, Mbanya J-C. Setting-up nurse-led pilot clinics for the management of non-communicable diseases at primary health care level in resource-limited settings of Africa. Pan Afr Med J. 2009;3:10.
32. Bovet P, Gervasoni J-P, Mkamba M, Balampama M, Lengeler C, Paccaud F. Low utilization of health services following screening for hypertension in Dar es Salaam (Tanzania): a prospective population-based study. BMC Public Health. 2008;8(1):407.
33. Gill GV, Price C, Shandu D, Dedicoat M, Wilkinson D. An effective system of nurse-led diabetes care in rural Africa. Diabet Med. 2008;25(5):606–11.
34. Bischoff A, Ekoe T, Perone N, Slama S, Loutan L. Chronic disease management in Sub-Saharan Africa: whose business is it? Int J Environ Res Public Health. 2009;6(8):2258–70.
35. World Health Organization. Task shifting to tackle health care worker shortage: HIV/AIDs Programme - strengtening health services to fight HIV/AIDS. Geneva: World Health Organization; 2007.
36. Zachariah R, Ford N, Philips M, Lynch S, Massaquoi M, Janssens V, et al. Task shifting in HIV/AIDS: opportunities, challenges and proposed actions for sub-Saharan Africa. Trans R Soc Trop Med Hyg. 2012;103(6):549–88.
37. Unwin N, Mugusi F, Aspray T, Whiting D, Edwards R, Mbanya JC, et al. Tackling the emerging pandemic of non-communicable diseases in sub-Saharan Africa: The essential NCD health intervention project. Public Health. 1999;113(3):141–6.
38. Maher D, Ford N, Unwin N. Priorities for developing countries in the global response to non-communicable diseases. Glob Health. 2012;8(1):1–8.
39. Libamba E, Makombe S, Harries A, Chimziz R, Salaniponi FM, Schouten EJ, Mpazanje R. Scaling up Antiretrovirla therapy in Malawi - implications for managing other chronic diseases in resource-limited countries. J Acquir Immune Defic Syndr. 2009;52 Suppl 1:14–6.
40. World Health Organization. World Health Statistics. Geneva: World Health Organization; 2011.
41. Levitt N, Steky K, Dave J, Bradshaw D. Chronic noncommunicable diseases and HIV-AIDS on a collision course: relevance for health care delivery, particularly in low-resource settings - insights from South Africa. Am J Clin Nutr. 2011;94(6):1690S–6.
42. Rabkin M, Kruk ME, El-Sadr WM. HIV, aging and continuity care: strengthening health systems to support services for noncommunicable diseases in low-income countries. AIDS. 2012;26 Suppl 1:77–83.
43. Olmen J, Schellevis F, Damme W, Kegels G, Rasschaert F. Management of chronic diseases in sub-Saharan Africa: cross-fertilisation between HIV/AIDS and diabetes care. J Trop Med. 2012;349312:97.
44. Rabkin M, Nishtar S. Scaling up chronic care systems: leveraging HIV programs to support noncommunicable disease services. J Acquir Immune Defic Syndr. 2011;57 Suppl 2:S87–90.
45. Brown TT, Cole SR, Li X, Kingsley LA, Palella FJ, Riddler SA, Visscher BR, Margolick JB, Dobs AS. Antiretroviral therapy and the prevalence and incidence of diabetes mellitus in the multicenter AIDS cohort study. Arch Intern Med. 2005;165(10):1179–84.
46. Snilstveit B, Oliver S, Vojtkova M. Narrative approaches to systematic review and synthesis of evidence for international development policy and practice. J Dev Eff. 2012;4(3):409–29.

19

Implementing multiple health behaviour change interventions for cardiovascular risk reduction in primary care

Samah Alageel*, Martin C. Gulliford, Lisa McDermott and Alison J. Wright

Abstract

Background: The implementation of multiple health behaviour change interventions for cardiovascular risk reduction in primary care is suboptimal. This study aimed to identify barriers and facilitators to implementing multiple health behaviour change interventions for cardiovascular disease (CVD) risk reduction in primary care.

Methods: Qualitative study using semi-structured interviews informed by the Theoretical Domains Framework. Interviews were conducted with a purposive sample of healthcare professionals working in the implementation of the NHS Health Check programme in London. Data were analysed using the Framework method.

Results: Thirty participants were recruited including ten general practitioners, ten practice nurses, seven healthcare assistants and three practice managers from 23 practices. Qualitative analysis identified three main themes: healthcare professionals' conceptualising health behaviour change; delivering multiple health behaviour change interventions in primary care; and delivering the health check programme. Healthcare professionals generally recognised the importance of health behaviour change for CVD risk reduction but were more sceptical about the potential for successful intervention through primary care. Participants identified the difficulty of sustained behaviour change for patients, the lack of evidence for effective interventions and limited access to appropriate resources in primary care as barriers. Discussing changing multiple health behaviours was perceived to be overwhelming for patients and difficult to implement for healthcare professionals with current primary care resources. The health check programme consists of several components that are difficult to fully complete in limited time.

Conclusions: Advancing the prevention agenda will require strategies to support the delivery of behaviour change interventions in primary care. Greater emphasis needs to be given to promoting behaviour change through supportive environmental context. Further research is needed to evaluate current external lifestyle services to improve the intervention outcomes.

Keywords: Behaviour change interventions, Primary care, Cardiovascular prevention, NHS health check, Intervention implementation

* Correspondence: samah.alageel@kcl.ac.uk
School of Population Health and Environmental Sciences, Faculty of Life Sciences and Medicine, King's College London, Addison House, Guy's Campus, London SE1 1UL, UK

Introduction

Cardiovascular risk management for the prevention of cardiovascular diseases (CVD) through multiple health behaviour change (MHBC) interventions and/or medication has the potential to reduce risk and provide health benefits. The potential for continuity of care in primary care presents an opportunity to support behaviour change interventions. In many countries, behaviour change interventions are being delivered by primary care professionals as part of their routine practice. However, there is only limited evidence for the effectiveness of MHBC interventions at reducing CVD risk and CVD risk factors or improving mortality outcomes among primary prevention populations [1–3]. A Cochrane systematic review evaluated the effect of multiple risk factor interventions on all cause and CVD mortality but did not find an effect on CVD-mortality (Odds Ratio = 0.99, CI = 0.92 to 1.07) [2]. We presently have limited understanding of factors influencing the effectiveness of MHBC interventions in primary care. Understanding providers' experiences may help to provide explanations for the apparently limited effectiveness of MHBC interventions.

A national health check programme was implemented in England in 2009, targeting individuals aged 40 to 74 years and estimating their risk of developing cardiovascular disease in the next 10 years [4]. After identifying individuals at elevated risk, a risk management intervention, tailored to the individual's behavioural risk factors, is provided. The risk management component focuses on MHBC intervention to address four behavioural areas: diet and weight management, smoking cessation, promoting physical activity and reducing excessive alcohol consumption [4]. MHBC interventions are defined by the Health Check programme as individual-level behaviour change interventions that can be delivered through brief advice, motivational interviewing and/ or referrals to external behaviour change services [4]. The intervention is delivered in primary care by several different healthcare professionals (HCPs). These include general practitioners (GPs), practice nurses (nurses based in GP surgeries, their main role involves health screening and promotion and managing patients with chronic diseases) and healthcare assistants (HCA) (assistants who help provide care, working under the guidance of a qualified healthcare professional, often a nurse) [5]. The NHS Health Check (NHSHC) programme provides an opportunity in terms of tackling multiple risk factors which, if successful, might reduce the risk of several diseases. However, several limitations were identified in relation to MHBC intervention implementation. A qualitative study examining the experience of high-risk individuals identified gaps in the promotion of behaviour change [6]. High-risk individuals were not always offered behaviour change interventions (especially for physical activity and alcohol consumption) [6]. Additionally, the implementation of behaviour change interventions, when offered, varied across general practices [5, 7]. Failure to deliver personalised behaviour change interventions to high-risk patients in some practices, decreases the likelihood that patients will change their behaviour and reduces any long-term impact of the health check programme [7]. Reported barriers in clinical practice include workload and lack of time, in addition to insufficient knowledge and skills to deliver behaviour change interventions [8, 9]. These barriers may have contributed to the lack of confidence in the effectiveness of behaviour change interventions [8, 9].

Psychological theories have often been used to understand, predict and generate behaviour change in HCPs [10–12]. However, the large number of overlapping psychological theories makes it difficult to select theoretical constructs or models for implementation research. In an attempt to address this problem, Cane et al. (2012) reviewed 128 theoretical constructs derived from 33 theories applicable to implementation behaviour, and grouped these constructs based on commonalities [13]. The Theoretical Domains Framework (TDF) was developed using a consensus approach with groups of experts including health services researchers and health psychologists [13, 14]. The aggregated nature of the TDF provides a programmatic framework for the explanation of HCPs' behaviours. It has been widely used to investigate perceived barriers and facilitators to HCPs' evidence-based implementation behaviour [15–17], and shown to be useful for providing explanations for implementation behaviour.

Although existing literature has investigated the experience of healthcare professionals in delivering single behaviour change interventions; further research is needed to understand barriers to the implementation of MHBC interventions. The extent of professionals' capability and motivation to promote multiple risk-reducing behavioural interventions to high-risk patients, together with the opportunities provided in primary care, influence the success of interventions in reducing CVD risk. This study aimed to explore HCPs experiences of, and views on, delivering MHBC interventions at health checks, in order to identify barriers and facilitators to implementing such interventions effectively in primary care.

Methods

This study employed qualitative methodology, applying framework analysis to data collected from semi- structured interviews with HCPs who were involved with MHBC interventions as part of the NHSHC programme. The study was approved by King's College London Research Ethics Committee (LRS- 15/16–2656).

Recruitment

A purposive sample, aiming to interview participants with a range of professional roles, was recruited from 23 general practices in two socioeconomically deprived and ethnically diverse inner-city London boroughs, Lambeth and Lewisham. The NHSHC uptake in Lewisham (38%) and Lambeth (28%) is below national average (45%) [18]. Of those who received the check, 4% in Lambeth and 8% in Lewisham were classified as at high risk of cardiovascular diseases [19, 20]. These two boroughs have a high proportion of smoking, obesity and excessive alcohol consumption, and high CVD mortality compared to London and England [21]. Most of the health checks conducted are provided in general practices [19, 20].

Potential participants were identified as all HCPs involved in the NHSHC programme implementation. Participants included GPs, practice nurses, HCAs, and practice managers. General practitioners, practice nurses and HCAs carry out the health check assessment, communicate the results and provide MHBC interventions to high risk individuals. Practice managers are involved in managing the business aspect of the practice and support HCPs with delivering patient services. Managers were included in this study as it has been suggested that their interest in and views about health promotion activities act as facilitator to implementation [22]. This heterogeneous sample enabled the identification of common themes across different experiences [23].

Interviews were conducted face-to-face between July and November 2016. Healthcare professionals were contacted via email and invited to take part in the study. Due to clinicians' busy schedules, the email message was followed by a visit to the general practice two weeks later to encourage participation and answer any enquiries related to the study. When clinicians agreed to participate, a mutually convenient time and place were decided, and consent was obtained before the beginning of each interview. Interviews were conducted by one researcher (SA), with training in qualitative research. Interviews lasted between 25 to 90 min. The length of the interviews varied depending on participants' experience with the NHSHC and available time. Interviews were audio recoded and transcribed verbatim. Recruitment continued until there were no further emerging themes and it was decided that saturation was reached. Participants were offered a fee for their participation in the study. This study was funded by the National Institute for Health Research (NIHR) Biomedical Research Centre at Guy's and St Thomas' NHS Foundation Trust and King's College London. The funding body had no role in study design, analysing the data or writing the manuscript.

Interview topic guide

The TDF [13] informed the development of the topic guide (Additional file 1) to identify barriers and enablers to implementing MHBC interventions in primary care. The TDF was developed and widely used for studying the implementation of evidence-based practice by identifying psychological and organizational theory related to clinicians' behaviour change [13]. The framework provides a robust theoretical basis for studies examining implementation behaviour, covering a broad range of individual and organizational theories [24], so limiting the possibility of missing important factors affecting the implementation of MHBC intervention. Using the TDF to examine barriers and facilitators of HCPs practice might enable the identification of factors that participants may not otherwise report [25].

Developing the topic guide was facilitated by a series of generic interview questions as developed by the originators of the TDF for each domain [13]. At the start of the interview, additional information was collected about participants' characteristics, such as job title and years of experience of the NHSHC programme. Hypothetical scenarios of high-risk patients were presented to the participants to stimulate the discussion of MHBC interventions. The topic guide was discussed and edited by three experts in the field with experience in using the TDF in qualitative research. It was then piloted with one participant, and the questions were rephrased and rearranged based on the participant's comments. The transcript from the pilot interview was not included in the analysis, as the aim of the pilot was to improve the topic guide.

Data analysis

Interview transcripts were managed using NVivo software. Interview data were analysed using Framework analysis [23], as this approach enables data to be compared and contrasted across and within cases until a coherent account emerge [23].

Framework analysis involves seven stages: transcription, familiarisation, coding, developing and applying the analytical framework, charting data into the framework matrix and data interpretation [23] . The familiarisation stage was conducted in parallel to the data collection process. As part of the familiarisation stage, two authors read through the transcripts before coding (SA, LM). The development of the coding framework and initial analysis of interview data was undertaken by the first author (SA) who conducted the interviews. A second author (LM) with expertise in qualitative methods checked all codes to ensure that codes reflected the data. Codes were then discussed, and amendments were made where appropriate until full agreement was reached.

Two authors (SA, AW) assessed and examined the data coded in relation to the TDF. Tables were produced to highlight key thematic content. Factors affecting intervention implementation were assigned to a relevant TDF domain or set of domains [24]. Face to face meetings ensured agreements between authors about charting TDF domains for each factor. Interpretations and over-arching themes were then identified and discussed with the research team.

Results

Thirty HCPs from 23 general practices in south London took part in the study. The sample included a broad cross section of HCPs, including GPs, practice nurses, HCAs and practice managers. The majority of the sample were female and had been working in delivering the programme since it was introduced. Participants' characteristics are presented in Table 1. No differences were observed in the experiences of HCPs based on gender, workplace geographical area or length of working in the NHSHC programme.

Three main themes emerged from the data as factors that HCPs viewed as affecting the implementation of MHBC interventions in primary care: 1) Conceptualising health behaviour change; 2) Delivering MHBC interventions in primary care; and 3) Delivering the health check programme. The relationship between themes and the TDF and further illustrative quotes are presented in Table 2.

Conceptualising health behaviour change

Complexity of behaviour change

Participants viewed health behaviour change as a challenging task for their patients. Patients' ability to change was perceived to be hindered by environmental context and resources (including cost, access to services and time), factors which were not always within patients' control. The fear of pressuring patients to change their behaviour, when change might not be within patients' abilities, acted as a barrier to implementing behaviour change interventions.

Table 1 Participants characteristics

Gender	
Male	6
Female	24
Job title	
GP	10
Practice nurse	10
Healthcare assistant	7
Manager	3
How long they have been involved with the NHS Health Check	
Since it was introduced in 2009	20
Less than a year	2
More than a year (1–3 years)	8
Borough	
Lewisham	20
Lambeth	10

> *"Environmental and societal factors hinder people from changing their behaviour, they're fighting a losing battle."* (Interview 21, GP).

Responsibility for enabling behaviour change was discussed. Participants emphasised that regulation at population-level could play a dominant role in facilitating individuals' behaviour change. Participants expressed the need to make the environment supportive of healthy behaviours, so that subsequently patients will be able to change their behaviour.

> *"Unhealthy behaviour is multi-factorial, the reasons why somebody becomes obese are just not as simple as because they eat too much or exercise too little. There are a whole host of socioeconomic and psychological factors. Behaviour change should be facilitated through laws."* (Interview 8, GP).

The nature of a "healthy behaviour"

Participants believed that most patients knew what constituted health-enhancing behaviours and the impact of risk behaviours on their health. Therefore, HCPs perceived little need to explain the importance of changing behaviour to patients.

> *"There's so many messages. I know you can ignore the messages, but people don't need to be told, "You need to exercise, you need to eat well," because we all know it."* (Interview 11, GP).

Some participants were concerned about what healthy lifestyle meant to them and how their own interpretation may be different to that of their patients. Even between HCPs, healthy behaviours were subjective.

> *"The definition of healthy behaviour is subjective. people have their own ideas about what good health is."* (Interview 15, Manager).

Health as a priority

For patients to engage in behaviour change, HCPs felt that a healthy lifestyle needed to be on patients' agendas and a priority in their lives. These goals were seen as a prerequisite to engaging in behaviour change. Healthcare professionals expressed the importance of not imposing their agendas over their patients' agendas, in order to

Table 2 Factors influencing the implementation of MHBC interventions for CVD risk reduction

Themes	Sub-themes	Theoretical domain (TDF)	Illustrative quote
Conceptualising health behaviour change	Complexity of health behaviour change	• Beliefs about patients' capabilities to change their behaviour. • Perceived patients' environmental context and resources.	"It's taking us a lifetime to form our behaviours, but they're expecting us to change overnight. It's not easy. So we know that changing these behaviours is not easy." (Interview 15, Manager)
	What is a "healthy behaviour"?	• Patients' and HCP's knowledge of health behaviour. • HCP's emotion towards behaviour change and health behaviour.	"There's a lot of different conflicting information, even for us in terms of the evidence, it's still very – so I have to say to my patients, "This is the best I can tell you at the moment, that's the best information I have." Will it change? Yes, well it may change. But, you know, we are not saying these are absolute absolutes. This is what we know for the moment."" (Interview 23, GP)
	Health as a priority	• Perceived patients' goals to change behaviour. • Perceived patients' intention to change behaviour.	"So I would kind of usually very much always approach it by kind of where he is at in terms of his attitude to his health and what he feels, you know, he needs to adapt before I even say to him, "Look, here are your figures," and take him through the meaning or the implications of them. So getting an idea of, of what his understanding is about his health and what concerns he has, to then build on them." (Interview 20, GP)
Delivering MHBC interventions in primary care	Beliefs about the intervention consequences	• Beliefs about the consequences of implementing behaviour change interventions. • HCPs emotions towards implementing behaviour change interventions. • Reinforcement to implement behaviour change interventions.	"But I think generally the impression I get is the only thing I could tell you is that it's a waste of time…But yes, generally felt that the brief intervention that you get, what's the point?" (Interview 29, GP)
	Multiple health behaviour change intervention	• Environmental context and resources that discourages or encourages the implementation of MHBC interventions. • Skills needed to implement MHBC intervention. • Goals.	"I think you can't obviously deal with everything at once... it would be up to the patient to decide what it is they would like to deal with in the first instance." (Interview 1, Manager)
	Who should implement health behaviour change interventions?	• Social/professional role and identity. • Social influences. • Skills.	"And I think, I think probably [HCA] because she does more of the health promotion, but she probably has learnt more ways of kind of motivating people and, and has a different relationship with them. So tends to find out a bit about them personally and their family and things. (Interview 24, GP)
	Skills to implement health behaviour change interventions	• HCPs perceived knowledge about MHBC interventions. • Skills needed to implement MHBC interventions. • HCP's beliefs about their capabilities to implement MHBC interventions.	"In terms of dietary requirements.... yes, it would be nice to just be more specific. Yes. I think, including me, we need more education on dietary advice, for sure." (Interview 5, HCA)
Delivering the health check programme	The NHSHC programme consists of several steps	• Environmental context and resources. • Skills needed to implement the health check. • Patients perceived knowledge. • Beliefs about capabilities.	"Time is always a major factor. Unfortunately, the GP-land, or practice nursing, as a rule, you're dealing with everything." (Interview 6, Nurse) "You can't give somebody advice if you're not sure what you're talking about." (Interview 14, HCA)
	The health check population	• Behavioural regulation. • Patients' views of the programme	'But I don't think that the health check scheme works, because I think it's

Table 2 Factors influencing the implementation of MHBC interventions for CVD risk reduction *(Continued)*

Themes	Sub-themes	Theoretical domain (TDF)	Illustrative quote
		social influences. • Knowledge.	targeting the wrong population and it's, it just - as I said, I think it's best done opportunistically when we see patients alongside other health issues, which might be more relevant even.' (Interview 8, GP)

TDF Theoretical Domains Framework, *NHSHC* NHS Health Check, *GP* general practitioner, *HCA* healthcare assistant

maintain good relationships with patients and to respond to their wants and needs.

'I think that the only way that I've experienced for people to actually make changes, is for them to come up with the ideas themselves...using their agenda, not mine.' (Interview 25, Nurse).

Delivering MHBC interventions in primary care

Beliefs about the consequences of MHBC interventions

Although all HCPs expressed the importance of promoting health behaviour, some were sceptical about the outcomes of MHBC interventions in primary care (see Table 2). The reasons for this scepticism included lack of evidence to support the success of such interventions in primary care and lack of confidence in patients making changes to their behaviour following the intervention.

"Whether it makes any difference at all to their lifestyle - as we know from the evidence, it doesn't. In fact, it makes things worse... it's just a waste of time." (Interview 8, GP).

The scepticism was more apparent among GPs, where some compared the success and ease of the "drug approach" in relation to the "non-drug approach".

"So I'm very open. I would prefer a non-drug approach to these problems. I think these problems are ultimately based in society and they are behavioural problems... And I know a tablet can't cure that. And yet the easiest thing for us to do is to prescribe a tablet. And when you do prescribe tablets, tablets do work." (Interview 4, GP).

Lack of confidence in the interventions' success was associated with feeling apathetic and frustrated about implementing MHBC interventions. In contrast, HCPs who were more optimistic about the intervention's outcomes felt a sense of achievement and satisfaction. Beliefs about the intervention's consequences were closely linked to HCPs emotions towards intervention implementation.

"I think we're slightly apathetic about it from a GP point of view, just because, I don't know, it's more soft work that we don't get a definite outcome from." (Interview 11, GP).

"I think you definitely get a sense, a good feeling of sense of achievement, whatever, if you feel that you've really been able to enthuse someone to make some lifestyle changes." (Interview 12, Nurse).

Healthcare professionals understanding of MHBC interventions had an impact on how optimistic they were about intervention outcomes. There was a considerable variation in how HCPs viewed the nature of MHBC interventions. Healthcare assistants often referred to behaviour change interventions as involving information sharing; which might explain their positive attitudes towards the intervention. However, GPs felt that patients knew what they needed to change, and therefore needed support to make that change happen, rather than more information. GPs sometimes questioned the long-term impact of behaviour change interventions in terms of maintaining change, which could explain their scepticism regarding the success of the intervention. Therefore, HCPs knowledge and understanding of the intervention and the skills needed to implement it influenced their beliefs about their capabilities and the consequences of implementing MHBC intervention.

"I'm confident with the information that I give to patients. And they always leave positive." (Interview 3, HCA).

"Is it useful? On an individual basis, it may be useful with a particular patient. But on a broader base, is it? I think that's what often we question. The time to do it, who does it and how well do they do it? In general, I'd say I'm fairly pessimistic because I think it's difficult." (Interview 16, GP).

Some participants felt advocating for behaviour change was an essential part of their job, which by itself was an enough of an incentive to implement MHBC interventions (personal incentive). However, monetary (external) incentives were often reported as the main reason to implement the health check among participants who were more sceptical about the intervention's effectiveness.

"We're only doing it, I think, because of the money, because if we don't, we get the money removed from us and we'll go under. So I think it is absolutely related to the money. It's nothing to do with us believing it works or it doesn't work." (Interview 8, GP).

Multiple health behaviour change (MHBC) interventions

Addressing MHBC was not always facilitated by primary care resources. Lack of sufficient time to deliver successful behaviour change interventions and to follow-up patients with continuing support were identified as barriers to implementing MHBC interventions.

"We don't have loads and loads of time to keep getting people back to give them more advice. But I mean we don't have a lot of time to do, you know, weight and dietary advice, just dietary advice. There's a lot of sick people that come in and have to be given a lot of time." (Interview 10, Nurse).

Discussing MHBC in one session was often viewed as overwhelming for patients. Participants felt that the best and most successful way to deal with MHBC was for the patient to decide on what to focus and discuss one behaviour change at a time. However, in practice, MHBC change was usually discussed in a single consultation due to contextual constraints (i.e. time and workload).

"I think in an ideal setting, you would want to tackle, you know, the multiple risk factors, each one of them separately. But there isn't time to bring patients back for multiple consultations. So you somehow try to discuss all of them." (Interview 18, GP).

Healthcare professionals expressed the importance of making referrals to external lifestyle services to support patients through the behaviour change process, but these services had difficulties with long waiting lists, budget cuts causing the discontinuation of some services and were not always offered at times that suited the working population.

"In terms of what's available to patients, I think it's very poor in the UK... And even when they are available, it's not so accessible, it's not so easy to negotiate. There's often a cost involved." (Interview 16, GP).

Who should implement behaviour change interventions?

Although GPs expressed the importance of behaviour change, they perceived behaviour change interventions as more suitably delivered by nurses and HCAs, who might have more time and appropriate skills, whereas GPs' time should be reserved for urgent and high-risk cases. Perceived professional role and identity was a barrier to implementing MHBC interventions among GPs.

"I think then the discussions of lifestyle interventions takes time, which obviously, in today's work environment, is difficult for GPs. But we do try to train nurses and healthcare assistants to be able to do that as well... I think it's probably better use of resources to be done by another clinician." (Interview 16, GP).

Some GPs were concerned about how promoting behaviour change could affect the balance of their relationship with their patients, which discouraged the initiation of the MHBC discussion. These concerns not clearly held by other HCPs.

"You have a one-to-one relationship with a patient. It's too much like the patient has done something wrong, or the patient is weak. It's interpreted as a weakness if they don't know how to reduce their diet, if they cannot reduce their smoking...It's, it becomes less relationship of equals and more relationship of parent-child, good parent, naughty child." (Interview 4, GP).

In some interviews, participants discussed how different clinicians influenced the success of behaviour change interventions. Some thought that if the intervention was delivered by a GP it would have a bigger influence on patients. Others argued that patients might be more open and engaged with interventions delivered by nurses and HCAs, due to the ease of the relationship. One manager thought that patients would be more open in community settings rather than with their healthcare provider.

"But often hearing these healthy lifestyle advices coming from a doctor, often people might value more than from a healthcare assistant." (Interview 16, GP).

"The doctor-patient relationship do affect that because in a community setting, you are in a different setting. The patient tends to be more open in terms of all the other factors that is affecting them, than when they sit in a clinical room." (Interview 15, Manager).

Skills to implement behaviour change interventions

GPs reported a lack of specific training to implement behaviour change interventions, but some GPs believed that they did not need special training to implement behaviour change interventions. It was viewed as being intrinsic to their medical training.

> *"And I think where people like me get really concerned about these questions, "Have you had any training?" Yes, so we've been medically trained. I've then been trained as a general practitioner. All of the skills required to do a health check are delivered to me. They do not depend on a one-day training programme."* (Interview 23, GP).

Lack of training was a concern to other HCPs who noted GPs' competency in managing ill health but not in delivering behaviour change interventions.

> *"Well I think clinicians are sort of culturally geared to deal with illness. And dealing with people's sort of illnesses that they come in with. And less geared up to deal with promoting health and promoting healthy behaviours."* (Interview 19, Manager).

Some participants described lack of training to deliver specific dietary interventions and individualised behaviour change interventions as barriers to implementation, which may have affected their perceived capabilities to implement the intervention. All HCPs discussed the absence of any guidance on implementing MHBC interventions. It was often perceived as a very individualised approach that should not be structured.

> *"You can't really have a template for the advice. It is kind of depending on each person."* (Interview 14, HCA).

Most HCPs expressed difficulty in delivering weight management interventions. The fear of offending and upsetting the patient and the difficulty of dealing with such a sensitive subject in limited time discouraged the implementation of weight management interventions. Some HCPs reflected on their own weight and how that affected the way they implemented weight management interventions, either by using themselves as an example to break barriers and facilitate the implementation of behaviour change intervention or that their weight might have inhibited the process.

> *"And they relate to me. You know, clearly I'm not thin. So when they sit down and I say, "You weigh a little bit more than is good for you," I say, "And you weigh a little bit more for you than is good for you, like I do." You know, "You're not the only one that has those problems.""* (Interview 25, Nurse).

Excessive alcohol consumption was also considered a difficult behaviour to tackle. Some HCPs thought patients would not easily discuss their alcohol consumption and its part in their social life. Issues around assessing patients' alcohol consumption accurately were also reported as barriers to implementing alcohol consumption interventions.

> *"The most difficult one I find is talking about the alcohol, because kind of some people aren't kind of upfront about the amount of alcohol.... So I find that the hardest really."* (Interview 9, HCA).

Delivering the health check programme

The programme consists of several steps

The majority of HCPs expressed difficulty in going through all the health check steps within one consultation.

> *"One of the problems has been, as with any service, by putting too many steps in, you can lose, you know, people get lost. So we want to try and tighten that up...One of the challenges of the health check, I think, is it's got complicated assessment. I think it's quite a big ask."* (Interview 1, Manager).

A further challenge was in discussing the results of the checks' several components, including CVD-risk score, in limited time. Comprehending CVD risk was perceived to be challenging for patients, where HCPs have expressed concerns over the inconsistency between patients' perceived risk and their actual risk.

> *"I think it's virtually an impossible explanation to give." To say somebody, "You have a risk in the next decade of dying," it's impossible. It's just impossible to say to somebody, "Your QRISK is...this is based on a population sample."* (Interview 8, GP).

The health check population

Patients who responded to the health check invitation were perceived to be healthy and at low risk. Healthcare professionals rarely identified high-risk patients through the health check invitation process, and patients checked opportunistically were perceived as the target group.

> *"I sometimes think we only get the ones booking, who want to do something - the 'worried well' I call them. Yes, whereas, I think the ones we pick up opportunistically are the more needy. And actually they're far harder to work with."* (Interview 12, Nurse).

Participants expressed concern over patients' perceptions of the programme (Table 2). Most patients who came for their check were thought to not understand the programme rationale. Patients' lack of knowledge about the programme's intended outcome of reducing risk was perceived as a barrier to patients' willingness to change their behaviour.

> *"And they often come in not quite sure what it's all about, but knowing that it's a health check... But yes, so patients will see it as a, 'just a check to see that I'm healthy, to see that I'm okay.'"* (Interview 10, Nurse).

Discussion

This study is among the first to examine HCPs' experiences of the implementation of MHBC interventions as part of cardiovascular health checks in primary care. The study identified several key domains that either facilitate or discourage the implementation of behaviour change interventions.

Healthcare professionals were concerned that behaviour change interventions delivered in primary care might be over-reliant on patients' individual agency, given many environmental factors can hinder efforts at behaviour change. They discussed the broader socioeconomic context in which behaviour change occurs and the need for supportive policies and regulation. The lack of a supportive wider context led to HCPs doubting the effectiveness of behaviour change interventions delivered in primary care and being less motivated to implement them. They also felt that such interventions may be an unfair imposition of HCPs' agendas on patients who were unable to change, given patients' circumstances. The importance accorded by HCPs to societal influences on behaviour contrasts with views of GPs in the same area of London over a decade ago, who saw obesity-related behaviour change as being chiefly the patient's responsibility [26]. There has been recent criticism of the public health interventions favoured by policymakers as over-reliant on individuals' ability to draw on personal resources to change. Critics have argued that interventions requiring a lower level of agency to benefit will be more effective and equitable [27]. Healthcare professionals may be more likely to be willing to promote behaviour change at an individual level when interventions in primary care are accompanied by efforts to make the wider environment more facilitative of health enhancing behaviour.

Healthcare professionals in our study questioned the effectiveness of behaviour change interventions delivered in primary care, especially in the long-term. These perceived lack of effectiveness of behaviour change was contrasted with the "drug approach" to risk reduction, which was seen as easier and more effective. However, when HCPs felt they had personal experience of successfully supporting patients to change behaviour, their sense of achievement motivated further efforts to deliver behaviour change interventions. In contrast, perceiving interventions as ineffective led to frustration and apathy. Although a recent systematic review did not find that MHBC interventions in primary care had quantitatively important effects on CVD risk factors [1], the included interventions often did not incorporate behaviour change techniques [28] now known to promote behaviour change. Sharing evidence about specific, effective behaviour change techniques, may increase HCPs' willingness to deliver behaviour change interventions that incorporate them. Several behaviour change techniques have been shown to be effective in changing behaviour in primary prevention populations and could be easily implemented in primary care setting. For example, prompting a plan to perform the behaviour (i.e. action planning) have been shown to increase physical activity [29, 30] and advice on stop smoking medications have been shown to facilitate smoking cessation [31]. The provision of smoking cessation medication is considered an effective strategy in sustaining smoking cessation, even among smokers who are not ready to quit smoking [32, 33]. In the present study, perceiving low effectiveness did not appear to deter HCPs completely from delivering health checks, due to the financial incentives for conducting the checks making an important contribution to GP practices' budgets. However, it may be harder for HCPs who feel doubtful about the effectiveness of behaviour change interventions to enthuse patients to change their behaviour.

Environmental context and resources were suggested to discourage the implementation and follow-up of MHBC interventions in primary care. Time constraints and workload pressures in general practice were viewed as barriers to implementation, as reported previously [22, 34]. In the NHSHC programme, clinicians are expected to assess people's risk, communicate the results and provide MHBC intervention in one session lasting at most 30 min. In contrast, HCPs felt that tackling one behaviour at a time, and being able to see patients for follow-up sessions, was more likely to promote behaviour change. Therefore, there is a need to develop and disseminate very brief behaviour change interventions that could be incorporated into health checks. For example, Pears and colleagues evaluated three very brief interventions to promote physical activity. The results suggested that providing a pedometer with instructions on how to use it and explanation of the recommended steps per day would take only five minutes and result in increased physical activity levels [35]. Technological solutions could enable patient follow-up without requiring further appointments. Many GP practices in England already use a text messaging system to contact patients with appointment reminders and cues for preventive health care. This system could also be used to further deliver brief behaviour change intervention components or follow-up on whether patients have met behavioural goals and provide suitable feedback. Providing HCPs with guidance on using technology-based methods of follow-up may facilitate intervention implementation. The usefulness of the guidance, however, is limited by professionals' beliefs of the importance of the implementation and effectiveness of such interventions [22].

Given the limited time available in primary care, referrals to community behaviour change services and resources may be provide a more suitable platform for behaviour change [36]. However, HCPs noted a number of difficulties with referring patients to these services. Some services had long waiting lists, or were even no longer available due to budget cuts, while others did not run at times convenient for a working age population. There is therefore a need to ensure these services are properly resourced and made available at times that reflect the availability of the working age health check population. However, as it would be difficult to offer community services at times to suit all eligible individuals, digital behaviour change interventions may provide an alternative, easily scalable and convenient solution. Therefore, research attention should also be paid to establishing the most effective digital interventions for the health check population.

Feeling one lacked the necessary skills and training made HCPs doubt their effectiveness at promoting particular types of behaviour change. Weight management interventions were inhibited by fears of upsetting patients, while alcohol reduction interventions were seen as difficult because patients might be uncomfortable disclosing the true extent of their drinking. Therefore, there is a need for further training and resources to enable clinicians to be more confident in tackling these two sensitive topics. In contrast, some HCPs felt that behaviour change was easy to promote. However, these HCPs seemed to view behaviour change as largely involving information provision. Therefore, there is a need to disseminate resources highlighting behaviour change techniques that are more effective than information provision but still brief.

Strengths and limitations

This study is among the first to present qualitative findings relating to HCP's experience in implementing MHBC interventions after health checks in primary care. It examined the views of a diverse group of clinicians and managers who work in the NHSHC programme. Using the TDF may have led participants to discuss the role of less conscious factors, such as emotions, that may influence their implementation behaviour [25]. The TDF synthesizes 33 theories of behaviour [13], so it is likely to be comprehensive in comparison to studies based on a single theory or using a conventional topic guide. The TDF enables looking beyond individual factors and considers environmental and social influences on implementation behaviour. The interviews were coded and analysed by two authors with experience in qualitative research and background in health psychology, which improves the reliability of this study interpretation [37].

The findings of this study may not be completely transferable beyond the current context. The results reflect the views of those who agreed to participate and who work in specific geographical area. Healthcare professionals who were not able to participate may have different experiences. Face to face interviews can produce social desirability bias [38], especially when discussing implementation behaviour. Ethnography could have provided the advantage of considering what HCPs do and whether it is similar (or not) to what they say they do. The interviewer was external to the practice and other related agencies, with no conflicting roles or affiliations, which is believed to help in accessing more private accounts and reducing socially desirable responses. Finally, it was difficult to reach theoretical saturation of themes representing the manager group, considering the limited number of managers in the two boroughs. However, it is believed that including this group provided further insights on possible factors that affect the implementation of MHBC interventions.

Conclusion

This study has identified several factors that may restrict the effective implementation of MHBC interventions for cardiovascular risk reduction. The implementation of MHBC interventions should be facilitated by the provision of suitable training in behaviour change techniques and specific approaches to very brief behaviour change interventions. Healthcare professionals should be supported with easy, efficient and effective guidance to implement MHBC interventions given limited resources. The use of technology-based interventions to facilitate behaviour change could also be considered. Greater emphasis on promoting behaviour change through supportive environments and external lifestyle services may improve behaviour change outcomes.

Abbreviations

CVD: Cardiovascular disease; GP: General practitioner; HCA: Healthcare assistant; HCP: Healthcare professional; MHBC: Multiple health behaviour change; NHS: National Health Services.; NHSHC: National Health Services Health Check; TDF: Theoretical Domains Framework

Acknowledgement
The authors would like to thank all participants for their participation in this study.

Funding
This work was supported by the National Institute for Health Research (NIHR) Biomedical Research Centre at Guy's and St Thomas' NHS Foundation Trust and King's College London. SA was supported by the Government of Saudi Arabia. The funders of the study had no role in study design, data collection, data analysis, data interpretation, or writing of the report.

Authors' contributions
SA, AW and MG conceptualized and designed the study. SA collected and analysed the data. AW and LM contributed to the coding and interpretation of the data. SA wrote the first draft of the manuscript. All authors contributed to the refinement of the manuscript. All authors read and approved the final manuscript.

Consent for publication
Not applicable.

Competing interests
The authors declare that they have no competing interests.

References

1. Alageel S, Gulliford MC, McDermott L, Wright AJ. Multiple health behaviour change interventions for primary prevention of cardiovascular disease in primary care: systematic review and meta-analysis. BMJ Open. 2017;7(6): e015375.
2. Ebrahim S, Taylor F, Ward K, Beswick A, Burke M, Davey Smith G. Multiple risk factor interventions for primary prevention of coronary heart disease. Cochrane Libr. 2011;1(1):CD001561.
3. Krogsbøll LT, Jørgensen KJ, Larsen CG, Gøtzsche PC. General health checks in adults for reducing morbidity and mortality from disease: Cochrane systematic review and meta-analysis. BMJ. 2012;345:e7191.
4. Public Health England. NHS Health Check: Best practic guidance. http://www.healthcheck.nhs.uk/commissioners_and_providers/guidance/national_guidance1/. Accessed 15 September 2017.
5. Nicholas JM, Burgess C, Dodhia H, Miller J, Fuller F, Cajeat E, Gulliford MC. Variations in the organization and delivery of the 'NHS health check'in primary care. Journal of Public Health. 2012;35(1):85–91.
6. McNaughton R, Shucksmith J. Reasons for (non) compliance with intervention following identification of 'high-risk'status in the NHS health check programme. Journal of Public Health. 2014;37(2):218–25.
7. Shaw RL, Pattison HM, Holland C, Cooke R, Be SMART. Examining the experience of implementing the NHS health check in UK primary care. BMC Fam Pract. 2015;16(1):1.
8. Riley R, Coghill N, Montgomery A, Feder G, Horwood J. Experiences of patients and healthcare professionals of NHS cardiovascular health checks: a qualitative study. Journal of Public Health. 2016;38(3):543–51.
9. Krska J, du Plessis R, Chellaswamy H. Views and experiences of the NHS health check provided by general medical practices: cross-sectional survey in high-risk patients. Journal of Public Health. 2014;37(2):210–7.
10. Eccles M, Grimshaw J, Walker A, Johnston M, Pitts N. Changing the behavior of healthcare professionals: the use of theory in promoting the uptake of research findings. J Clin Epidemiol. 2005;58(2):107–12.
11. Godin G, Bélanger-Gravel A, Eccles M, Grimshaw J. Healthcare professionals' intentions and behaviours: a systematic review of studies based on social cognitive theories. Implement Sci. 2008;3(1):36.
12. Francis JJ, Stockton C, Eccles MP, Johnston M, Cuthbertson BH, Grimshaw JM, Hyde C, Tinmouth A, Stanworth SJ. Evidence-based selection of theories for designing behaviour change interventions: using methods based on theoretical construct domains to understand clinicians' blood transfusion behaviour. Br J Health Psychol. 2009;14(4):625–46.
13. Cane J, O'Connor D, Michie S. Validation of the theoretical domains framework for use in behaviour change and implementation research. Implement Sci. 2012;7(1):37.
14. Michie S, Johnston M, Abraham C, Lawton R, Parker D, Walker A. Making psychological theory useful for implementing evidence based practice: a consensus approach. BMJ Quality & Safety. 2005;14(1):26–33.
15. Beenstock J, Sniehotta FF, White M, Bell R, Milne EM, Araujo-Soares V. What helps and hinders midwives in engaging with pregnant women about stopping smoking? A cross-sectional survey of perceived implementation difficulties among midwives in the north east of England. Implement Sci. 2012;7(1):36.
16. Bussières AE, Patey AM, Francis JJ, Sales AE, Grimshaw JM. Identifying factors likely to influence compliance with diagnostic imaging guideline recommendations for spine disorders among chiropractors in North America: a focus group study using the theoretical domains framework. Implement Sci. 2012;7(1):82.
17. Islam R, Tinmouth AT, Francis JJ, Brehaut JC, Born J, Stockton C, Stanworth SJ, Eccles MP, Cuthbertson BH, Hyde C. A cross-country comparison of intensive care physicians' beliefs about their transfusion behaviour: a qualitative study using the theoretical domains framework. Implement Sci. 2012;7(1):93.
18. Public Health England Data - People taking up an NHS Health Check invite. https://fingertips.phe.org.uk/profile/nhs-health-check-detailed/data#page/3/gid/1938132726/pat/6/par/E12000007/ati/102/are/E09000022/iid/91116/age/219/sex/4. Accessed October 2017.
19. Public Health in Lambeth and Southwark http://moderngov.southwarksites.com/documents/s59342/Appendix%201%20Public%20Health%20Report.pdf. Accessed 20 October 2017.
20. Lewisham Clinical Commissioning Group Public Sector Equality Duty Annu Rep January 2016 – January 2017. http://councilmeetings.lewisham.gov.uk/documents/s33258/06B%20Reducing%20Cardiovascular%20Disease%20in%20Lewisham.pdf. Accessed 20 October 2017.
21. Reducing Cardiovascular Disease in Lewisham. http://councilmeetings.lewisham.gov.uk/documents/s33258/06B%20Reducing%20Cardiovascular%20Disease%20in%20Lewisham.pdf. Accessed 20 October 2017.
22. Rubio-Valera M, Pons-Vigués M, Martínez-Andrés M, Moreno-Peral P, Berenguera A, Fernández A. Barriers and facilitators for the implementation of primary prevention and health promotion activities in primary care: a synthesis through meta-ethnography. PLoS One. 2014;9(2):e89554.
23. Ritchie J, Lewis J, Nicholls CM, Ormston R, editors. Qualitative research practice: A guide for social science students and researchers. London: Sage; 2013.
24. Atkins L, Francis J, Islam R, O'Connor D, Patey A, Ivers N, Foy R, Duncan EM, Colquhoun H, Grimshaw JM. A guide to using the theoretical domains framework of behaviour change to investigate implementation problems. Implement Sci. 2017;12(1):77.
25. Dyson J, Lawton R, Jackson C, Cheater F. Does the use of a theoretical approach tell us more about hand hygiene behaviour? The barriers and levers to hand hygiene. J Infect Prev. 2011;12(1):17–24.
26. Epstein L, Ogden J. A qualitative study of GPs' views of treating obesity. Br J Gen Pract. 2005;55(519):750–4.
27. Adams J, Mytton O, White M, Monsivais P. Why are some population interventions for diet and obesity more equitable and effective than others? The role of individual agency PLoS Medicine. 2016;13(4):e1001990.
28. Michie S, Richardson M, Johnston M, Abraham C, Francis J, Hardeman W, Eccles MP, Cane J, Wood CE. The behavior change technique taxonomy (v1) of 93 hierarchically clustered techniques: building an international consensus for the reporting of behavior change interventions. Ann Behav Med. 2013;46(1):81–95.
29. Olander EK, Fletcher H, Williams S, Atkinson L, Turner A, French DP. What are the most effective techniques in changing obese individuals' physical activity self-efficacy and behaviour: a systematic review and meta-analysis. Int J Behav Nutr Phys Act. 2013;10(1):29.
30. Webb T, Joseph J, Yardley L, Michie S. Using the internet to promote health behavior change: a systematic review and meta-analysis of the impact of theoretical basis, use of behavior change techniques, and mode of delivery on efficacy. J Med Internet Res. 2010;12(1):e4.
31. West R, Walia A, Hyder N, Shahab L, Michie S. Behavior change techniques used by the English stop smoking services and their associations with short-term quit outcomes. Nicotine Tob Res. 2010;12(7):742–7.

32. Asfar T, Ebbert JO, Klesges RC, Relyea GE. Do smoking reduction interventions promote cessation in smokers not ready to quit? Addict Behav. 2011;36(7):764–8.
33. Moore D, Aveyard P, Connock M, Wang D, Fry-Smith A, Barton P. Effectiveness and safety of nicotine replacement therapy assisted reduction to stop smoking: systematic review and meta-analysis. BMJ. 2009;338:b1024.
34. Krska J, du Plessis R, Chellaswamy H. Views of practice managers and general practitioners on implementing NHS health checks. Primary health care research & development. 2016;17(2):198–205.
35. Pears S, Bijker M, Morton K, Vasconcelos J, Parker RA, Westgate K, Brage S, Wilson E, Prevost AT, Kinmonth A-L. A randomised controlled trial of three very brief interventions for physical activity in primary care. BMC Public Health. 2016;16(1):1033.
36. Brandling J, House W. Social prescribing in general practice: adding meaning to medicine. Br J Gen Pract. 2009;59(563):454–6.
37. Green J, Thorogood N. Qualitative methods for health research. London: Sage; 2013.
38. Holbrook AL, Green MC, Krosnick JA. Telephone versus face-to-face interviewing of national probability samples with long questionnaires: comparisons of respondent satisficing and social desirability response bias. Public Opinion Quarterly. 2003;67(1):79–125.

20

Factors contributing to patient safety incidents in primary care: a descriptive analysis of patient safety incidents in a French study using CADYA (categorization of errors in primary care)

M. Chaneliere[1,2,3*], D. Koehler[1], T. Morlan[1], J. Berra[2], C. Colin[2,3], I. Dupie[4] and P. Michel[2,3]

Abstract

Background: Patient safety incidents (PSIs) frequently occur in primary care and are often considered to be preventable. Better knowledge of factors contributing to PSIs is required to build safer care. The aim of this work was to describe the underlying factors, specifically the human factors, that are associated with PSIs in primary care using CADYA ("CAtégorisation des DYsfonctionnements en Ambulatoire" or "Categorization of Errors in Primary Care").

Methods: We followed a mixed method with content analysis and coding in CADYA of PSIs reported in the ESPRIT study, a French cross-sectional survey of primary care. For each incident, a main contributing factor (MD) and, if applicable, a secondary contributing factor (SD) were identified. Several descriptive keywords from an incremental glossary have been suggested to describe each identified human factor (attitudes or behaviours). A descriptive statistical analysis was then conducted.

Results: Among the 482 PSIs reported in the ESPRIT study, from 13,438 acts reported by 127 participating general practitioners (GPs), we identified 590 contributing factors (482 MDs and 178 SDs). Overall, 35% were related to the care process, 30% to human factors, 22% to the healthcare environment and 13% to technical factors. The contributing factors, in decreasing order of frequency, were communication errors (13.7%), human factors related to healthcare providers (12.9%) and human factors related to patients (12.9%). The human factors were mainly related to 'lack of attention', 'stress', 'anger' and 'fatigue'.

Conclusions: Our results tend to prove that human factors are often involved in PSIs in primary care, with GPs and patients being equally responsible. Beyond the identification of communication errors, often found in other international research, we have described the attitudes and behaviours contributing to unsafe care. Further research exploring the links between working conditions and human factors is required.

Keywords: Patient safety, Primary care, Patient safety incident, Contributing factors, Human factor

* Correspondence: marc.chaneliere@univ-lyon1.fr
[1]Family Medicine Department, Université Claude Bernard Lyon 1, 8 avenue Rockefeller, 69008 LYON, France
[2]Hospices Civils de Lyon, 3 quai des Célestins, 69002 Lyon, France
Full list of author information is available at the end of the article

Background

Patient safety incidents (PSIs) have been reported in primary care under various names [1]. Fifteen years ago, the report 'To err is human' led to an international awareness of the frequency and gravity of PSIs [2]. In 2007 [3], the frequency of PSIs in primary care was estimated to be from 2 to 240 incidents per 1000 encounters, and 45–76% were considered to be preventable. The wide range in PSI frequencies can be explained by the type of study (prospective or retrospective), the data collection methods, the multiple proposed definitions of PSIs and the trend of underreporting [3, 4]. In France, two prospective studies [5, 6] have estimated the frequency of PSIs in primary care to be between 0.5 and 1 event per day per general practitioner (GP). PSIs in the primary care setting significantly differ from those in hospitals [7–9] regarding their contributing factors [10]. To classify PSIs, several taxonomies, both specific and not specific to primary care, exist [11–18]. The World Health Organization (WHO) classification [18] is the most universal, but the consequent number of items that compose this taxonomy limits its current use. The first results of the French national survey on PSIs in primary care (ESPRIT) study [5] were based on the Threats to Australian Patient Safety (TAPS) version of the International Taxonomy of Medical Error in Primary Care [12] (ITME-PC) and the Tempos classification [14]. The TAPS Taxonomy [12] describes the nature of the incident according to 2 main types of errors: errors related to the care process with 5 sublevels and errors of knowledge or skills of the actors with 2 sublevels (diagnosis and patient management). The Tempos classification [14] uses time in classifying factors contributing to incidents according to five categories: the tempo of illness and treatment, the tempo of the physician, the tempo of the office, the tempo of the patient and the tempo of the health system. CADYA (Additional file 1: Appendix S1), which can be translated as Categorization of Errors in Primary Care, is a French taxonomy [17] that provides a complementary approach by describing more accurately the factors contributing to PSIs, especially the human factors, as suggested by research in aeronautics [19]. Four main levels are explored: technical factors, the environment (action background), processes related to the decision or care process (skills), and human factors (physical conditions, psycho-relational elements, attitudes or behaviours).

The main objective of the present study was to describe the incidents of the ESPRIT study [5] using the CADYA taxonomy to have better knowledge of their contributing factors.

Methods

A mixed method approach, combining qualitative analysis (content analysis) and quantitative analysis (descriptive analysis), has been used. Because the work is based on the results of the ESPRIT study [5], we only present the most relevant methodological elements.

ESPRIT study's methodological aspects

The ESPRIT study [5] was a cross-sectional study. Its aim was to describe the incidence and nature of PSIs in primary care general practice settings. The incidence was defined as the ratio of the number of medical encounters (or patient contacts) with one PSI and the total number of medical encounters included during the study period.

The target population was all of the patients seen or contacted by GPs working in France. The source population in the ESPRIT study [5] was composed of all of the patients seen or contacted by a GP from the GROG (Groupes régionaux d'observation de la grippe). The GROG was a nationwide network for influenza surveillance in France that included more than 800 volunteer GPs. The GROG was considered sufficiently representative of the French GPs to support several epidemiological studies in general practice in France and Europe. The sample was composed of GPs that were randomly selected from the GROG physicians. A minimum sample size of 120 GPs, with a gender distribution consistent with the national distribution (70 men and 50 women), was achieved. The GPs were invited to participate in the study by telephone. The GROG coordination team trained all participating GPs on the study protocol and on the data collection method by phone and by a written procedure sent by mail. A specific training on PSIs in primary care was also provided by phone or by web with a video (available on the study website). The aim was to ensure that all GPs had a same understanding of what constituted an incident to be reported in an effort to reduce the selection bias and reporting bias.

Data collection method

Data collection for each GP occurred for one week, which was chosen by the GP within the six-week data collection period from May 2013–June 2013. The definition of an incident was proposed by focus groups and approved by consensus among primary care experts and GP representatives. An incident was defined as "an event or circumstance that could have resulted, or did result, in harm to a patient, and which should not be repeated again" [20]. An "act" was defined as any patient contact, including a consultation, visit, or intervention, in a nursing home or by telephone. Participating GPs completed a daily PSI reporting webform throughout the data collection period. That form was developed by the ESPRIT study expert group after a literature review. Three forms were used: a GP profile form, a register of acts (all acts during the collection week) and a PSI reporting form containing 25 questions capturing a description of each PSI along with contributing factors and consequences. The data that were collected were compiled on a secure website; data quality was reviewed by an expert group (eight GPs competent in the patient safety field and two epidemiologists). At the end of the data collection process, each reported event was reviewed during an expert group seminar to verify the situation as a PSI. The data quality control process was thus carried out in several stages.

Ethical aspects

No nominative, sensitive or personal health data concerning patients were systematically collected. The ESPRIT study [5] was therefore not, strictly speaking, in the field of biomedical research (fields of application of the French reference methodology MR 001), nor was it within the framework of Chapter X of the French Data Protection Act. For this practice-oriented study, the only nominative data collected were GP profile data that were available in a database declared to the French CNIL (number 1684220). GPs provided their written informed consent to participate by email. The National Council of the French Medical Association was also informed due to the indemnification of the participating GP. All ethical approvals of the study were given by the Ile-de-France Paris III committee and by the CNIL (French Data Protection Authority).

Work methodological aspects

Recruiting coders

Two GPs from the Family Medicine Department of the Claude Bernard University Lyon 1 (DK and TM) volunteered to analyse the ESPRIT study PSIs. An expert GP (MC) who was involved in patient safety in primary care trained the two recruiting coders to reach a shared understanding of, and a similar level of expertise on, the root cause analysis and the use of CADYA.

Coding process

All of the PSIs related to a patient were extracted from the ESPRIT study database. For each PSI, the investigators were required to independently search for the underlying factors contributing to their occurrence according to a qualitative approach (content analysis). Then, the investigators had to select a main contributing factor (MD), called "dysfunction" in French, and, if relevant, a secondary contributing factor (SD) in CADYA [17]. The choice between designating the factor as a MD or SD depended on the estimated impact of the contributing factor to the PSI. In the case of a factor related to a human attitude or behaviour, the investigators had to specify a keyword to describe its nature (e.g., "anger", "stress" or "tiredness") according to an incremental glossary (a keyword that was already identified, or, if necessary, a new keyword). The investigators had to describe the human factor with as much accuracy as possible. They regularly compared their coding after every 50 reports. In cases of disagreement, the investigators were required to reach a consensus. At the end of data extraction, all coding was approved by the expert GP (MC). The review of each investigator, the consensus and the expert final review were compiled into a single Excel® file. Finally, the investigators checked, for a second time, that there were no redundant keywords in the thesaurus. If necessary, they gathered redundant keywords into a single consensual keyword to obtain a reduced, but more precise, thesaurus.

Statistical analysis

Descriptive data analysis was conducted according to the dimensions of CADYA. The frequencies of agreements between the two coders and between coders and experts were estimated. The inter-rater reliability was analysed with a kappa coefficient [21], which was expressed as follows: (% observed agreement - % agreement due to chance) / (1 -% agreement due to chance). The interpretation of the calculated kappa coefficients followed the six classes by Landis and Koch [22].

Results

Main ESPRIT study results [5]

A total of 13,438 acts were recorded by the 127 participating GPs; 82% ($n = 11{,}023$) were office consultations, 8% ($n = 1090$) were telephone contacts, 8% ($n = 1022$) were home visits and 2% ($n = 303$) were visits at nursing homes. The GPs in the sample were older and worked more often in groups and more often in rural areas than the population of GPs in France (Table 1). The average number of patient encounters per day was 21. The average age of the patients was 48 years, and 4013 patients (30%) had a chronic or long-term condition.

A total of 694 events were reported by the participating GPs, 674 (97%) of which were reported as being related to a patient and 20 (3%) of which were reported as being not related to a particular patient. Additionally, of these 694 PSIs, 212 (31%) were not PSIs as defined. Thus, 482 (69%) PSIs were validated by experts, 475 (99%) of which were related to one patient and 7 (1%) of which were non-patient related (usually computer glitches affecting a whole range of medical encounters). Of these 475 PSIs, 52% occurred in the office, 37% occurred in patients' homes and 12% occurred in nursing homes. Additionally, 55% of the patients were women. The average age of the patients was 56 years (standard deviation: 25 years), with a range from zero years (four patients) to 100 years (one patient). Nearly half of the patients (40%) were retirees.

There were no clinical consequences for 73% of PSIs, and for 25%, there was a temporary disability. Only 2% of the PSIs were serious in the ESPRIT study ($n = 9$), being associated with a life-threatening or permanent disability (i.e., 0.07% of the 13,438 patient encounters observed in the study).

Table 1 Description of the participant GPs

Variables	Answers	French National Data	ESPRIT study data (%)	*p*-value
Gender	Men Women	66% 34%	60% 40%	NS
Average act per week		102	100	NS
Average age		51 years	54 years	< 0.05
Mode of practice	Solo Group practice	52% 48%	40% 60%	< 0,05
Area of practice	Rural Urban	15% 85%	17% 83%	< 0,05

General data

The investigators reviewed the 482 validated PSI reports. They excluded 74 incidents due to unpredictable adverse drug reactions (no identifiable contributing factors). Therefore, 408 reports were ultimately included for review. The investigators identified 408 MDs and 182 SDs (ratio of 0.45) for a total of 590 factors (TDs).

Frequency and nature of contributing factors

Table 2 shows the distributions of the MDs, SDs and TDs according to the CADYA items.

Table 3 shows some examples of the factors identified by the dimensions and sub-dimensions of CADYA.

Figures 1 and 2 show the distributions of the 590 contributing factors according to the main dimensions and sub-dimensions of CADYA, ranked in order of frequency.

Analysis of main contributing factors (Fig. 3)

The MDs were related primarily to the care process (39%), communication errors (14.5%) and cognitive aspects (13.8, 6.4% of which were due to training defects) and secondarily to environmental factors (22.8%) and human factors (21.8%). Regarding the environmental factors, the management of workload (5.4%) and the occurrence of a disruptive element (6.6%), such as a phone call during the consultation, were responsible for more than half of these MDs. Human factors were more often related to the patient (11%) than to the health professionals (8.6%). When these factors were due to a technical factor (16.4%), it was mainly related to issues in the information system (8.3% due to missing or incorrect data in the medical chart).

Secondary contributing factors (Fig. 4)

Almost half of the SDs were related to human factors (47.3%) and were linked more frequently to the GP (22.5%) than to the patient (17%). More than one quarter (27.5%) of the errors in the care process were identified as being from SDs, including communication errors (15%). Technical factors were still relatively low (4.9%), while those related to the environment (20.3%), including workload (6.6%) and place of care (4.4%), remained stable.

Nature of human factors

Overall, we identified 175 factors related to human attitudes or behaviours, divided similarly between MDs ($n = 89$) and SDs ($n = 86$), consisting of more than a quarter of all of the TDs (29.7%). These factors represented more than one-fifth of all MDs (21.8%) and almost half of all SDs (47.3%). In total, human factors related to either the GP or the patient constituted 87% of all the identified human factors (13% due to a third party and other caregivers). Figures 5 and 6 display the frequencies of keywords used to describe the human factors that are linked to the patient and to the GP, respectively. Table 4 shows a glossary of 15 keywords resulting from semantic harmonization by the investigators. Overall, 5 keywords represented 2/3 of all the human factors: 'lack of attention', 'stress', 'lack of involvement', 'nervousness' and 'tiredness'.

Reproducibility analysis

The levels of agreement between the investigators were 64.5% for the main dysfunctions (311 of 482) and 67.4% for the secondary dysfunctions (325 of 482). The kappa coefficient for agreement between the investigators at the first level of CADYA (main dimensions) was estimated to be 0.685, suggesting a strong agreement. The statistical analysis was completed with the calculation of the kappa coefficient for the agreement between the investigators and the expert. The result was 0.028, which corresponds to a very low agreement.

Discussion

Key results

If we consider the overall contributing factors, our results suggest that errors in care processes are frequent. As highlighted in other research, communication errors are indeed of primary importance. More remarkably, our analysis has identified several attitudes and behaviours that contribute to unsafe care. Those attitudes and behaviours regard both professionals and patients and could often be described with only a 15-word glossary.

Table 2 Distributions of the main (MD), secondary (SD) and total number of (TD) contributing factors

Dimensions	Main contributing factor *n* (% of MD)	Secondary contributing factor *n* (% of SD)	Total contributing factor *n* (% of TD)
ENVIRONMENTAL FACTORS	93 (22.8)	37 (20.3)	130 (22)
PATIENT'S SOCIAL CONTEXT	5 (1.2)	5 (2.7)	10 (1.7)
BACKGROUND OF CARE	38 (9.3)	20 (11)	58 (9.8)
Unplanned consultation	10 (2.4)	0 (0)	10 (1.7)
Place of care	6 (1.5)	8 (4.4)	14 (2.4)
Workload management	22 (5.4)	12 (6.6)	34 (5.7)
DISRUPTIVE ELEMENT	27 (6.6)	7 (3.9)	34 (5.7)
HEALTH SYSTEM	23 (5.7)	5 (2.7)	28 (4.7)
Healthcare service	20 (5)	2 (1)	22 (3.7)
Financial or administrative issue	3 (0.7)	3 (1.7)	6 (1)
HUMAN FACTORS	89 (21.8)	86 (47.3)	175 (29.7)
LINKED TO THE PATIENT	45 (11)	31 (17)	76 (12.9)
LINKED TO THE PROVIDER	35 (8.6)	41 (22.5)	76 (12.9)
LINKED TO OTHER PROVIDERS	4 (1)	7 (3.9)	11 (1.9)
LINKED TO A THIRD PARTY	5 (1.2)	7 (3.9)	12 (2)
TECHNICAL FACTORS	67 (16.4)	9 (4.9)	76 (12.9)
EQUIPMENT	21(5.2)	2 (1)	23 (3.9)
Failure, malfunction, unavailability	19 (4.7)	1 (0.5)	20 (3.4)
Incorrect use	2 (0.5)	1 (0.5)	3 (0.5)
INFORMATION SYSTEM	46 (11.3)	7 (3.9)	53 (8.9)
Incorrect or missing data	34 (8.3)	4 (2.2)	38 (6.4)
Failure of the communication system	12 (3)	3 (1.7)	15 (2.5)
PROCESS OF CARE	159 (39)	50 (27.5)	209 (35.4)
COGNITIVE DIMENSION	56 (13.8)	9 (5)	65 (11)
Lack in initial training	26 (6.4)	3 (1.7)	29 (4.9)
Incorrect recall (after training)	13 (3.2)	2 (1)	15 (2.5)
Incorrect synthesis	17 (4.2)	4 (2.2)	21 (3.6)
CARE PROCEDURE	34 (8.3)	14 (7.7)	48 (8.1)
Inappropriate or unachieved procedure	31 (7.6)	13 (7.1)	44 (7.5)
Lack of protocol	3 (0.7)	1 (0.6)	4 (0.6)
CARE COORDINATION	69 (16.9)	27 (14.8)	96 (16.3)
Communication failure	59 (14.5)	22 (12.1)	81 (13.7)
Lack of (or incorrect) monitoring	9 (2.2)	5 (2.7)	14 (2.4)
Lack of response after feedback	1 (0.2)	0 (0)	1 (0.2)
TOTAL	408 (100)	182 (100)	590 (100)

Process of care

Among the contributing factors related to the process of care, miscommunication between healthcare professionals constitutes a main source of errors, as suggested by several international studies [11, 23–25]. This result suggests the need to develop communication training for health professionals (students or graduates). 'Good communication skills' is one of the seven pillars of a safety culture according to Sammer et al. [26]. For that reason, we think that it may be useful to share some training programmes among all students across all health disciplines. The students could then better understand the mutual roles of all primary care professionals. Other actions should be implemented and evaluated, e.g., promoting learning via games and simulations during medical studies to develop relationship skills in healthcare. To train primary care professionals to better

Table 3 Examples of contributing factors by the dimensions and sub-dimensions of CADYA

Item	Examples of patient safety incidents (in the ESPRIT study)
ENVIRONMENTAL FACTORS	
Patient's social context	Elderly, suffering from dementia, unsuitable assistance plan
Background of care	
Unplanned consultation	A woman took an appointment just for herself and came with her son
Place of care	Incomplete medical examination because the patient was seen at home
Workload management	Workload increased by adding too many consultations
Disruptive element	Phone call caused the physician to dismiss his patient
Health system	
Healthcare service	A medical specialist was required but unavailable on weekends
Financial or administrative issue	No general practitioner declared to social security
HUMAN FACTORS	
Linked to the patient	Aggressive patient (who felt rejected by her physician)
Linked to the provider	Stressed physician (bad news needed to be announced)
Linked to other providers	Pharmacist distracted when dispensing treatment
Linked to a third party	Indiscretion of the mother of a patient regarding her daughter
TECHNICAL FACTORS	
Equipment	
Failure, malfunction, unavailability	Failure of the computer server
Incorrect use	Wound following the inappropriate use of pedicure equipment
Information system	
Incorrect or missing data	Lack of discharge letter after hospitalization of a patient
Failure of the communication system	Ultrasound result was unreadable over the internet
PROCESS OF CARE	
Cognitive dimension	
Lack of initial training	Ignorance of drug contraindication
Incorrect recall (after training)	Insufficient exploration of thromboembolic risk
Wrong synthesis	Minimization of a chronic kidney disease
Care procedure	
Inappropriate or unachieved procedure	Coronary patient who stopped the statin on her own
Lack of protocol	Medical appointment for an emergency assigned too late by the secretary
Care coordination	
Communication failure	The nurse did not call the physician despite an unusual dosage
Lack of (or incorrect) monitoring	Lack of specialized ophthalmic monitoring despite serious uveitis
Lack of response after feedback	Diabetes mellitus non-equilibrated, without medical appointment, for several months despite several blood tests

structure their communication (especially oral), some standardized tools such as 'SBAR' ('Situation-Background–Assessment-Recommendation') [27], which is already used in some hospitals, could be deployed. Patients should also play a leading role in their safety. They should have access to similar tools to better communicate with professionals [28]. If these standardized communication tools were implemented in primary care, such tools could reduce the number of PSIs [29].

Contributing factors related to cognitive dimensions have been more frequently identified as being MDs rather than SDs. This difference seems to be related to the importance of the cognitive processes themselves. Indeed, even a small error at this level can produce a diagnostic or therapeutic issue, sometimes serious [30]. This issue leads to more frequent identification as a MD. In the ESPRIT study [5], 17% of the PSIs were related to 'knowledge and skill errors' according to the taxonomy of Makeham [12]

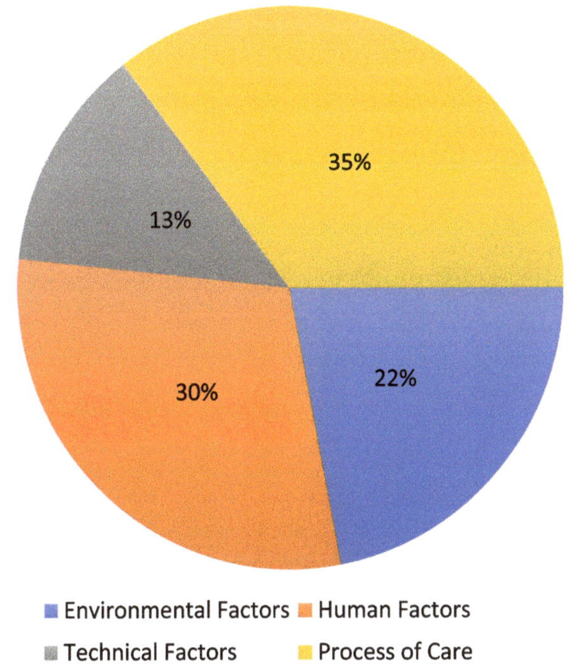

Fig. 1 Distribution (%) of the total contributing factors by the main dimensions of CADYA

and 30% to a 'lack of knowledge or skills' with the Tempos method [14]. Our analysis using CADYA is consistent with these results. As a consequence, to improve the quality and safety of primary care, it seems necessary to strongly promote the continuing education of all health professionals.

Missing or incorrect protocols constituted a marginal source of error in our research. However, GPs in the ESPRIT study [5] and, more broadly, French GPs do not write protocols in their daily practices. To explain the flaws in procedure executions, we must consider the independence in primary care of patients and professionals. The patient may choose to not take or insufficiently take the prescribed treatment, as shown by several studies [31], or they may defer an examination or new appointment. A health care professional may not always follow all of the guidelines, even if he or she knows that they exist. However, it is not necessarily a question of resistance to change [31, 32] but may be an evidence-based medicine approach [33]. Thus, decisions are also made in relation to the patient's expectations and wishes, as well as to the caregiver's context of care and representations.

Human factors

Unsafe attitudes and behaviours have frequently been found and may be due to the particular patient-provider relationship in primary care. In French healthcare, as in many countries, the patient chooses professionals with more freedom in the primary care setting than in the hospital. CADYA distinguishes cognitive processes from other types of human factors. Other tools, such as the ALARM method (Association of Litigation And Risk Management) [34], have included these human factors in cognitive or decision process levels. The literature does not provide a definitive answer as to which is the best option. CADYA has been designed for educational purposes, e.g., university trainings, where the identification of unsafe attitudes and behaviours of healthcare workers is important for the development of a proper safety culture.

Overall, analysis of the glossary of terms used to describe the nature of human factors (GP and patient) showed three main types of factors: first, those related to a physical or mental impairment (e.g., 'stress', 'extreme tiredness', 'worry', or 'distraction'); second, those related to a mental disorder (e.g., 'aggressiveness', 'extreme nervousness', or 'addictive disease'); and finally, attitudes of relatively conscious disengagement of individuals during care ('negligence', 'lack of commitment', or 'lack of compliance and absence of authority').

It is tempting to establish a link between some human factors, especially those designating impaired performances, with unfavourable conditions of care. The 'stress' of GP and the 'nervousness' and 'aggressiveness' of some patients were sometimes secondary to a significant delay in the schedule of the appointments. Currently, providers in primary care are often confronted with multiple, sometimes paradoxical, injunctions, e.g., 'to provide fewer appointments but with sufficient time to allow for patient-centred care' but also 'to open appointment access to have more consultations so that more patients can consult'. Therefore, human factors likely contribute to other factors, especially those related to cognitive processes.

Environmental factors: Importance of favourable care conditions

Two elements are quite significant: an inadequate management of the workload and the existence of a "parasitic" or "disruptive element". There is a wide variety of disruptive elements, including the interruption of the consultation by a third party in the office or by a phone call. The effect of this disruptive element is twofold. On the one hand, this disruption causes a break during the consultation, which can potentially alter the care provider's reasoning process (blackout). On the other hand, it can induce "human impairment", e.g., during the consultation, the GP answers the phone and learns of the death of a patient; this can induce a considerable emotional charge that is stressful for the healthcare provider. It seems logical, then, to limit the risk for disturbance during care, but there is a paradox: if they are unreachable or less easily reachable, the providers are less able to manage emergencies. In the ESPRIT study

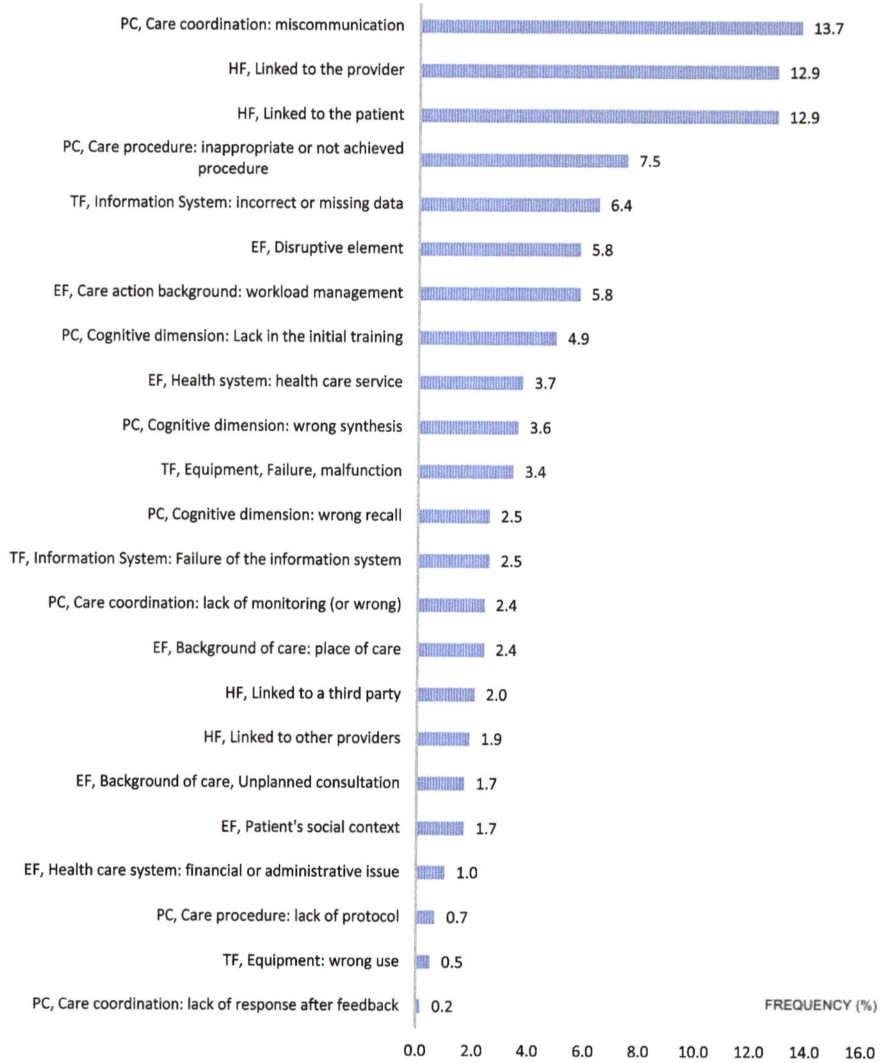

Fig. 2 Distribution of all the identified contributing factors in CADYA (% of the total number). Legend: PC: Process of Care; HF: Human Factors; TF: Technical Factors; EF: Environmental Factors

[5], unexpected emergencies were seldom identified because they were probably responsible for problems in the workload. This situation is consistent with the limited number of "true" emergencies in primary care [35] in modern health systems, where these acute events are ideally supported by dedicated services. To our knowledge, no study has specifically quantified the impact of an improvement in the environment of care on safety. However, this seems pragmatic, as it is known that anything that impairs communication within a team is likely to generate PSIs [36].

Technical factors: First, gaps in information systems

GPs perform a small number of technical acts, which is consistent with a rather low frequency of 'purely technical' errors. Moreover, with the development of communication technologies in the past twenty years, many doubt that this type of error is experiencing a substantial decrease. The widespread use of secured software (including prescription-assistance modules) and electronic patient records help to limit some errors (e.g., illegible handwritten prescriptions), but this has also contributed to other issues, e.g., common 'click' errors in medication lists.

CADYA

CADYA is complementary to the taxonomy of Makeham [12] and to the Tempos method [14], as it specifically explores processes related to medical decision-making and the unsafe attitudes and behaviours of actors. Regarding the main dimensions, the strong coefficient kappa between investigators argues for the robustness of CADYA.

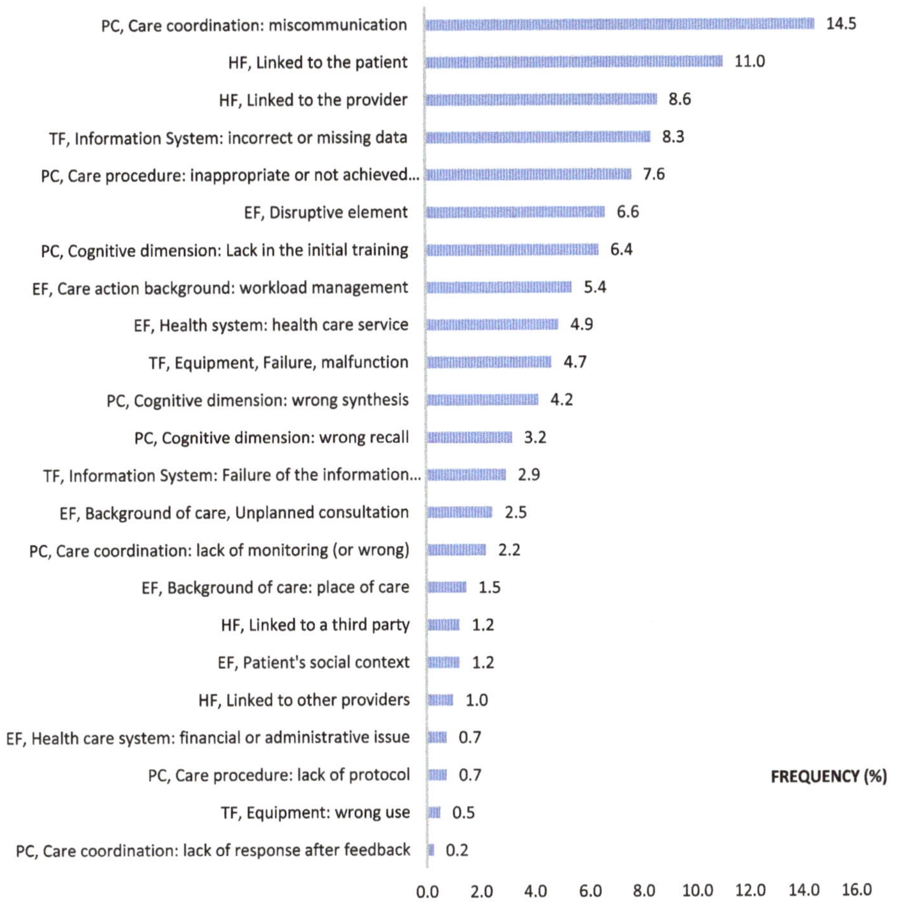
PC, Care coordination: miscommunication 14.5
HF, Linked to the patient 11.0
HF, Linked to the provider 8.6
TF, Information System: incorrect or missing data 8.3
PC, Care procedure: inappropriate or not achieved... 7.6
EF, Disruptive element 6.6
PC, Cognitive dimension: Lack in the initial training 6.4
EF, Care action background: workload management 5.4
EF, Health system: health care service 4.9
TF, Equipment, Failure, malfunction 4.7
PC, Cognitive dimension: wrong synthesis 4.2
PC, Cognitive dimension: wrong recall 3.2
TF, Information System: Failure of the information... 2.9
EF, Background of care, Unplanned consultation 2.5
PC, Care coordination: lack of monitoring (or wrong) 2.2
EF, Background of care: place of care 1.5
HF, Linked to a third party 1.2
EF, Patient's social context 1.2
HF, Linked to other providers 1.0
EF, Health care system: financial or administrative issue 0.7
PC, Care procedure: lack of protocol 0.7
TF, Equipment: wrong use 0.5
PC, Care coordination: lack of response after feedback 0.2
FREQUENCY (%)
0.0 2.0 4.0 6.0 8.0 10.0 12.0 14.0 16.0

Fig. 3 Distribution of the main contributing factors in CADYA (% of the total number). Legend: PC: Process of Care; HF: Human Factors; TF: Technical Factors; EF: Environmental Factors

The poor kappa between the investigators and the expert seems paradoxical. This result is explained by the paradox of Feinstein and Ciccheti [37]: with a similar level of observed agreement, the estimated kappa is lower when the symmetrical balance is perfect. Despite a very high level of agreement, we obtained an abnormally low kappa coefficient.

CADYA is used in France by several morbidity and mortality review groups [17] and was supported by the French High Health Authority. It was also used during specific trainings on patient safety at Claude Bernard University Lyon 1, especially in those on Family Practice.

In its first version, CADYA did not provide a glossary to describe human factors related to attitudes and behaviours, and users could use any descriptive terms they wished. However, this flexibility created a limitation for a more standardized use. In addition, some users regretted the absence of a glossary that would facilitate the identification of human factors. The Glossary of human factors constitutes a useful upgrade in the most recent version of CADYA. This version is currently being used as part of the ongoing PRisM national study, which is dedicated to the assessment of a multifaceted programme on risk management in primary care. A full and validated English adaptation of CADYA is in progress, following the recommendations of the WHO [38].

Strengths and limitations

Some limitations are inherent to the ESPRIT study [5]. The GPs were randomly selected within a network that was potentially biased towards reporting. According to us, this strategy was preferable to improve the number of PSIs reported by GPs and to have a better data collection quality. Yet, there is no indication that physicians enrolled in GROG are more concerned by issues related to patient safety. For that reason, we think that the findings - based on over 12,000 medical encounters - were not necessarily affected by this choice and the generalizability still remains acceptable. More than 200 events of the 694 incidents reported by GPs were deemed to not be PSIs by the expert group. This finding

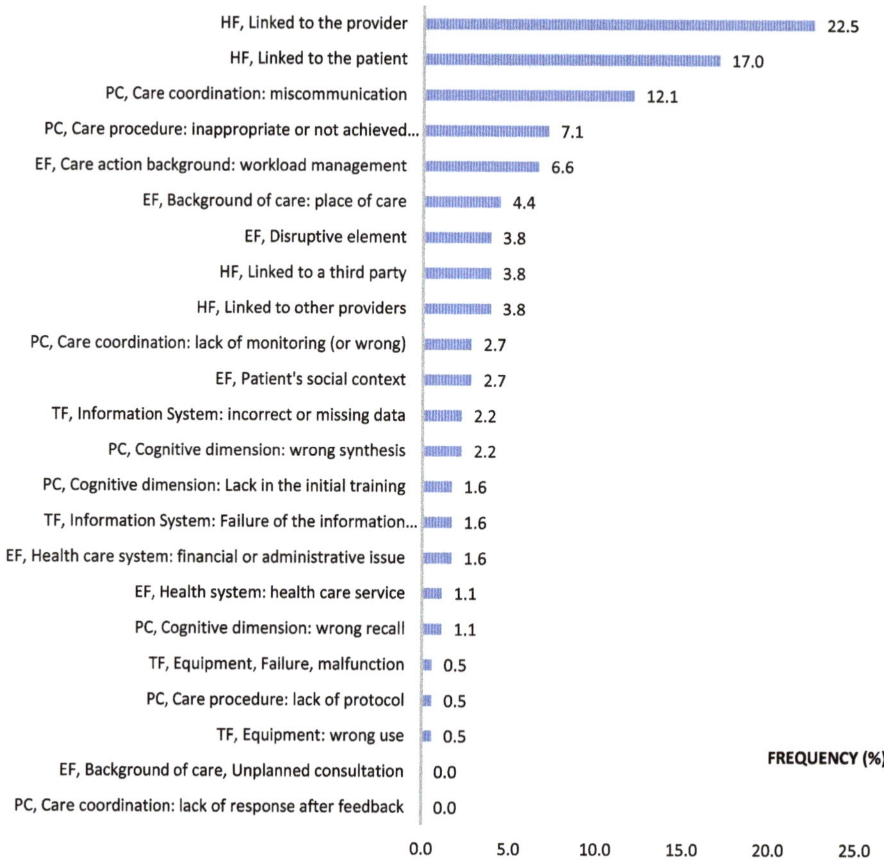

Fig. 4 Distribution of the secondary contributing factors in CADYA (% of the total number). Legend: PC: Process of Care; HF: Human Factors; TF: Technical Factors; EF: Environmental Factors

suggests that the level of understanding of the definition of PSI by participant GPs was not high, despite the time spent in GP training. This issue has been already described in previous studies [3, 4]. The main limitation of the ESPRIT study is that information on the patient health statuses remains limited. However, the literature on PSIs in primary care has already shown that factors such as an older patient age and an increased number of comorbidities have been associated with an increased risk for adverse events.

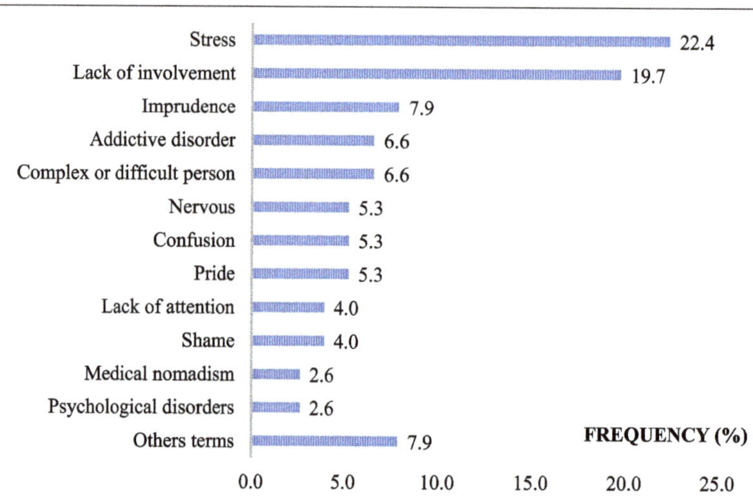

Fig. 5 Keywords used to describe the human factors linked with the patient, as ranked by the frequency of use (%)

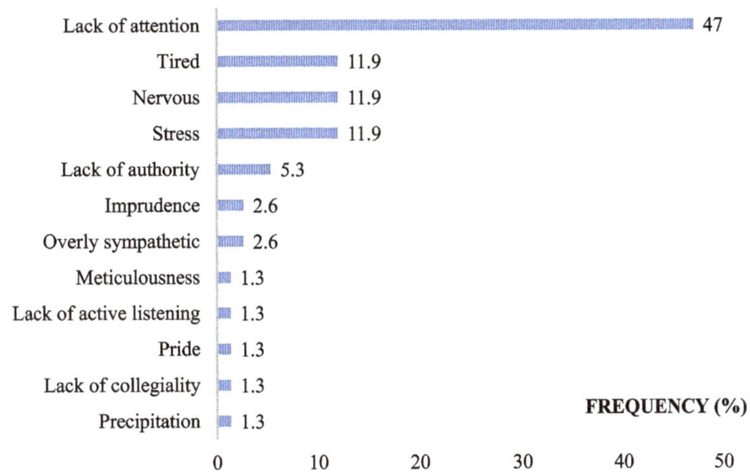

Fig. 6 Keywords used to describe the human factors linked with the GP, as ranked by the frequency of use (%)

Regarding our work, the coding of the PSIs was performed by only 2 investigators. However, they have been previously trained to use the CADYA grid, and they regularly compared their coding results. The lack of information in some clinical descriptions, as well as the absence of time constraints to code the PSIs, may have also constituted a subjective bias in coding. For that reason, an expert validated the consistency of all the codes. The number of contributing factors identified was consistent with the limited information reported by the GPs in the ESPRIT study [5]. Thus, the reported events have often been reduced to one sentence or a few words. The investigators were instructed to only consider information without interpreting it to limit the

Table 4 Keywords related to the human factor descriptions (glossary)

KEYWORDS AFTER SEMANTIC WORK	KEYWORDS IN THE STUDY	GLOBAL FREQUENCY OF USE IN GLOSSARY (% of all tags)
LACK OF ATTENTION	Lack of attention, Lapse in concentration, Absent-mindedness	27.5
STRESS	Anxiety, Stress, Anguish, Fear	15.5
LACK OF INVOLVEMENT	Lack of medical observance, Non-involvement, Refusing care, Lag (to consult), Lack of active listening	10.3
NERVOUSNESS	Anger, Irritation, Violence, Aggressiveness	8
TIREDNESS	Tiredness, Asthenia	5.7
IMPRUDENCE	Negligence, Clumsiness	5.1
COMPLEX OR DIFFICULT PERSON	Grouchy, Child-King, Claims	3.4
ADDICTIVE DISORDER	Addictive disorder	2.9
PRIDE	Self-love, Pride, Overconfidence, Vanity	2.9
LACK OF AUTHORITY	Lack of authority, Lack of bravery	2.2
MISUNDERSTANDING	Confusion, Misunderstanding	2.2
SHAME	Shame, Inconvenience, Shyness	1.7
PSYCHOLOGICAL DISORDERS	Psychological disorders	1.1
OVERLY SYMPATHETIC	Sympathetic, Overly empathic	1.1
IMPATIENCE	Impatience, Precipitation	1.1
OTHER WORDS	Falsehood, Medical nomadism, Impairment, Indiscretion, Meticulousness, Verbal comprehension issue, Personal emergency, Recklessness, Abusive request, Lack of collegiality	9.3
	TOTAL (%)	100

risk of bias. Finally, the glossary consists of only 15 keywords; our experience is that attitudes and behaviours can, most of the time, be described with these keywords.

Conclusions

PSIs are common in primary care, and research is needed to better understand them, as they differ from those in hospitals. We conducted an original study on a French national cohort of several hundred PSIs identified by GPs to describe their contributing factors. Our work confirms that, while there is a wide variety of contributing factors, the factors related to the process of care (in particular miscommunication) and the human factors related to unsafe attitudes and behaviours (e.g., stress, tiredness, etc.) represent major sources of PSIs.

We propose a 15-keyword glossary to describe these human factors. This glossary is applicable to all the actors, patients and caregivers alike engaged in care and can be useful in the initial training of medical students and in the continuing education of health providers. It remains, however, necessary to explore the links between these human factors and the working conditions of healthcare providers (e.g., the influence of the number of daily appointments and the influence of access without an appointment for patients), the patient's life context and the healthcare system to improve patient safety in primary care.

Abbreviations

ALARM: Association of Litigation And Risk Management; CADYA: CAtégorisation des DYsfonctionnements en Ambulatoire (or Categorization of Errors in Primary Care); CNIL: Commission Nationale de L'informatique et des Libertés; GP: General practitioner; GROG: Groupes régionaux d'observation de la grippe; ITME-PC: International Taxonomy of Medical Error in Primary Care; MD: Main contributing factor; PSI: Patient safety incident; SD: Secondary contributing factor; TAPS: Threats to Australian Patient Safety; WHO: World Health Organization

Acknowledgements

We would like to thank AJE for their contribution in the revision of the English version of this manuscript.

Funding

With respect to the ESPRIT study, funds were provided by the Direction Générale de l'Offre de Soins, from the French Ministry of Health. The funder had no role in research design, data collection and analysis, decision to publish, or preparation of the manuscript. No other funding was provided for this research.

Authors' contributions

MC, DK and TM contributed to the design of the research (extracting data, coding); MC, DK, TM, JB, PM, and CC contributed to the analysis of the results; MC, PM and ID contributed to the writing and revising of the manuscript. All the authors have approved the manuscript for submission.

Consent for publication

Not applicable.

Competing interests

Competing interests are limited to the membership of the authors (MC, PM, ID) on the ESPRIT study advisory board. The other authors have declared that no competing interests exist.

Author details

[1]Family Medicine Department, Université Claude Bernard Lyon 1, 8 avenue Rockefeller, 69008 LYON, France. [2]Hospices Civils de Lyon, 3 quai des Célestins, 69002 Lyon, France. [3]University of Lyon, Université Claude Bernard Lyon 1, Université Saint-Etienne, HESPER EA 7425 69008 LYON, F-42023 Saint-Etienne, France. [4]Société de Formation Thérapeutique du Généraliste, 233 Bis Rue de Tolbiac, 75013 Paris, France.

References

1. Schimmel EM. The hazards of hospitalization. Ann Intern Med. 1964;60:100–10.
2. Institute of Medicine. To err is human: building a safer health system. Washington DC: National Academies Press; 2000.
3. Dovey S, Makeham M, Runciman W, Larizgoitia I. Variation in safety incidents: a systematic review of primary care patient safety research 2007. http://www.who.int/patientsafety/research/methods_measures/makeham_dovey_full.pdf. Accessed 13 May 2018.
4. Elder NC, Vonder Meulen M, Cassedy A. The identification of medical errors by family physicians during outpatient visits. Ann Fam Med. 2004;2:125–9.
5. Michel P, Brami J, Chanelière M, Kret M, Mosnier A, Dupie I, et al. Patient safety incidents are common in primary care: a national prospective active incident reporting survey. PLoS One. 2017;12:e0165455. https://doi.org/10.1371/journal.pone.0165455.
6. Chaneliere M, Proboeuf T, Letrilliart L, Zerbib Y, Colin C. La iatrogénie observée en médecine générale. Exercer. 2014;114:173–80.
7. Michel P, Lathelize M, Quenon JL, Bru-Sonnet R, Domecq S, Kret M. Comparaison des deux Etudes Nationales sur les Evénements Indésirables graves liés aux Soins menées en 2004 et 2009. Rapport final à la DREES (Ministère de la Santé et des Sports), Paris. 2011. http://drees.solidarites-sante.gouv.fr/IMG/pdf/serieetud109.pdf. Accessed 13 May 2018.
8. de Vries EN, Ramrattan MA, Smorenburg SM, Gouma DJ, Boermeester MA. The incidence and nature of in-hospital adverse events: a systematic review. Qual Saf Health Care. 2008;17:216–23.
9. Wachter RM. Is ambulatory patient safety just like hospital safety, only without the "stat"? Ann Intern Med. 2006;145:547–9.
10. Reason J. Human error : models and management. West J Med. 2000;172:393–6.
11. Dovey SM, Meyers DS, Phillips RL Jr, Green LA, Fryer GE, Galliher JM, et al. A preliminary taxonomy of medical errors in family practice. Qual Saf Health Care. 2002;11:233–8.
12. Makeham MAB, Stromer S, Bridges-Webb C, Mira M, Saltman DC, Cooper C, et al. Patient safety events reported in general practice: a taxonomy. Qual Saf Health Care. 2008;17:53–7.
13. Fernald DH, Pace WD, Harris DM, West DR, Main DS, Westfall JM. Event reporting to a primary care patient safety reporting system: a report from the ASIPS collaborative. Ann Fam Med. 2004;2:327–32.
14. Amalberti R, Brami J. 'Tempos' management in primary care: a key factor for classifying adverse events, and improving quality and safety. BMJ Qual Saf. 2012;21:729–36.
15. Kostopoulou O, Delaney B. Confidential reporting of patient safety events in primary care: results from a multilevel classification of cognitive and system factors. Qual Saf Health Care. 2007;16:95–100.
16. Rubin G, George A, Chinn DJ, Richardson C. Errors in general practice: development of an error classification and pilot study of a method for detecting errors. Qual Saf Health Care. 2003;12:443–7.
17. Chanelière M, Oriol J-M, Senez B, Keriel-Gascou M, Fanjat H, Blanc M-D, et al. Un outil pour analyser des incidents en soins primaires. Risqual. 2014;12:34–40.

18. World Alliance For Patient Safety Drafting Group. Sherman H, Castro G, fletcher M; world alliance for patient safety, Hatlie M, Hibbert P, Jakob R, Koss R, Lewalle P, Loeb J, Perneger T, Runciman W, Thomson R, van Der Schaaf T, Virtanen M. Towards an international classification for patient safety: the conceptual framework. Int J Qual Health Care. 2009 Feb;21(1):2–8.
19. Wilf-Miron R, Lewenhoff I, Benyamini Z, Aviram A. From aviation to medicine: applying concepts of aviation safety to risk management in ambulatory care. Qual Saf Health Care. 2003;12:35–9.
20. Keriel-Gascou M, Brami J, Chanelière M, Haeringer-cholet A, Larrieu C, Villebrun F, et al. Définition et Taxonomie pour une étude épidémiologique Française sur les événements indésirables associés aux soins primaires. Rev Epidemiol S Publ. 2014;62:41–52.
21. Cohen J. A coefficient of agreement for nominal scales. Educ Psychol Meas. 1960;20:37–46.
22. Landis JR, Koch GG. The measurement of observer agreement for categorical data. Biometrics. 1977;33:159–74.
23. Kripalani S, LeFevre F, Phillips CO, Williams MV, Basaviah P, Baker DW. Deficits in communication and information transfer between hospital-based and primary care physicians: implications for patient safety and continuity of care. JAMA. 2007;297:831–41. https://doi.org/10.1001/jama.297.8.831.
24. O'Beirne M, Sterling PD, Zwicker K, Hebert P, Norton PG. Safety incidents in family medicine. BMJ Qual Saf. 2011;20:1005–10.
25. Rosser W, Dovey SM, Bordman R, White D, Crighton E, Drummond N. Medical errors in primary care: results of an international study of family practice. Can Fam Phys. 2005;51:386–7.
26. Sammer CE, Lykens K, Singh KP, Mains DA, Lackan NA. What is patient safety culture? A review of the literature. J Nurs Scholarsh. 2010;42:156–65.
27. Pope BB, Rodzen L, Spross G. Raising the SBAR: how better communication improves patient outcomes. Nursing. 2008;38:41–3.
28. Denham CR. SBAR for patients. J Patient Saf. 2008;4:38–48.
29. Raduma-Tomàs MA, Flin R, Yule S, Williams D. Doctors' handovers in hospitals: a literature review. BMJ Qual Saf. 2011;20:128–33.
30. Wachter RM. Why diagnostic errors don't get any respect–and what can be done about them. Health Aff (Millwood). 2010;29:1605–10. https://doi.org/10.1377/hlthaff.2009.0513.
31. Butler C, Rollnick S, Stott N. The practitioner, the patient and resistance to change: recent ideas on compliance. CMAJ. 1996;154:1357–62.
32. Mittman BS, Tonesk X, Jacobson PD. Implementing clinical practice guidelines: social influence strategies and practitioner behavior change. Qual Rev Bull. 1992;18:413–22.
33. Evidence-Based Medicine Working Group. A new approach to teaching the practice of medicine. JAMA. 1992;268:2420–5. https://doi.org/10.1001/jama.1992.03490170092032.
34. Vincent C, Taylor-Adams S, Chapman EJ, Hewett D, Prior S, Strange P, et al. How to investigate and analyse clinical incidents: clinical risk unit and association of litigation and risk management protocol. BMJ. 2000;320:777–81.
35. Pronovost PJ, Nolan T, Zeger S, Miller M, Rubin H. How can clinicians measure safety and quality in acute care? Lancet. 2004;363:1061–7.
36. Leonard M, Graham S, Bonacum D. The human factor: the critical importance of effective teamwork and communication in providing safe care. Qual Saf Health Care. 2004;13(1):i85–90.
37. Feinstein AR, Cicchetti DV. High agreement but low kappa: I. The problems of two paradoxes. J Clin Epidemiol. 1990;43:543–9.
38. Wild D, Grove A, Martin M, Eremenco S, McElroy S, Verjee-Lorenz A, et al. Principles of good practice for the translation and cultural adaptation process for patient-reported outcomes (PRO) measures: report of the ISPOR task force for translation and cultural adaptation. Value Health. 2005;8:94–104.

21

Association of general psychological factors with frequent attendance in primary care

André Hajek*, Jens-Oliver Bock and Hans-Helmut König

Abstract

Background: Whereas several studies have examined the association between frequent attendance in primary care and *illness-specific* psychological factors, little is known about the relation between frequent attendance and *general* psychological factors. Thus, the aim of this study was to investigate the association between being a frequent attender in primary care and general psychological factors.

Methods: Data were used from a large, population-based sample of community-dwelling individuals aged 40 and above in Germany in 2014 ($n = 7,446$). Positive and negative affect, life satisfaction, optimism, self-esteem, self-efficacy, and self-regulation were included as general psychological factors. The number of self-reported GP visits in the past twelve months was used to quantify frequency of attendance; individuals with more than 9 visits (highest decile) were defined as frequent attenders.

Results: Multiple logistic regressions showed that being a frequent attender was positively associated with less life satisfaction [OR: 0.79 (0.70–0.89)], higher negative affect [OR: 1.38 (1.17–1.62)], less self-efficacy [OR: 0.74 (0.63–0.86)], less self-esteem [OR: 0.65 (0.54–0.79)], less self-regulation [OR: 0.74 (0.60–0.91)], and higher perceived stress [OR: 1.46 (1.28–1.66)], after adjusting for sociodemographic factors, morbidity and lifestyle factors. However, frequent attendance was not significantly associated with positive affect and self-regulation.

Conclusions: The present study highlights the association between general psychological factors and frequent attendance. As frequent GP visits produce high health care costs and are potentially associated with increased referrals and use of secondary health care services, this knowledge might help to address these individuals with high needs.

Keywords: Primary health care, General Practitioners, Health Care Utilization, Health Services Needs and Demand

Background

Only a small proportion of patients account for large number of encounters to general practices [1]. Since these frequent attenders consume a large share of health care resources [2], many studies have tried to characterize them, particularly focusing on certain physical, psychological and social factors [3]. This cited literature review found, for example, a high illness level, low social support, unemployment or divorce to be associated with frequent attendance to general practices. Thereby, analyses of psychological factors were restricted to mental health disorders or, more generally, mental problems, which were an equally important factor for frequent attendance [3].

In general, studies analyzing health care use or, more specifically, frequent attendance often base their analysis on Andersen's Behavioral model. This model distinguishes predisposing factors, like general demographics, enabling resources like income or health insurance, and need factors such as perceived and evaluated illness level as determinants of health care use [4].

* Correspondence: a.hajek@uke.de
Department of Health Economics and Health Services Research, Hamburg Center for Health Economics, University Medical Center Hamburg-Eppendorf, Hamburg, Germany

This model has been modified several times including a version for health care use of vulnerable people [5]. The modified version of the model also refers to psychological factors as predisposing factors and include constructs, such as coping or self-esteem. Yet, despite that, little is known about the association of general psychological factors and frequent attendance in primary care. This is despite the fact that some previous studies indicated that general psychological factors, like satisfaction with life, self-esteem, self-efficacy, etc., might play an important role for a better understanding of frequent attendance in primary care. Thus, for example, a cross-sectional study showed that frequent attenders (109 frequent attenders at a general practice surgery) differed substantially compared to a control group (86 individuals) with regard to the personality trait of neuroticism [6]. Furthermore, another cross-sectional observational study (suburban teaching practice with 12,400 patients, UK) showed that frequent attenders ($n = 132$ patients) and controls ($n = 102$ age and sex-matched control patients) differed significantly in all considered dimensions of well-being, such as energy, emotional reactions or social isolation [7]. Another psychological construct associated with frequent attendance is perceived susceptibility to and severity of illnesses. These findings were made by a cross-sectional observational study conducted in Spain (public Health Centre in Granada, 236 frequent attenders and 420 controls, matched by sex and age) [8].

In addition, in a case control study (100 regular and 100 normal attenders; England) it has been shown that one reason of frequent attendance in primary care could be somatization [9], which is the presence of somatic complaints that cannot be explained by organic findings [10]. This stresses the importance of psychological dimensions of frequent attendance, as somatization is highly associated with psychological factors, such as negative affect or illness behavior [11]. More generally, as stated in a literature review, because different persons perceive identical organic symptoms completely differently, consultation rates do not only rely on need factors, but moreover on the way a person perceives his body and arising symptoms [12]. This means that frequent attenders might be characterized by certain character traits or general psychological constructs.

However, *comprehensive* investigations of well-established psychological concepts with regard to frequent attendance are missing. Therefore, the aim of this study was to determine associations of the well-established psychological factors of life satisfaction, positive and negative affect, optimism, self-efficacy, self-esteem, self-regulation, as well as perceived stress with frequent attendance in a population-based sample of Germans aged 40 and older. Consequently, the present study adds new insights into the relation between general psychological factors and frequent attendance. Unlike other studies, general psychological factors were used and data were gathered from a large representative sample of individuals in the second half of life. Knowing psychological factors associated with frequent attendance might help to address these individuals with high needs.

Subjective well-being (positive and negative affect, and life satisfaction) were included in our study because it has been demonstrated that it is associated with health-related behavior [13], which in turn is related to frequent attendance. Furthermore, it has been shown that stress [14] as well as optimism [15] are positively associated with neuroticism, which is known to be associated with an increase in health care use [16]. Therefore, these factors were included in our study. In addition, it has been found that optimism is related to physical and mental health [17], which is associated with frequent attendance [18]. Furthermore, it appears plausible that self-regulation is related to frequent attendance because individuals scoring high in self-regulation might be more willing to visit GP more often in order to achieve the goal of good health. Besides, individuals scoring high in self-efficacy believe in their skills to achieve goals. Consequently, they might believe that frequent physician visits are not required to reach their goals. Self-esteem was included in our study because individuals scoring low in self-esteem tend to be more anxious and had poor physical functioning [19] – factors that are associated with an increased likelihood of frequent attendance [20, 21].

Methods

Sample

Cross-sectional data were derived from the fifth wave (2014) of the German Ageing Survey (DEAS), funded by the Federal Ministry for Family Affairs, Senior Citizens, Women and Youth (BMFSFJ). The DEAS study is a representative survey among community-dwelling older adults (aged 40 and above). Since 1996, data were collected about social exclusion, income, occupation, health and various other issues. While more than 4,000 individuals have already been interviewed in former waves (response rate: 61%), about 6,000 participants from the birth cohorts 1929 to 1974 were interviewed for the first time in the fifth wave (response rate: 25%). In wave 5, 7,446 individuals filled out the drop-off questionnaire and delivered data on GP visits. Klaus and Engstler [22] provided more details with regard to the fifth wave as well as the sampling frame and sample composition. We focused on the fifth wave of the DEAS study as our main interest lay in investigating the association between frequent attendance and psychological factors such as self-regulation and perceived stress, which were only collected in this wave. Moreover, the exact number for all GP visits were solely reported in the fifth wave.

Dependent variable

To measure the number of GP visits in the drop-off questionnaire of the German Ageing Survey, individuals were asked whether (no; yes) and, if so, how often they had visited GPs in the past twelve months. In this questionnaire, the individuals should include house calls. Solely collecting a prescription was not considered as a visit in the drop-off questionnaire.

In main analysis, frequent attendance (=1) was defined as the 10% of patients with most frequent contacts (i.e. the number of GP visits was ≥ 10 in our study). This definition is in accordance with many previous studies [3].

To test the robustness of our results, highest quartile (GP visits ≥ 5) and the highest 5% (GP visits ≥ 12) were also used to quantify frequent attendance in additional analysis.

Independent variables: psychological variables

The widely used and well-validated [23] positive and negative affect schedule (PANAS) [24] was used to measure negative affect (emotions such as anger or fear) and positive affect (emotions such as joy or excitement), consisting of ten items (ranging from 1 = "very slightly or not at all" to 5 ="extremely"). The index score (1–5) for positive affect as well as negative affect was computed by averaging the score of the corresponding items (higher values reflect higher positive affect/negative affect; Cronbach's Alpha for the PANAS was .87).

The Satisfaction with Life Scale (SWLS) [25] which has very good psychometric properties [26] was used to assess life satisfaction (reflecting the cognitive evaluation of one's life as a whole). The SWLS consists of five items (ranging from 1 = "strongly agree" to 5 = "strongly disagree"). The higher the index score (1-5) is, the higher is the life satisfaction (Cronbach's Alpha was .86).

Brandstädter and Wentura [27] created the validated optimism scale (reflecting the perspectives about the future). The scale comprises five items, each ranging from 1 = "strongly agree" to 4 = "strongly disagree". An index score (1–4) was created by averaging the items (higher values representing higher optimism; Cronbach's Alpha was .84).

Perceived stress (reflecting the degree to which situations in one's life are considered as stressful) was quantified by using a scale which was developed by Cohen et al. [28]. The scale covers four items and the index score ranges from 1 to 5 (higher values represent higher perceived stress; Cronbach's Alpha was .70).

Schwarzer and Jerusalem [29] developed a scale to quantify self-efficacy (reflecting the ability that an individual has to do a certain action), with five items ranging from 1 = "strongly agree" to 4 = "strongly disagree". The higher the index score (1-4) is, the higher is the self-efficacy (Cronbach's Alpha was .75).

Based on the theory of selection, optimization, and compensation (SOC), self-regulation (reflecting the ability to withstand competing attractions) was assessed. The validated scale [30] has four items (1-5). The index value (1-5) was generated by averaging the items. Higher values correspond to higher self-regulation (Cronbach's Alpha was .78).

Self-esteem (reflecting the conscious feeling of self-worth and acceptance) was measured by the widely used and validated Rosenberg scale [31] which consists of ten items (from 1 = "strongly agree" to 4 = "strongly disagree"). An index score (1-4) was computed by averaging the items, with higher values reflecting higher self-esteem (Cronbach's Alpha was .84).

Independent variables: control variables

In addition to psychological variables, control variables were included, namely age, family status (married, living together with spouse, and others (married, living separated from spouse; divorced; widowed; never married), as well as employment status (working; retired; not employed). Furthermore, the region (West and East Germany), and individual log monthly net equivalence income in Euro (new OECD scale) was included. In addition, the number of physical illnesses (yes; no) such as cancer, diabetes, bladder problems, bad circulation or insomnia was included to measure morbidity (ranging from 0 to 11). Four lifestyle factors were also included. The days with alcohol consumption (e.g., spirits, long drinks, wine or beer) was used (daily alcohol consumption, and others (several times a week, once a week, 1 to 3 times a month, less often and never)). In addition, the smoking status (no; yes) and self-reported Body Mass Index (BMI) was included. Furthermore, physical activities such as hiking, soccer, swimming or gymnastics were assessed (at least once a week (daily; several times a week; once a week) vs. less than once a week (1-3 times a month; less often)).

There is evidence that frequent attendance in primary care is associated with depression.[7, 20, 21] Consequently, in additional analysis, the main model was extended by adding depression (1 if Center for Epidemiological Studies Depression Scale (15 items, 0-45) ≥ 18 [32]) to test the robustness of our results. Depression was omitted in the main models since it is correlated with the psychological factors.

Statistical analysis

First, bivariate comparisons between non-frequent attenders and frequent attenders were conducted using Chi^2-tests and independent t-tests for categorical and continuous data, respectively. Second, multiple logistic regressions were performed. The criterion for statistical significance was set at $p < .05$. All analyses were conducted using Stata 14.0 (StataCorp, College Station, Texas, USA). Since the general psychological factors are strongly associated with each other, they were included separately in the regression models.

More importantly, the main motivation why the general psychological factors were included separately in the regression models was to show that whenever one of these general psychological variables is available, future studies of frequent attendance should include this factor as explanatory variable. This is because we hypothesized that these factors are significantly associated with frequent attendance, after adjustment for a full set of potential confounders (e.g., sociodemographic variables, lifestyle factors and morbidity).

Results

Bivariate associations

Mean GP visits were 3.9 (±5.2), ranging from 0 to 120 visits. Median GP visits were 3. The highest quartile had at least 5 GP visits, whereas the highest decile had 10 or more GP visits. In addition, the top 5% had 12 or more GP visits (these results are not shown in Table 1).

Sample characteristics are displayed in Table 1, separated by status (non-frequent attenders vs. frequent attenders). Compared to non-frequent attenders, frequent attenders (= highest decile in GP visits) had a significant higher age, a lower income, a higher BMI and a higher number of physical illnesses. Moreover, frequent attendance was significantly associated with employment status, marital status, sports, and alcohol consumption, whereas it was not significantly associated with sex, region, and smoking status. Furthermore, frequent attenders had a lower satisfaction with life, less positive affect, higher negative affect, less optimism, less self-efficacy, less self-esteem, less self-regulation and higher perceived stress.

Furthermore, it is worth noting that psychological variables were associated from r = -.22 (self-regulation and negative affect as well as self-regulation and social exclusion) to .61 (life satisfaction and optimism as well as self-esteem and optimism).

Regression analysis: main analysis

The results of multiple logistic regressions (determinants of frequent attendance) are displayed in Table 2 (highest decile; main model), Table 3 (highest quartile; additional analysis) and Table 4 (highest 5%; additional analysis). In

Table 1 Sample characteristics, by status (non-frequent attenders vs. frequent attenders) ($n = 7{,}446$)

Variables	Non-frequent attenders ($n = 6{,}700$)	Frequent attenders ($n = 746$)	*p*-value	Missings (%)
Female (Ref.: Male): N (%)	3,385 (50.5)	399 (53.5)	ns	0.0
Age in years: Mean (SD); Range	64.1 (11.2); 40–95	67.8 (11.3); 40–93	<.001	0.0
Employment status: N (%)			<.001	0.0
Working	2,576 (38.5)	150 (20.1)		
Retired	3,549 (53.0)	505 (67.7)		
Not employed	572 (8.5)	91 (12.2)		
Married, living together with spouse (Ref.: Others): N (%)	4,745 (70.9)	460 (62.0)	<.001	0.2
Monthly net equivalence income in Euro: Mean (SD); Range	1,976.2 (1,415.1); 80–33,333.3	1,579.9 (828.3); 122.0–7,018.0	<.001	5.3
East Germany (Ref.: West Germany): N (%)	2,238 (33.4)	228 (30.6)	ns	0.0
Sports at least once a week (Ref.: Sports less than once a week): N (%)	3,693 (55.1)	331 (44.4)	<.001	0.0
Body-Mass-Index (BMI): Mean (SD); Range	26.7 (4.4); 13.2–55.8	28.5 (5.5); 16.4–60.9	<.001	1.7
Current smoker (Ref.: No): N (%)	1,178 (17.7)	122 (16.5)	ns	0.8
Daily alcohol consumption (Ref.: Less than daily alcohol consumption): N (%)	818 (12.2)	70 (9.4)	<.05	0.2
Number of physical illnesses: Mean (SD); Range	2.5 (1.8); 0–11	4.0 (2.0); 0–11	<.001	1.5
Life satisfaction (Pavot/Diener 1993): Mean (SD); Range	3.8 (0.7); 1–5	3.5 (0.9); 1–5	<.001	0.9
Positive affect (Watson, Clark & Tellegen, 1988): Mean (SD); Range	3.6 (0.5); 1–5	3.4 (0.5); 1.4–5	<.001	0.9
Negative affect (Watson, Clark & Tellegen, 1988): Mean (SD); Range	2.1 (0.5); 1–5	2.2 (0.6); 1–4.6	<.001	0.9
Optimism (Brandstädter & Wentura, 1994): Mean (SD); Range	3.0 (0.5); 1–4	2.8 (0.6); 1–4	<.001	0.3
Self-efficacy (Schwarzer & Jerusalem, 1999): Mean (SD); Range	3.1 (0.4); 1–4	2.9 (0.5); 1-4	<.001	0.4
Self-esteem (Rosenberg 1965): Mean (SD); Range	3.4 (0.4); 1.4–4	3.3 (0.5); 1.2–4	<.001	0.1
Self-regulation (Freund & Baltes, 2002): Mean (SD); Range	4.0 (0.5); 2-5	3.9 (0.5); 2–5	<.01	2.0
Perceived stress (Cohen et al., 1983): Mean (SD); Range	2.3 (0.6); 1–5	2.6 (0.7); 1–4.8	<.001	1.5

ns not significant, *N* number, *SD* standard deviation; Comparisons between the two groups were done using *t*-test and chi-square procedures

Table 2 Predictors of frequent attenders (0 = Non-frequent attenders; 1 = Frequent attenders; cut-off at the highest decile). Results of multiple logistic regressions[a]

	(1)	(2)	(3)	(4)	(5)	(6)	(7)	(8)
Independent variables	Frequent attenders	Frequent attenders	Frequent attenders	Frequent attenders	Frequent attenders	Frequent attenders	Frequent attenders	Frequent attenders
Potential confounders	✓	✓	✓	✓	✓	✓	✓	✓
Life satisfaction	0.79***							
	(0.70 – 0.89)							
Positive affect		0.87+						
		(0.73 – 1.02)						
Negative affect			1.38***					
			(1.17 – 1.62)					
Optimism				0.74***				
				(0.63 – 0.86)				
Self-efficacy					0.65***			
					(0.54 – 0.79)			
Self-esteem						0.74**		
						(0.60 – 0.91)		
Self-regulation							0.93	
							(0.79 – 1.10)	
Perceived stress								1.46***
								(1.28 – 1.66)
Constant	0.24+	0.34	0.07**	0.45	0.56	0.46	0.30	0.05***
	(0.05 – 1.19)	(0.06 – 1.75)	(0.01 – 0.41)	(0.09 – 2.24)	(0.11 – 2.92)	(0.09 – 2.42)	(0.06 – 1.59)	(0.01 – 0.25)
Observations	6,730	6,725	6,724	6,764	6,760	6,778	6,662	6,692
Pseudo R^2	0.110	0.107	0.110	0.110	0.111	0.107	0.104	0.113

[a]All estimations include age, (log) equivalence income, number of chronic diseases, Body-Mass-Index, as well as dummy-variables for sex, marital status, employment status, region, sports, alcohol consumption and smoking status as potential confounders. Odds ratios were reported; 95% confidence intervals in parentheses; ***$p < 0.001$, **$p < 0.01$, *$p < 0.05$, + $p < 0.10$. Life satisfaction (SWLS, Pavot & Diener, 1993); Positive and negative affect (PANAS, Watson et al., 1988); Optimism (Brandtstädter & Wentura, 1994); Self-efficacy (Schwarzer & Jerusalem, 1999); Self-esteem (Rosenberg, 1965); Self-regulation (Freund & Baltes, 2002); Perceived stress (Cohen et al., 1983). The Wald test was used to test the significance of each parameter

all multiple logistic regressions, we adjusted for age, (log) equivalence income, number of chronic diseases, BMI, as well as dummy-variables for sex, marital status, employment status, region, sports, alcohol consumption and smoking status.

Adjusting for several potential confounders, logistic regressions revealed that frequent attendance was associated with less life satisfaction [OR: 0.79 (0.70–0.89)], higher negative affect [OR: 1.38 (1.17–1.62)], less self-efficacy [OR: 0.74 (0.63–0.86)], less self-esteem [OR: 0.65 (0.54–0.79)], less self-regulation [OR: 0.74 (0.60–0.91)], and higher perceived stress [OR: 1.46 (1.28–1.66)], whereas the outcome measure was not significantly associated with positive affect and self-regulation.

When general psychological factors were *not* included in the regression model (i.e. only controlling for potential confounders noted above), it is worth noting that Pseudo R^2 was .106 (main model: highest decile), .102 (first additional model: highest quartile), and .119 (second additional model: highest 5%), respectively. When general psychological factors were included in the respective regression model, Pseudo R^2 values can be found in the Tables 2 to 4.

Regression analysis: additional analysis

Compared with our main model (Table 2), our additional models (Table 3; highest quartile) showed similar results in terms of significance and effect sizes. Contrarily, the association between being a frequent attender and positive affect as well as self-regulation became significant in this model specification. Furthermore, our additional models with a cut-off at the highest 5% (Table 4) showed similar results when compared with our main model. However, the association between self-esteem and the outcome measure became insignificant.

Moreover, our main model was extended by additionally controlling for depression. In terms of effect sizes and significance, findings were similar (please see Additional file 1, Additional file 2 and Additional file 3). However, the association between self-esteem and the outcome measure vanished.

Table 3 Predictors of frequent attenders (0 = Non-frequent attenders; 1 = Frequent attenders; cut-off at the highest quartile). Results of multiple logistic regressions[a]

Independent variables	(1) Frequent attenders	(2) Frequent attenders	(3) Frequent attenders	(4) Frequent attenders	(5) Frequent attenders	(6) Frequent attenders	(7) Frequent attenders	(8) Frequent attenders
Potential confounders	✓	✓	✓	✓	✓	✓	✓	✓
Life satisfaction	0.77***							
	(0.71 – 0.84)							
Positive affect		0.74***						
		(0.66 – 0.84)						
Negative affect			1.40***					
			(1.24 – 1.58)					
Optimism				0.70***				
				(0.63 – 0.78)				
Self-efficacy					0.64***			
					(0.55 – 0.73)			
Self-esteem						0.74***		
						(0.64 – 0.86)		
Self-regulation							0.82***	
							(0.73 – 0.92)	
Perceived stress								1.48***
								(1.35 – 1.63)
Constant	0.46	0.87	0.13***	0.86	1.16	0.85	0.73	0.09***
	(0.15 – 1.47)	(0.26 – 2.85)	(0.04 – 0.43)	(0.27 – 2.76)	(0.35 – 3.81)	(0.26 – 2.79)	(0.22 – 2.45)	(0.03 – 0.30)
Observations	6,730	6,725	6,724	6,764	6,760	6,778	6,662	6,692
Pseudo R^2	0.109	0.106	0.107	0.108	0.108	0.104	0.104	0.112

[a]All estimations include age, (log) equivalence income, number of chronic diseases, Body-Mass-Index, as well as dummy-variables for sex, marital status, employment status, region, sports, alcohol consumption and smoking status as potential confounders. Odds ratios were reported; 95% confidence intervals in parentheses; ***$p < 0.001$, **$p < 0.01$, *$p < 0.05$, + $p < 0.10$. Life satisfaction (SWLS, Pavot & Diener, 1993); Positive and negative affect (PANAS, Watson et al., 1988); Optimism (Brandtstädter & Wentura, 1994); Self-efficacy (Schwarzer & Jerusalem, 1999); Self-esteem (Rosenberg, 1965); Self-regulation (Freund & Baltes, 2002); Perceived stress (Cohen et al., 1983). The Wald test was used to test the significance of each parameter

Discussion

The present study aimed at investigating the association between frequent attendance in primary care and general psychological factors in a large, population-based sample of community-dwelling individuals aged 40 and over in Germany. In the main model (10%), negative affect is positively associated with frequent attendance, while positive affect is only close to reach the level of statistical significance. Negative affect is more closely related to, for example, physical complaints and perceived stress [33]. In addition, negative affect is associated with anxiety and depression, whereas positive affect with anxiety only [34]. Furthermore, it has been shown that satisfaction with life is associated with health-related behavior [13], which is linked to frequent attendance. Hence, our results appear plausible.

In our study, frequent attendance in primary care was positively associated with increased perceived stress and a decreased optimism. Both results might be explained by the fact that stress [14] as well as optimism [15] is positively associated with neuroticism which is related to an increased health care use [16]. Moreover, optimism generally affects physical and mental health [17], with an inferior mental health status being known to be a key characteristic of frequent attenders [18]. Yet as associations of optimism and frequent attendance persisted after controlling for depression status, considering optimism adds insights into the psychological characteristics of frequent attenders as an independent factor.

In our main model, self-regulation was not associated with frequent attendance. A possible explanation might be that individuals scoring high in self-regulation do *not* believe in the fact that *frequent* doctor visits are important for their functional status. Nevertheless, doctor visits and self-regulation might be correlated to some extent because patients with higher self-regulation might be more willing to visit the GP more often to satisfy the long-term goal of staying healthy. Yet, at high levels of physician visits, this association apparently disappears.

Table 4 Predictors of frequent attenders (0 = Non-frequent attenders; 1 = Frequent attenders; cut-off at the highest 5%). Results of multiple logistic regressions[a]

	(1)	(2)	(3)	(4)	(5)	(6)	(7)	(8)
Independent variables	Frequent attenders	Frequent attenders	Frequent attenders	Frequent attenders	Frequent attenders	Frequent attenders	Frequent attenders	Frequent attenders
Potential confounders	✓	✓	✓	✓	✓	✓	✓	✓
Life satisfaction	0.79***							
	(0.68 – 0.91)							
Positive affect		0.83+						
		(0.68 – 1.02)						
Negative affect			1.34**					
			(1.10 – 1.63)					
Optimism				0.74**				
				(0.62 – 0.89)				
Self-efficacy					0.71**			
					(0.56 – 0.89)			
Self-esteem						0.81+		
						(0.63 – 1.03)		
Self-regulation							1.05	
							(0.86 – 1.28)	
Perceived stress								1.37***
								(1.18 – 1.61)
Constant	0.14*	0.21	0.05**	0.26	0.33	0.23	0.13*	0.04**
	(0.02 – 0.94)	(0.03 – 1.58)	(0.01 – 0.37)	(0.04 – 1.79)	(0.05 – 2.37)	(0.03 – 1.72)	(0.02 – 1.00)	(0.00 – 0.29)
Observations	6,730	6,725	6,724	6,764	6,760	6,778	6,662	6,692
Pseudo R^2	0.124	0.121	0.123	0.123	0.123	0.120	0.118	0.125

[a]All estimations include age, (log) equivalence income, number of chronic diseases, Body-Mass-Index, as well as dummy-variables for sex, marital status, employment status, region, sports, alcohol consumption and smoking status as potential confounders. Odds ratios were reported; 95% confidence intervals in parentheses; ***$p < 0.001$, **$p < 0.01$, *$p < 0.05$, + $p < 0.10$. Life satisfaction (SWLS, Pavot & Diener, 1993); Positive and negative affect (PANAS, Watson et al., 1988); Optimism (Brandtstädter & Wentura, 1994); Self-efficacy (Schwarzer & Jerusalem, 1999); Self-esteem (Rosenberg, 1965); Self-regulation (Freund & Baltes, 2002); Perceived stress (Cohen et al., 1983). The Wald test was used to test the significance of each parameter

Frequent attendance in primary care was negatively associated with self-efficacy in our study. This appears plausible because individuals with high self-efficacy believe in their *own* capabilities to achieve aims. Thus, these individuals might think that frequent doctor visits are not necessary to stay healthy. In addition, frequent attendance in primary care was negatively associated with self-esteem in our study. This might be explained by the fact that individuals with a low self-esteem tend to be, e.g., more anxious, more maladjusted or had poor functioning [19]. These factors are in turn associated with frequent GP visits [20, 21]. In sum, while previous studies focused on (illness-) specific psychological factors, the current study extends this literature by a broader perspective on general psychological factors characterizing frequent attendance in primary care.

A major strength of our study was that data were gathered from a large, population-based study of community-dwelling individuals aged 40 and above in Germany. Furthermore, the general psychological factors were quantified using well-validated scales. In addition, we used different cut-offs to quantify frequent attendance, revealing similar results. Consequently, our results were robust against the definition of frequent attenders. However, this is a cross-sectional study and therefore the temporal relationship between psychological factors and the outcome measure cannot be assessed. In our study, self-reported GP visits in the past 12 months were used. Thus, a recall bias cannot be ruled out. Given the long recall period used in the current study, under-reporting is likely to occur. If this inaccuracy is associated with variables of interest (e.g., life satisfaction or negative affect), this bias might be somewhat stronger. However, it remains an open question whether variables of interest are associated with recall of GP visits in our study. In addition, generally speaking, this recall bias might be rather small [35]. However, future studies should use, as far as data are available, objective measures of health care attendance. Moreover, sample selection bias is a limiting factor of this study. Thus, it might be difficult to generalize our findings to individuals with subjective poor skills in the German language and individuals with low education. However, in total, the sample selection bias is supposed to be rather small [36]. In addition, our findings might not be generalizable to individuals living in institutional settings.

Conclusions

Beyond various characteristics related to the domain of in particular mental and physical health, frequent attenders of primary care setting can be characterized by various well-established psychological constructs. As frequent GP visits produce high health care costs and are potentially associated with increased referrals and the use of secondary health care services [37], this knowledge might help to address these individuals with high needs. Specific interventions are available to improve the provision of care for or to decrease the service use of these high users [38, 39]. Future interventions might additionally benefit from the insights into their psychological constitution and can identify these specific target groups better.

Abbreviations

BMFSFJ: Federal ministry for family affairs senior citizens women and youth; BMI: Body mass index; DEAS: German ageing survey; GP: General practitioner; OECD: Organization for economic Co-operation and development; PANAS: positive and negative affect schedule; SOC: selection, optimization, and compensation; SWLS: Satisfaction with life scale

Acknowledgements

None.

Funding

None.

Authors' contributions

AH, JOB, HHK: Design and concept of analyses, preparation of data, statistical analysis and interpretation of data, preparing of the manuscript. All authors critically reviewed the manuscript, provided significant editing of the article and approved the final manuscript.

Competing interests

The authors declare that they have no competing interests.

Consent for publication

Not applicable.

References

1. van den Bussche H, Kaduszkiewicz H, Schäfer I, Koller D, Hansen H, Scherer M, Schön G. Overutilization of ambulatory medical care in the elderly German population?-An empirical study based on national insurance claims data and a review of foreign studies. BMC Health Serv Res. 2016;16(1):1.
2. Von Korff M, Ormel J, Katon W, Lin EH. Disability and depression among high utilizers of health care: a longitudinal analysis. Arch Gen Psychiatry. 1992;49(2):91–100.
3. Vedsted P, Christensen MB. Frequent attenders in general practice care: a literature review with special reference to methodological considerations. Public Health. 2005;119(2):118–37.
4. Andersen R, Newman JF: Societal and individual determinants of medical care utilization in the United States. Milbank Mem Fund Q Health Soc. 1973;51(1): 95-124.
5. Gelberg L, Andersen RM, Leake BD. The behavioral model for vulnerable populations: application to medical care use and outcomes for homeless people. Health Serv Res. 2000;34(6):1273-302.
6. Westhead J. Frequent attenders in general practice: medical, psychological and social characteristics. JR Coll Gen Pract. 1985;35(276):337–40.
7. Heywood P, Blackie GC, Cameron I, Dowell A. An assessment of the attributes of frequent attenders to general practice. Fam Pract. 1998;15(3):198–204.
8. Bellon J, Delgado A, Luna JDD, Lardelli P. Psychosocial and health belief variables associated with frequent attendance in primary care. Psychol Med. 1999;29(06):1347–57.
9. Morriss R, Kai J, Atha C, Avery A, Bayes S, Franklin M, George T, James M, Malins S, McDonald R. Persistent frequent attenders in primary care: costs, reasons for attendance, organisation of care and potential for cognitive behavioural therapeutic intervention. BMC Fam Pract. 2012;13(1):39.
10. De Gucht V, Maes S. Explaining medically unexplained symptoms: toward a multidimensional, theory-based approach to somatization. J Psychosom Res. 2006;60(4):349–52.
11. Duddu V, Isaac MK, Chaturvedi SK. Somatization, somatosensory amplification, attribution styles and illness behaviour: a review. Int Rev Psychiatry. 2006;18(1):25–33.
12. Campbell SM, Roland MO. Why do people consult the doctor? Fam Pract. 1996;13(1):75–83.
13. Koivumaa-Honkanen H, Honkanen R, Viinamäki H, Heikkilä K, Kaprio J, Koskenvuo M. Self-reported life satisfaction and 20-year mortality in healthy Finnish adults. Am J Epidemiol. 2000;152(10):983–91.
14. Flett GL, Hewitt PL, Dyck DG. Self-oriented perfectionism, neuroticism and anxiety. Personal Individ Differ. 1989;10(7):731–5.
15. Scheier MF, Carver CS, Bridges MW. Distinguishing optimism from neuroticism (and trait anxiety, self-mastery, and self-esteem): a reevaluation of the life orientation test. J Pers Soc Psychol. 1994;67(6):1063-78.
16. Friedman B, Veazie PJ, Chapman BP, Manning WG, Duberstein PR. Is personality associated with health care use by older adults? Milbank Q. 2013;91(3):491–527.
17. Taylor SE, Stanton AL. Coping resources, coping processes, and mental health. Annu Rev Clin Psychol. 2007;3:377–401.
18. Williams ER, Guthrie E, Mackway-Jones K, James M, Tomenson B, Eastham J, McNally D. Psychiatric status, somatisation, and health care utilization of frequent attenders at the emergency department: a comparison with routine attenders. J Psychosom Res. 2001;50(3):161–7.
19. Leary MR, Tambor ES, Terdal SK, Downs DL. Self-esteem as an interpersonal monitor: The sociometer hypothesis. J Pers Soc Psychol. 1995;68(3):518-30.
20. Dowrick C, Bellon J, Gomez M. GP frequent attendance in Liverpool and Granada: the impact of depressive symptoms. Br J Gen Pract. 2000;50(454):361–5.
21. Menchetti M, Cevenini N, De Ronchi D, Quartesan R, Berardi D. Depression and frequent attendance in elderly primary care patients. Gen Hosp Psychiatry. 2006;28(2):119–24.
22. Klaus D, Engstler H: Daten und Methoden des Deutschen Alterssurveys. In: Altern im Wandel: Zwei Jahrzehnte Deutscher Alterssurvey (DEAS). edn. Edited by Mahne K, Wolff JK, Simonson J, Tesch-Römer C. Berlin: Springer; 2016:25-42.
23. Crawford JR, Henry JD. The Positive and Negative Affect Schedule (PANAS): Construct validity, measurement properties and normative data in a large non-clinical sample. Br J Clin Psychol. 2004;43(3):245–65.
24. Watson D, Clark LA, Tellegen A. Development and validation of brief measures of positive and negative affect: the PANAS scales. J Pers Soc Psychol. 1988;54(6):1063–70.
25. Pavot W, Diener E. Review of the satisfaction with life scale. Psychol Assess. 1993;5(2):164–72.
26. Glaesmer H, Grande G, Braehler E, Roth M. The German version of the satisfaction with life scale (SWLS). Eur J Psychol Assess. 2011;27(2):127–32.
27. Brandtstädter J, Wentura D: Veränderungen der Zeit-und Zukunftsperspektive im Übergang zum höheren Erwachsenenalter: entwicklungspsychologische und differentielle Aspekte. Z Entwicklungspsychol Padagog Psychol. 1994;26:2-21.
28. Cohen S, Kamarck T, Mermelstein R. A global measure of perceived stress. J Health Soc Behav. 1983;24:385–96.
29. Schwarzer R, Jerusalem M. Skalen zur Erfassung von Lehrer- und Schülermerkmalen. Dokumentation der psychometrischen Verfahren im Rahmen der Wissenschaftlichen Begleitung des Modellversuchs Selbstwirksame Schulen. Berlin: Freie Universität Berlin; 1999.
30. Ziegelmann JP, Lippke S. Selbstregulation in der Gesundheitsverhaltensänderung: Strategienutzung und Bewältigungsplanung im jungen, mittleren und höheren Alter. Z Gesundheitspsychol. 2006;14(2):82–90.

31. Rosenberg M. Society and the adolescent self-image. Princetion: Princeton University Press; 1965.
32. Lehr D, Hillert A, Schmitz E, Sosnowsky N. Screening depressiver störungen mittels allgemeiner depressions-skala (ADS-K) und state-trait depressions scales (STDS-T) eine vergleichende evaluation von Cut-off-werten. Diagnostica. 2008;54(2):61–70.
33. Watson D. Intraindividual and interindividual analyses of positive and negative affect: their relation to health complaints, perceived stress, and daily activities. J Pers Soc Psychol. 1988;54(6):1020-30.
34. Watson D, Clark LA, Carey G. Positive and negative affectivity and their relation to anxiety and depressive disorders. J Abnorm Psychol. 1988;97(3):346-53.
35. Bhandari A, Wagner T. Self-reported utilization of health care services: improving measurement and accuracy. Med Care Res Rev. 2006;63(2):217–35.
36. Schiel S, Knerr P, Dickmann C, Aust F. Deutscher alterssurvey (DEAS): methodenbericht zur durchführung der fünften erhebungswelle 2014. Bonn: infas; 2015.
37. Reid S, Wessely S, Crayford T, Hotopf M. Frequent attenders with medically unexplained symptoms: service use and costs in secondary care. Br J Psychiatry. 2002;180(3):248–53.
38. Bellón JÁ, Rodríguez-Bayón A, de Dios LJ, Torres-González F. Successful GP intervention with frequent attenders in primary care: randomised controlled trial. Br J Gen Pract. 2008;58(550):324–30.
39. Matalon A, Nahmani T, Rabin S, Maoz B, Hart J. A short-term intervention in a multidisciplinary referral clinic for primary care frequent attenders: description of the model, patient characteristics and their use of medical resources. Fam Pract. 2002;19(3):251–6.

Permissions

All chapters in this book were first published in FP, by BioMed Central; hereby published with permission under the Creative Commons Attribution License or equivalent. Every chapter published in this book has been scrutinized by our experts. Their significance has been extensively debated. The topics covered herein carry significant findings which will fuel the growth of the discipline. They may even be implemented as practical applications or may be referred to as a beginning point for another development.

The contributors of this book come from diverse backgrounds, making this book a truly international effort. This book will bring forth new frontiers with its revolutionizing research information and detailed analysis of the nascent developments around the world.

We would like to thank all the contributing authors for lending their expertise to make the book truly unique. They have played a crucial role in the development of this book. Without their invaluable contributions this book wouldn't have been possible. They have made vital efforts to compile up to date information on the varied aspects of this subject to make this book a valuable addition to the collection of many professionals and students.

This book was conceptualized with the vision of imparting up-to-date information and advanced data in this field. To ensure the same, a matchless editorial board was set up. Every individual on the board went through rigorous rounds of assessment to prove their worth. After which they invested a large part of their time researching and compiling the most relevant data for our readers.

The editorial board has been involved in producing this book since its inception. They have spent rigorous hours researching and exploring the diverse topics which have resulted in the successful publishing of this book. They have passed on their knowledge of decades through this book. To expedite this challenging task, the publisher supported the team at every step. A small team of assistant editors was also appointed to further simplify the editing procedure and attain best results for the readers.

Apart from the editorial board, the designing team has also invested a significant amount of their time in understanding the subject and creating the most relevant covers. They scrutinized every image to scout for the most suitable representation of the subject and create an appropriate cover for the book.

The publishing team has been an ardent support to the editorial, designing and production team. Their endless efforts to recruit the best for this project, has resulted in the accomplishment of this book. They are a veteran in the field of academics and their pool of knowledge is as vast as their experience in printing. Their expertise and guidance has proved useful at every step. Their uncompromising quality standards have made this book an exceptional effort. Their encouragement from time to time has been an inspiration for everyone.

The publisher and the editorial board hope that this book will prove to be a valuable piece of knowledge for researchers, students, practitioners and scholars across the globe.

List of Contributors

Jane Murray Cramm and Anna Petra Nieboer
Erasmus School of Health Policy & Management, Erasmus University, Rotterdam, The Netherlands

Mieke van der Biezen
Radboud university medical center, Radboud Institute for Health Sciences, IQ healthcare, Scientific Center for Quality of Healthcare, Nijmegen 6500 HB, The Netherlands

Michel Wensing
Radboud university medical center, Radboud Institute for Health Sciences, IQ healthcare, Scientific Center for Quality of Healthcare, Nijmegen 6500 HB, The Netherlands
Department of General Practice and Health Services Research, Heidelberg University, INF- Marsilius Arkaden, Im Neuenheimer Feld 130.3, Heidelberg 69120, Germany

Miranda Laurant
Radboud university medical center, Radboud Institute for Health Sciences, IQ healthcare, Scientific Center for Quality of Healthcare, Nijmegen 6500 HB, The Netherlands
HAN University of Applied Sciences, Faculty of Health and Social Studies, Nijmegen 6503 GL, The Netherlands

Abebaw Fekadu
Center for Innovative Drug Development and Therapeutic Trials for Africa (CDT-Africa), Addis Ababa University, College of Health Sciences, Addis Ababa, Ethiopia
Department of Psychiatry, Addis Ababa University, College of Health Sciences, School of Medicine, Addis Ababa, Ethiopia
Department of Psychological Medicine, Centre for Affective Disorders, King's College London, Institute of Psychiatry, Psychology and Neuroscience, London, UK

Medhin Selamu and Atalay Alem
Department of Psychiatry, Addis Ababa University, College of Health Sciences, School of Medicine, Addis Ababa, Ethiopia

Charlotte Hanlon
Department of Psychiatry, Addis Ababa University, College of Health Sciences, School of Medicine, Addis Ababa, Ethiopia
King's College London, Institute of Psychiatry, Psychology and Neuroscience, Health Services and Population Research Department, London, UK

Girmay Medhin
Aklilu Lemma Institute of Pathobiology, Addis Ababa University, Addis Ababa, Ethiopia

Tedla W. Giorgis
Federal Ministry of Health, Addis Ababa, Ethiopia

Crick Lund
Alan J Flisher Centre for Public Mental Health, Department of Psychiatry and Mental Health, University of Cape Town, Cape Town, South Africa

Martin Prince
King's College London, Institute of Psychiatry, Psychology and Neuroscience, Health Services and Population Research Department, London, UK

Ellen Keizer, Paul Giesen, Michel Wensing, Femke Atsma and Marleen Smits
Scientific Center for Quality of Healthcare (IQ healthcare), Radboud Institute for Health Sciences, Radboud University Medical Center, 6500, HB, Nijmegen, The Netherlands

Peter Bakker
Scientific Center for Quality of Healthcare (IQ healthcare), Radboud Institute for Health Sciences, Radboud University Medical Center, 6500, HB, Nijmegen, The Netherlands
Department of Primary and Community Care, Radboud Institute for Health Sciences, Radboud University Medical Center, 6500, HB, Nijmegen, The Netherlands

Maria van den Muijsenbergh
Department of Primary and Community Care, Radboud Institute for Health Sciences, Radboud University Medical Center, 6500, HB, Nijmegen, The Netherlands
Pharos, Centre of Expertise of Health Disparities, 3507, LH, Utrecht, The Netherlands

Marek Oleszczyk, Anna Krztoń-Królewiecka and Adam Windak
Department of Family Medicine, Chair of Internal Medicine and Gerontology, Jagiellonian University Medical College, 4 Bochenska St., 31-061, Krakow, Poland

Willemijn L. A. Schäfer and Wienke G. W. Boerma
NIVEL, Netherlands Institute for Health Services Research, 3500, BN, Utrecht, the Netherlands

Kirti D. Doekhie, Martina Buljac-Samardzic and Mathilde M. H. Strating
Erasmus School of Health Policy and Management (ESHPM), Erasmus University Rotterdam, Rotterdam 3000, DR, The Netherlands

Jaap Paauwe
Erasmus School of Health Policy and Management (ESHPM), Erasmus University Rotterdam, Rotterdam 3000, DR, The Netherlands
Department of Applied Economics, Erasmus University Rotterdam , Rotterdam 3000, DR, The Netherlands
Department of Human Resource Studies, Tilburg University, Tilburg 5000, LE, The Netherlands

Yogarabindranath Swarna Nantha
Non-Communicable Disease Clinic, Seremban Primary Care Clinic, Jalan Rasah, 70300 Seremban, Negeri Sembilan, Malaysia

Lei Hum Wee and Caryn Mei-Hsien Chan
Faculty of Health Sciences, Universiti Kebangsaan Malaysia, 50586 Kuala Lumpur, Malaysia

Bobbi Jo H. Yarborough, Scott P. Stumbo, Nancy A. Perrin and Carla A. Green
Kaiser Permanente Northwest Center for Health Research, 3800 N. Interstate Avenue, Portland, OR 97227, USA

Ginger C. Hanson
Johns Hopkins School of Nursing, 525 N. Wolfe Street, Baltimore, MD 21205, USA

John Muench
Oregon Health & Science University, 3181 S.W. Sam Jackson Park Road, Portland, OR 97239, USA

Stefan Bösner, Sonja Schwarm, Paula Grevenrath, Laura Schmidt, Kaja Hörner, Dominik Beidatsch, Milena Bergmann, Annika Viniol, Annette Becker and Jörg Haasenritter
Department of General Practice / Family Medicine, University of Marburg, Karl-von-Frisch-Str, 435043 Marburg, Germany

Liam G. Glynn, Fergus Glynn and Monica Casey
Graduate Entry Medical School and Health Research Institute, University of Limerick, Limerick, Ireland

Louise Gaffney Wilkinson
Southampton University Medical School, Southampton University, Southampton, UK

Patrick S. Hayes and Andrew W. M. Murphy
Discipline of General Practice, National University of Ireland, Galway, Ireland

David Heaney
Centre for Rural Health, University of Aberdeen, Inverness, Scotland

Souhel Flayeh Beneyto
Centre d'Atenció Primària Gran Sol, Gerència d'Àmbit d'Atenció Primària Metropolitana Nord, Institut Català de la Salut, Avinguda del Doctor Bassols, 112 - 130, 08914 Badalona, Spain

David Lacasta Tintorer
Centre d'Atenció Primària Gran Sol, Gerència d'Àmbit d'Atenció Primària Metropolitana Nord, Institut Català de la Salut, Avinguda del Doctor Bassols, 112 - 130, 08914 Badalona, Spain
Unitat de Suport a la Recerca Metropolitana Nord, IDIAP Jordi Gol. CAP El Maresme, Camí del Mig, 36 planta 4a, 08303 Mataró, Spain
Universitat Autònoma de Barcelona, Plaça Cívica, s/n, 08193 Bellaterra, Cerdanyola del Vallès, Spain

Josep Maria Manresa Domínguez
Unitat de Suport a la Recerca Metropolitana Nord, IDIAP Jordi Gol. CAP El Maresme, Camí del Mig, 36 planta 4a, 08303 Mataró, Spain
Universitat Autònoma de Barcelona, Plaça Cívica, s/n, 08193 Bellaterra, Cerdanyola del Vallès, Spain

Xavier Mundet Tuduri
Universitat Autònoma de Barcelona, Plaça Cívica, s/n, 08193 Bellaterra, Cerdanyola del Vallès, Spain

Enriqueta Pujol-Rivera
Institut Universitari d'Investigació en Atenció Primària (IDIAP Jordi Gol), Gran Via Corts Catalanes, 587, àtic, 08007 Barcelona, Spain

Francesc Saigí-Rubió
Facultyof Health Sciences, Universitat Oberta de Catalunya, Barcelona. Av. Tibidabo, 39-43, 08035 Barcelona, Spain

Stephanie Aboueid
School of Public Health and Health Systems, Faculty of Applied Health Sciences, University of Waterloo, 200 University Avenue West, Waterloo, ON N2L 3G1, Canada

Ivy Bourgeault
Department of Health Systems, Telfer School of Management, University of Ottawa, 55 Laurier Avenue East, Ottawa, ON K1N6N5, Canada

Isabelle Giroux
School of Nutrition Sciences, Faculty of Health Sciences, University of Ottawa, 25 University Private, Ottawa, ON K1N6N5, Canada

Ian Litchfield and Sheila Greenfield
Institute of Applied Health Research, College of Medical and Dental Sciences, University of Birmingham, Birmingham, UK

Paramjit Gill
Warwick Medical School - Social Science and Systems in Health, University of Warwick, Coventry, UK

Tony Avery and Kate Marsden
School of Medicine, Division of Primary Care, University of Nottingham, Nottingham, UK

Stephen Campbell and Katherine Perryman
Centre for Primary Care, Division of Population Health, Health Services Research and Primary Care, University of Manchester, Manchester, UK

Simon Schwill, Katja Krug, Frank Peters-Klimm, Gunter Laux, Joachim Szecsenyi and Michel Wensing
Department of General Practice and Health Services Research, University Hospital Heidelberg, Heidelberg, Germany

Jan van Lieshout
Radboud Institute of Health Sciences, Radboud University Medical Centre, Nijmegen, Netherlands

D. Koehler and T. Morlan
Family Medicine Department, Université Claude Bernard Lyon 1, 8 avenue Rockefeller, 69008 LYON, France

M. Chaneliere
Family Medicine Department, Université Claude Bernard Lyon 1, 8 avenue Rockefeller, 69008 LYON, France
Hospices Civils de Lyon, 3 quai des Célestins, 69002 Lyon, France
University of Lyon, Université Claude Bernard Lyon 1, Université Saint-Etienne, HESPER EA 7425 69008 LYON, F-42023 Saint-Etienne, France

J. Berra
Hospices Civils de Lyon, 3 quai des Célestins, 69002 Lyon, France

C. Colin and P. Michel
Hospices Civils de Lyon, 3 quai des Célestins, 69002 Lyon, France
University of Lyon, Université Claude Bernard Lyon 1, Université Saint-Etienne, HESPER EA 7425 69008 LYON, F-42023 Saint-Etienne, France

I. Dupie
Société de Formation Thérapeutique du Généraliste, 233 Bis Rue de Tolbiac, 75013 Paris, France

Emmy Derckx
Foundation for Development of Quality Care in General Practice, Tilburgseweg-West 100, Eindhoven 5652 NP, The Netherlands

Samah Alageel, Martin C. Gulliford, Lisa McDermott and Alison J. Wright
School of Population Health and Environmental Sciences, Faculty of Life Sciences and Medicine, King's College London, Addison House, Guy's Campus, London SE1 1UL, UK

Danielle M. Nash
ICES, London, Ontario, Canada
Department of Health Research Methods, Evidence, and Impact, McMaster University, Hamilton, Ontario, Canada

Amit X. Garg
ICES, London, Ontario, Canada
Department of Health Research Methods, Evidence, and Impact, McMaster University, Hamilton, Ontario, Canada
Department of Medicine, University of Western Ontario, London, Ontario, Canada
The Ontario Renal Network, Toronto, Ontario, Canada

Maureen Markle-Reid
Department of Health Research Methods, Evidence, and Impact, McMaster University, Hamilton, Ontario, Canada
School of Nursing, McMaster University, Hamilton, Ontario, Canada

K. Scott Brimble
The Ontario Renal Network, Toronto, Ontario, Canada
Department of Medicine, McMaster University, Hamilton, Ontario, Canada. 6School of Nursing, McMaster University, Hamilton, Ontario, Canada

Jordi Real
Primary Healthcare University Research Institute IDIAP-Jordi Gol, Barcelona, Spain
Epidemiologia i Salut Pública, Universitat Internacional de Catalunya, Sant Cugat, Spain

Caroline S. Clarke, Kate Walters, Kalpa Kharicha and Steve Iliffe
Department Primary Care & Population Health, University College London (UCL), Royal Free Campus, Rowland Hill St, London NW3 2PF, UK

Claire Goodman and Melanie Handley
Centre for Research in Primary and Community Care, University of Hertfordshire, College Lane, Hatfield AL10 9AB, Hertfordshire, UK

Jill Manthorpe
Social Care Workforce Research Unit, King's College London, Strand, London WC2B 4LL, UK

Mima Cattan
University of Northumbria, Sutherland Building Newcastle-upon-Tyne, Newcastle NE1 8ST, UK

Steve Morris and Jeff Round
Department of Applied Health Research, UCL, 1-19 Torrington Place, London WC1E 7HB, UK

Jennifer Kane and Amy Nolen
Department of Family and Community Medicine, University of Toronto, Toronto, ON, Canada

Sumeet Sodhi and Megan Landes
Department of Family and Community Medicine, University of Toronto, Toronto, ON, Canada
Dignitas International, 2 Adelaide Street West, Suite 200, Toronto M5H 1L6, Canada

Christopher Carroll
Health Economics and Decision Science (HEDS), School of Health and Related Research (ScHARR), University of Sheffield Regent Court, Regent Street, Sheffield S1 4DA, UK

José-Luis Del Val, Mar Domingo, Ester Calero and Nuria Soldevila-Bacardit
Institut Català de la Salut, Barcelona, Spain
Primary Healthcare University Research Institute IDIAP-Jordi Gol, Barcelona, Spain

Miguel-Angel Muñoz, Xavier Mundet-Tuduri and José-María Verdú-Rotellar
Institut Català de la Salut, Barcelona, Spain
Primary Healthcare University Research Institute IDIAP-Jordi Gol, Barcelona, Spain
Universitat Autònoma de Barcelona, Bellaterra, Spain

Ernest Vinyoles
Institut Català de la Salut, Barcelona, Spain
Primary Healthcare University Research Institute IDIAP-Jordi Gol, Barcelona, Spain
Universitat de Barcelona, Barcelona, Spain

Caterina Checa
Primary Healthcare University Research Institute IDIAP-Jordi Gol, Barcelona, Spain
EAP Dreta de l'Eixample, Barcelona, Spain

André Hajek, Jens-Oliver Bock and Hans-Helmut König
Department of Health Economics and Health Services Research, Hamburg Center for Health Economics, University Medical Center Hamburg-Eppendorf, Hamburg, Germany

Index

CPSIA information can be obtained
at www.ICGtesting.com
Printed in the USA
LVHW060859030122
707669LV00002B/247

9 781639 274512